KU-113-993

THE YEAR BOOK

of

ANESTHESIA

1971

Distributed in the United Kingdom & Europe by: ₨S

LLOYD-LUKE (MEDICAL BOOKS) LTD

49 NEWMAN STREET

LONDON, W1P 4BX

THE PRACTICAL MEDICINE YEAR BOOKS

Medicine: DAVID E. ROGERS, M.D.; CARL MUSCHENHEIM, M.D.; PAUL HELLER, M.D.; T. JOSEPH REEVES, M.D.; NORTON J. GREENBERGER, M.D.; PHILIP K. BONDY, M.D.; FRANKLIN H. EPSTEIN, M.D.

Surgery: SEYMOUR I. SCHWARTZ, M.D.; JOHN S. NAJARIAN, M.D.; ERLE E. PEACOCK, JR., M.D.; G. TOM SHIRES, M.D.; WILLIAM SILEN, M.D.; FRANK C. SPENCER, M.D.

Anesthesia: JAMES E. ECKENHOFF, M.D.

Drug Therapy: DALE G. FRIEND, M.D.

Obstetrics & Gynecology: J. P. GREENHILL, M.D.

Pediatrics: SYDNEY S. GELLIS, M.D.

Radiology: WALTER M. WHITEHOUSE, M.D.; HOWARD B. LATOURETTE, M.D.

Ophthalmology: WILLIAM F. HUGHES, M.D.

Ear, Nose & Throat: JOHN A. KIRCHNER, M.D.

Neurology & Neurosurgery: RUSSELL N. DE JONG, M.D.; OSCAR SUGAR, M.D.

Psychiatry & Applied Mental Health: FRANCIS J. BRACELAND, DOUGLAS D. BOND, M.D.; M.D.; DANIEL X. FREEDMAN, M.D.; ARNOLD J. FRIEDHOFF, M.D.; LAWRENCE C. KOLB, M.D.; REGINALD S. LOURIE, M.D.

Dermatology: FREDERICK D. MALKINSON, M.D.; RODGER W. PEARSON, M.D.

Urology: JOHN T. GRAYHACK, M.D.

Orthopedics & Traumatic Surgery: H. HERMAN YOUNG, M.D.

Plastic & Reconstructive Surgery: NEAL OWENS, M.D.; KATHRYN STEPHENSON, M.D.

Endocrinology: THEODORE B. SCHWARTZ, M.D.

Pathology & Clinical Pathology: WILLIAM B. WARTMAN, M.D.

Nuclear Medicine: JAMES L. QUINN, III, M.D.

Cancer: RANDOLPH LEE CLARK, M.D.; RUSSELL W. CUMLEY, Ph.D.

Cardiovascular Medicine & Surgery: EUGENE BRAUNWALD, M.D.; W. PROCTOR HARVEY, M.D.; JOHN W. KIRKLIN, M.D.; ALEXANDER S. NADAS, M.D.; OGLESBY PAUL, M.D.; ROBERT W. WILKINS, M.D.; IRVING S. WRIGHT, M.D.

Library of Congress Catalog Card Number: 63-25215

There are twenty YEAR BOOKS in various fields of medicine and one in dentistry. Publication of these annual volumes has been continuous since 1900. The YEAR BOOKS make available in detailed abstract form the working essence of the cream of recent international medicoscientific literature. Selection of the material is made by distinguished editors who critically review each year more than 500,000 articles published in the world's foremost journals.

TABLE OF CONTENTS

The material covered in this volume represents literature reviewed up to May, 1971.

PHILOSOPHY, LOGISTICS AND UTILIZATION

The Normality of the Abnormal is discussed by William W. Mushin[1] (Cardiff, Wales). The practice of anesthesia is now dominated by a desire to maintain a "normal" state; "homeostasis" has become a key work in present practice. When the range of the physiologic functions of importance is considered, considerable differences are found on either side of an imaginary ideal state of health, but they are quantitative rather than qualitative. Some wide variations in function occur for no apparent reason, some from habits and others from natural factors such as age. The concept of "normality" as a fairly sharp physiologic point should be abandoned. Variation is the essential characteristic of living things. Surgical populations may be different from others in many respects. A great many surgically treatable conditions are associated with physiologic disturbances that are mostly compensatory or resultant, rather than causal in nature.

Postoperative personality disorders in aging patients may result from vigorous hyperventilation by an anesthesiologist attempting to maintain some form of homeostasis in terms of Pco_2. Various effects of smoking may be important to the anesthesiologist, such as elasticity of the lung and a reduction in surfactant. The numbers that smoke make these changes "normal." Obesity is another matter on which an epidemiologic outlook must be developed. Circadian rhythm may modify the effects of anesthesia and surgery. Some of the difficulties or successes of induced hypothermia may be due to cyclic variations in temperature control. Circadian variations in blood pressure and in sensitivity of the central nervous system to various stimuli also occur. Persons who take sedatives may react differently than others to anesthesia. Age is important in reactions of patients to anesthetic procedures. Degeneration of aging affects neuronal tissue and also the blood supply to the central nervous system. Blood pressure changes with age may be of significance as may altering dose-effect ratios for drugs.

Programed anesthesia is expected in the future, with automated control of anesthetic gases modified by feedback of monitored physiologic events as they occur during anesthesia. Char-

(1)   Anesth. & Analg. 49:667-679, Sept.-Oct., 1970.

acteristics of the "whole patient" must be identified, so that individual patients will not be matched against a theoretic, often unattainable physiologic idea to their possible disadvantage, but rather against a prototype drawn from actual knowledge of the particular defined population groups to which they belong.

▶ [We usually forget, and many never accept, that what is acknowledged as normal is but the average of the observations between the extreme.—Eds.]

Analysis of Manpower in Anesthesiology is presented by J. S. Gravenstein, J. E. Steinhaus and P. P. Volpitto.[2] Additional anesthesia services will be required as our medical resources are made available to the underprivileged. Anesthesiologists are assuming more responsibilities for patients in intensive care units, pulmonary care centers and obstetric services. It is not feasible to place an anesthesiologist with every patient requiring an anesthetic. Distinction may be made between simple standardized tasks, routine tasks responsive to general or specific direction, semiroutine tasks responsive to general direction, nonroutine tasks performed under little supervision and nonroutine tasks performed without supervision. Procedures vary in the degree of medical judgment required and the activities observed. Difficulties are more prone to arise during induction than during maintenance of anesthesia. Tasks have not yet been weighed in simulation experiments. Experience suggests that simple standardized tasks should be combined with routine tasks performed in response to general or specific directions. Semiroutine tasks may also be combined, as in the functions of nurses or nurse-anesthetists. Both nurse-anesthetists and anesthesiologists often perform tasks at lower levels than those who require their services.

Often the nurse-anesthetist is placed in an unfair position when asked to work independently or under the direction of a physician with little training in anesthesiology. Only a few anesthesia aides or technicians are presently available for tasks at the lowest level. The role of these persons must be better defined. A person should be able to rise to higher levels of responsibility as capability and desire permit or move laterally into related areas. Training of anesthesia technologists is directed at the increased use of technology in medicine, specifically, toward further use of physiologic measurement in anesthesiology. It is planned that the master technologist in anesthesi-

   (2)   Anesthesiology 33:350-357, September, 1970.

ology will complement the aide, nurse-anesthetist and anesthesiologist. An alternate approach is the training of assistants and associates in anesthesiology for specific tasks at the lower levels.

Arterial Punctures by Nurses were evaluated by Marvin A. Sackner, Wilbur G. Avery and Jean Sokolowski[3] (Mt. Sinai Hosp., Miami Beach, Fla.). Requests for arterial blood gas studies have risen markedly, and physicians in small hospitals have found it difficult to obtain such analyses readily as interns and residents are often unavailable. An attempt was made to train registered nurses to perform arterial punctures. Two nurses have performed 1,541 punctures since 1969 without morbidity or complications.

PROCEDURE.—With the patient supine or semirecumbent and the wrist extended, the area over the radial artery $1/2$-1 in. above the wrist is cleansed and infiltrated with xylocaine. The artery is palpated with one hand. With the other hand, the needle is advanced into the artery at a 45-degree angle. A 3-5-ml. sample of blood is withdrawn. The brachial or femoral artery can be punctured if radial artery blood cannot be obtained.

Nurses were instructed for 1 week and have generally been able to perform all arterial punctures. Sampling usually required less than 2 minutes. The punctures done in 1969-70 included 127 brachial and 67 femoral punctures. No vasovagal reaction has occurred. The only morbidity was occasional minimal superficial hematoma formation over the puncture site.

Arterial punctures can be performed safely by nurses and ultimately by paramedical personnel, relieving the house staff of this burden. Local anesthesia should be used before arterial puncture. It reduces the tendency of patients to hold their breath or hyperventilate, interfering with a steady state, and reduces the frequency of vasovagal reactions. Nurses must be taught to ask about reactions to the "caine" type of drugs and to treat sensitivity reactions.

▶ [We suspect this will be greeted with cries of anguish by some. It makes sense to the editors.—Eds.]

BIOCHEMISTRY AND PHYSICAL CHEMISTRY

Influence of Arterial Hypoxemia upon Labile Phosphates and upon Extracellular and Intracellular Lactate and Pyruvate Concentrations in the Rat Brain. B. K. Siesjö and L. Nilsson[4] (Univ. of Lund) studied the effects of varying degrees of hy-

(3) Chest 59:97-98, January, 1971.
(4) Scandinav. J. Clin. & Lab. Invest. 27:83-96, February, 1971.

poxia on cerebral energy metabolism in male Wistar rats by relating arterial oxygen tension to brain tissue contents of phosphocreatine, ATP, adenosine diphosphate (ADP), adenosine monophosphate adenylic acid and inorganic phosphorus, as well as the cerebrospinal fluid lactate and pyruvate levels. Components of the glutamate-α-ketoglutarate equilibrium were also analyzed in most brains.

Cisternal cerebrospinal fluid was sampled from animals anesthetized with divinyl ether and nitrous oxide. Hypoxia was induced for 30 minutes by reducing the oxygen flow at constant ventilation. Attempts were made to minimize variations in factors other than oxygen tension. The blood pressure tended to fall at a Pao_2 below about 25 mm. Hg; below 20 mm. Hg it almost always declined, and the exposure to hypoxia had to be reduced to 15 minutes.

Progressive monrespiratory acidosis developed with a Pao_2 below 45-50 mm. Hg. The whole blood lactate concentration and the lactate-pyruvate ratio increased with a Pao_2 below about 50 mm. Hg. A fall in base excess was correlated with these changes. Similar changes occurred in cisternal cerebrospinal fluid at low PO_2 levels. Brain phosphocreatine levels fell significantly and inorganic phosphorus increased with a PO_2 below about 35 mm. Hg. The ATP-ADP ratio fell moderately at a PO_2 below about 25 mm. Hg; changes were more pronounced in hypotensive animals.

Intracellular lactate levels increased at a Pao_2 not associated with significant changes in labile phosphates (35-45 mm. Hg). Cerebrospinal fluid changes exceeded those occurring in the intracellular space at low Pao_2 levels. At extremely low levels the greatest lactate accumulation was intracellular. The tissue α-ketoglutarate content did not decrease until the PO_2 fell below 20 mm. Hg, and the drop was most marked in animals with hypotension.

The earliest tissue changes with arterial hypoxemia were increased in the intracellular lactate concentration and the lactate-pyruvate ratio. The energy metabolism of the brain is remarkably resistant to pure hypoxemia. The finding that cerebrospinal fluid changes were less marked than those in the cells at extreme degrees of hypoxemia may have been due to an insufficient equilibration time.

▶ [Interpretation of intracellular metabolic events is difficult even under the best circumstances. This study documents a disparity between intracellular and cerebrospinal fluid lactate-pyruvate ratios and draws attention to the limitations of extracellular lactate-pyruvate measurements as indicators of intracellular hypoxia. More importantly, however, tissue levels of high energy phosphate compounds were well maintained in markedly hypoxemic states. The brain tolerated a Pao_2 of 30 mm. Hg or less without causing major changes in cerebral energy reserves and without evidence of threat to viability of cerebral cells, provided hypotension did not occur. It appears that maintenance of cardiovascular function is the critical factor in severely hypoxemic states.—Eds.]

Reduced Red Cell Glycolysis, 2,3-Diphosphoglycerate and Adenosine Triphosphate Concentration and Increased Hemoglobin-Oxygen Affinity Caused by Hypophosphatemia were studied by Marshall A. Lichtman, Denis R. Miller, Jules Cohen and Christine Waterhouse[5] (Univ. of Rochester). The red blood cell glycolytic rate and glycolytic intermediates are intimately related to red blood cell survival in the circulation and to the function of hemoglobin as an oxygen donor at tissue partial pressures of oxygen. Extracellular organic phosphate can influence the red cell glycolytic rate.

A woman aged 52 was seen for progressive peripheral neuropathy and intractable steatorrhea. An intestinal biopsy specimen indicated a sprue-like disorder, but there was no response to gluten proscription or high doses of prednisone. Intravenous feedings with 12% glucose and 4% casein hydrolysate were given. Positive nitrogen balance was observed during the period of parenteral feeding. The patient died of infection and gastrointestinal bleeding after 5 months. There was extensive necrosis of the gastrointestinal mucosa. Red cell metabolism was examined during the illness.

Plasma inorganic phosphate levels fell to extremely low levels when parenteral nutrition was instituted and were below 1 mg./100 ml. by 72-96 hours. Urinary phosphorus excretion fell to zero. There was a 60% drop in red cell glucose utilization and in lactate production. Lactate-glucose ratios remained constant. The red cell 2,3-diphosphoglycerate (2,3-DPG) level fell to 45% and the ATP level fell to 52% of baseline, corresponding temporally to the fall in the glycolytic rate. Phosphate infusion intravenously increased glucose utilization and lactate production, and the 2,3-DPG and ATP levels increased to normal in close parallel with the increase in plasma phosphate concentration. The low glycolytic rate of the red cells from the patient was partly corrected when the red cells were placed in normal plasma. The glycolytic rate of normal red cells declined in the plasma from the patient. No important blood pH changes were noted. Oxygen affinity of hemoglobin was reduced in normophosphatemia and increased during protracted hypophosphatemia. Over half the red cells were spherocytes during protracted hypophosphatemia. Moderate anemia and slight reticulocytosis were present during the period of parenteral feeding. A direct Coombs test was negative.

Extracellular phosphate is important in modulating the glycolytic rate and the red cell ATP and 2,3-DPG levels in vivo. Red cell energy stores are critically reduced during marked hypophosphatemia, threatening red cell survival. Tissue oxygen delivery may be impaired under these circumstances.

▶ [The work of Benesch and Benesch on the regulatory effects of intracellular organic phosphate on oxygen release by hemoglobin is assuming greater clinical significance. Both 2,3-DPG and ATP bind to hemoglobin and decrease the affinity of hemoglobin for oxygen over the physiologic range of oxygen tensions. Since there is about 3 times as much 2,3-DPG in the red cell, its effect on Hb-O_2 binding is more important. In this case the observed hypophosphatemia was accompanied by a decrease in red blood cell 2,3-DPG, which in turn interfered with the ability of hemoglobin to release oxygen at the tissue level.—Eds.]

Effect of Chronic Intake of Ethanol on Pentobarbital Metabolism was studied by H. Kalant, J. M. Khanna and Joan Marshman.[6] Ethanol was given for 2 weeks to male rats on a liquid diet; ethanol constituted 5.1% of the diet and provided 36% of the total calories. The daily intake of ethanol was 10-12 Gm./kg. Control animals received an equicaloric amount of sucrose instead. Liquid diets were replaced by tap water 24 hours before the study. Phenobarbital sodium was given in a daily dose of 100 mg./kg. for a week, by gastric intubation, as a 1% aqueous solution. Sleep time was determined after the injection of pentobarbital, 30 mg./kg. in saline intraperitoneally; the interval between loss and return of the righting reflex was recorded. Plasma and brain levels of pentobarbital were determined. Pentobarbital metabolism also was studied in liver slices.

Ethanol-treated and control rats had similar growth. Sleep was of slower onset and shorter duration in the ethanol group. At 15 minutes after a pentobarbital dose, plasma and brain pentobarbital levels were lower in the study group, but the blood-brain ratios were almost identical in the two groups of rats. Pentobarbital disappearance in plasma or brain did not differ 30-60 minutes after administration. The rate of pentobarbital metabolism was 33% lower in liver slices from the ethanol group than in those from control animals. Pretreatment with phenobarbital for a week led to a significant increase in the rate of pentobarbital metabolism by liver slices.

The changes seen in pentobarbital sleep time after chronic ethanol administration result primarily from changes in nervous system sensitivity, rather than from changes in the distribution or metabolism of pentobarbital.

► [Is this altered reactivity restricted to the brain or does it happen in other excitable tissues, is it dose dependent, is it reversible? These and many other questions require answers if we are to deal rationally with the large number of alcoholic patients encountered in practice.—Eds.]

Comparison of In Vivo and In Vitro Partition Coefficients for Nitrous Oxide and Cyclopropane. Theoretical prediction of the uptake and distribution of inhaled anesthetics requires knowledge of their tissue solubilities or tissue-gas partition coefficients. Almost all values for coefficients of anesthetics have been obtained in in vitro studies. D. E. Evans, Valerie Flook and W. W. Mapleson[7] (Cardiff, Wales) attempted to determine whether there is significant discrepancy between coefficients determined in vitro and in vivo in a given individual. Studies were done in rabbits anesthetized with pentobarbitone and lignocaine. A plate of skull bone was marked out, and cannulas were placed in carotid and jugular vessels. Nitrous oxide was given with oxygen, approximately 70-30%. Cyclopropane was given as 14% in air. Skeletal muscle, brain, kidney, liver and heart were sampled at the end of the study. In vitro coefficients were determined by equilibrating tissue homogenates with known partial pressures of anesthetic agent and vacuum extracting the dissolved agent from samples of homogenate.

The extraction apparatus showed mean recoveries of 98.7% for nitrous oxide and 100.7% for cyclopropane. For nitrous oxide, the mean of differences of all available pairs of observations was 6% of the mean of all coefficients, a three-way cross-classification analysis of variance showed this difference to be significant. For cyclopropane, the mean difference between technics for tissues other than brain was less than for nitrous oxide and not significant. For brain, the mean difference was large, but a two-way analysis of variance showed it not to be significant.

The possibility of real differences between in vivo and in

(7)   Brit. J. Anaesth. 42:1028-1032, December, 1970.

vitro partition coefficients for nitrous oxide and cyclopropane cannot be excluded, but the differences are unlikely to exceed about 10%, except perhaps for cyclopropane in brain, and they are probably less than 5%. For the agents studied, greater confidence can be placed in in vitro coefficients that have been published, and there appears to be no need to attempt to measure partition coefficients in vivo in man. There remains the possibility of differences with other agents; work is in progress on halothane as a representative of the volatile anesthetics.

▶ [This indicates that in vitro measurement of partition coefficients is an adequate estimate in the living subject. Harry Lowe has data showing considerable variation in partition coefficients for volatile agents among different subjects.—Eds.]

PHARMACOLOGY

Effects of Anesthetic Agents on Respiration

Effects of Halothane and Atropine on Total Respiratory Resistance in Anesthetized Man. Allan L. Brakensiek and Norman A. Bergman[8] (Salt Lake City, Utah) measured respiratory resistance in male patients scheduled for elective operations with general anesthesia, aged 34-76 years. Subjects were premedicated with pentobarbital. Anesthesia was induced with thiopental. Tubocurarine was given for intubation. Anesthesia was maintained initially with 60% nitrous oxide, 40% oxygen and supplemental doses of thiopental. Ventilation was controlled with a Manley ventilator and a nonrebreathing circuit at a minute volume of about 8 L. per minute. The end-expiratory Pco_2 was maintained at 32-35 mm. Hg. Some patients were then given 0.5-1.0% halothane followed by 0.8 mg. atropine intravenously about halfway through the experimental period (group A). Others received 0.8 mg. atropine, followed by halothane after about 20-25 minutes, which was continued for an additional 20-25 minutes (group B). The pulse and/or blood pressure was reduced by halothane in all subjects. Operation was begun at various times in the sequence.

One of 10 group A patients had a significant reduction in respiratory resistance following halothane, and a further decrease after atropine. Halothane reduced resistance significantly in a second patient, but atropine had no effect in this case.

(8) Anesthesiology 33:341-344, September, 1970.

Both these patients had signs of chronic obstructive airway disease and high initial resistance values. Resistance and compliance did not change clinically during the course of anesthesia. No group B patient had significant change in respiratory resistance during the study. End-expiratory Pco_2 did not vary more than 1.5 mm. Hg in any subject during the study.

These results suggest that the reported beneficial effects of halothane in preventing and treating bronchospastic episodes are probably related to its anesthetic actions in blocking reflex responses to stimuli that elicit bronchospasm in susceptible persons. A direct effect of halothane on respiratory resistance in man under usual clinical conditions could not be demonstrated in this study.

▶ [These results will surprise many who have taught and believed that halothane decreased airway resistance.—Eds.]

Effects of Halothane on Respiratory and Cardiovascular Responses to Hypoxia in Dogs: Dose-Response Study. The extent to which the depth of anesthesia attenuates cardiorespiratory responses has not been documented despite the importance of signs such as hyperventilation and hypertension in recognizing hypoxia. David J. Cullen and Edmond I. Eger, II[9] (Univ. of California) studied the effects of hypoxia in dogs at several concentrations of halothane anesthesia.

Respiratory responses to hypoxia were measured during spontaneous ventilation in 6 dogs (group 1) anesthetized with halothane and oxygen. Halothane concentrations were 1.25, 1.5, 1.75 and 2%. The Pao_2 was reduced to about 45 torr using nitrogen as the end-tidal halothane level was reduced to 1% and a second dose-response curve was recorded. Measurements were repeated at a Pao_2 of 30 torr and 0.75% halothane. Cardiovascular function was studied during assisted or controlled respiration in 6 other dogs (group 2). The $Paco_2$ was maintained at 25-34 torr in these animals. Measurements were made at hyperoxia and moderate hypoxia in 3 dogs from 1 to 2% and in the other 3 dogs from 2 to 1% halothane. Severe hypoxia started at 0.75% halothane.

In group 1 studies the $Paco_2$ rose with increasing halothane concentration but was significantly lower than the 100% oxygen value for each level of halothane. The significant rise in minute ventilation during moderate hypoxia resulted from tachypnea alone. Cardiac output was increased in moderate hy-

(9)   Anesthesiology 33:487-496, November, 1970.

poxia at every level of halothane anesthesia in group 2 studies due both to tachycardia and increased stroke volume. The response was well preserved to 2% halothane, with cardiac output greater than that during 1% halothane in oxygen.

In severe hypoxia, cardiorespiratory function was stimulated at lower halothane levels in both groups. At 0.75-1.25% halothane, a 0.25% increment rapidly converted hyperventilation and cardiovascular stimulation to respiratory or cardiac arrest. Oxygen transport did not meet the needs of oxygen consumption during moderate or severe hypoxia. Slight metabolic acidosis developed during moderate hypoxia, progressing to severe metabolic acidosis at 0.75% halothane during severe hypoxia.

The cardiorespiratory stimulus of moderate hypoxia persists to deep levels of halothane anesthesia. Halothane probably interferes with all the factors leading to the circulatory response to hypoxia without anesthesia, including a direct vasodilatory effect, a direct depressant effect on myocardial function, reflex pressor responses from chemoreceptor stimulation, central sympathetic excitation and catecholamine effects.

Cardiorespiratory stimulation may also result from too light a plane of anesthesia; failure to distinguish this from hypoxia may be hazardous. A halothane level that is safe under normal circumstances can be fatal during severe hypoxia.

► [Cardiorespiratory stimulation during halothane may be from light anesthesia or hypoxia. The treatment of the two conditions is not the same.—Eds.]

EFFECTS OF ANESTHETIC AGENTS ON CIRCULATION

Effects of β-Adrenergic Blockade on Cardiopulmonary Response to Ketamine. Daniel L. Traber, Roy D. Wilson and Lawrence L. Priano[1] (Galveston, Texas) studied the effect of β-adrenergic blockade with propranolol and practolol on the cardiopulmonary responses to ketamine. Studies were done on unanesthetized dogs implanted with cardiac catheters through femoral incisions and then allowing the animals to recover from the anesthetic. Eighteen dogs were given ketamine, 5 mg./kg., intravenously. At about 2 hours, when the dogs had recovered from the dissociative anesthetic, 8 dogs were given propranolol, 0.25 mg./kg. intravenously, and 10 were given practolol, 2 mg./kg. intravenously, a cardioselective β-adrenergic

_____
(1)   Anesth. & Analg. 49:604-613, July-Aug., 1970.

blocker. A second dose of ketamine, 5 mg./kg., was given after the cardiovascular system was stable.

Ketamine elicited a significant rise in arterial pressure before and after practolol. The positive chronotropic response persisted after practolol. The cardiac output was elevated by ketamine before and after practolol. Maximum left ventricular dp/dt was elevated similarly before and after the blocker was given. Ketamine reduced the left ventricular end-diastolic before and elevated it after practolol. Changes in arterial pressure, heart rate and cardiac output were similar before and after propranolol. The response of maximal left ventricular dp/dt was not significantly different from control values before or after propranolol administration. Ketamine elevated the left ventricular end-diastolic pressure after, but not before, propranolol.

It is concluded that neither the sympathetic innervation to the heart nor circulating catecholamines that might have been released from the adrenal are responsible for the cardiostimulatory effects of ketamine.

▶ [The cardiac response to ketamine is not blocked by β-blockers but the cardiovascular response is blocked by ganglionic blockade. Does this suggest an α-response?—Eds.]

Sodium Nitroprusside as Hypotensive Agent in General Anesthesia. Sodium nitroprusside is a potent hypotensive agent with an evanescent action. It can only be safely given by continuous infusion with careful regulation of the infusion rate, making it ideal for use by anesthetists. T. H. Taylor, M. Styles and A. J. Lamming[2] (London), evaluated sodium nitroprusside in 83 cases of induced hypotension during general anesthesia. The patients had transsphenoid hypophysectomy for the pain of terminal carcinoma and were poor operative risks or had hypophysectomy for pituitary tumors. Pleural effusions were drained in the carcinoma patients on the day of operation. Premedication was with pethidine and promethazine. Anesthesia was induced with thiopental and maintained with halothane in oxygen after intubation. Patients were flat or at a 5-degree head-up tilt. Nitroprusside was infused as a solution of 10 mg. in 100 ml. dextrose-saline. Patients received 3.1 to 166 mg. in 1 hour. The infusion rate was varied to produce a "dry field"; a particular pressure level was not sought. Infusion was stopped at the end of operation.

(2) Brit. J. Anaesth. 42:859-864, October, 1970.

No postoperative sequelae were attributable to the infusion of nitroprusside. The blood pressure level varied with the infusion rate during operation, usually in a highly precise manner. One patient did not respond completely satisfactorily. Sodium nitroprusside is considered to be a safe hypotensive agent that is easy to administer and has a rapid, reversible action, with a complete absence of side effects. Further trials are justified where controlled hypotension during anesthesia is desired.

▶ [John Homi of Northwestern University's Anesthesia Department has had extensive experience with nitroprusside and believes it is the agent of choice for deliberate hypotension.—Eds.]

Local Anesthetic and Antiarrhythmic Actions of Alprenolol Relative to Its Effect on Intracellular Potentials and Other Properties of Isolated Cardiac Muscle. Alprenolol is a β-adrenoceptor blocking drug reported to have the same potency as propranolol in vitro and in vivo. B. N. Singh and E. M. Vaughan Williams[3] (Oxford Univ.) compared the concentrations of alprenolol required to depress depolarization in frog nerve and isolated cardiac muscle and tested its in vivo efficacy in protecting anesthetized guinea pigs from ouabain-induced cardiac arrhythmias. Action potentials of a frog sciatic nerve were measured on stimulation with and without alprenolol present. Ouabain was infused into guinea pigs anesthetized with urethane. Intracellular potentials were recorded in isolated rabbit atria.

Alprenolol was a powerful local anesthetic for frog nerve, having four times the potency of procaine on a molar basis. Alprenolol was about three times more effective than propranolol in protecting anesthetized guinea pigs against ventricular fibrillation induced by ouabain. Weak positive inotropic and chronotropic actions of alprenolol were evident in the isolated rabbit atrium at low concentrations. A concentration less than 3 μM. had no significant "nonspecific" depressant effect; this concentration is 200 times greater than that required to double the median effective dose of isoprenaline in augmenting the contractions of isolated rabbit papillary muscle. Alprenolol did not affect the resting potential of isolated rabbit atria. The rate of rise of the action potential was reduced by the drug; the effect was highly significant even with a concentration of 0.525×10^{-6}M.

A dose of 5 mg. alprenolol given intravenously to human

(3)   Brit. J. Pharmacol. 38:749-757, April, 1970.

subjects partially blocked the chronotropic effects of isoprena-line for a 2-hour period. The plasma concentrations achieved are well above those needed to reduce the maximum rate of de-polarization in vitro. If alprenolol interferes with the relation-ship between membrane voltage and the time of return of ex-citability, the generation of abnormal impulses could well be prevented by concentrations lower than those needed to reduce the maximum rate of depolarization at a normal frequency of impulse formation.

► [The ability to block β-receptor sites and also to produce classic local anesthesia is worthy of pursuit.—Eds.]

Reflections on β-Adrenergic Blockade in Anesthetics are presented by M. Johnstone[4] (Royal Infirm., Manchester, Eng-land). Whereas the β-blocking drugs increase the protective-ness of surgical anesthesia, they may enhance its hazards if not used with a full appreciation of their pharmacology. Mod-ern anesthetic technics combining blockade of the vasoconstric-tive reaction to surgical trauma and insulation of the heart from autonomic influences place control of the circulation vir-tually in the hands of the anesthetist. A β-blocking drug com-petitively antagonizes the beta effects of catecholamines. Some of the agents have intrinsic sympathomimetic activity. Pro-pranolol has no such activity.

Patients treated with β-blocking drugs who acquire surgical disease may have altered cardiovascular reactions to anesthetic and surgical stress. β-Blockade is helpful in controlling the un-desirable cardiac reactions to the adrenergic stress of anesthesia and operation. Vagolytic drugs such as atropine and gallamine increase the susceptibility of the heart to adrenergic influences. Some anesthetics, such as halothane and cyclopropane, increase the sensitivity of the β-adrenergic receptors.

β-Adrenergic blockade may be used preoperatively to con-trol the cardiac dysfunction of thyrotoxicosis, especially in pa-tients sensitive to antithyroid drugs. Combined with α-blockers, β-blockers are helpful in patients with pheochromocytoma. They are also effective in anxious patients and those with digi-talis intoxication. β-Blockade is indicated for cardiac dysrhyth-mia provoked by catecholamine injection or by intraperitoneal CO_2 insufflation and possibly with operations in the region of the 4th cranial ventricle. Postoperative thyrotoxic crisis has been successfully treated with β-blockers.

(4) Brit. J. Anaesth. 42:262-268, March, 1970.

The dangers of β-blockers are essentially those of β-adrenergic blockade. They include negative inotropism and vagal inhibition of the heart in anesthetized patients. The latter is avoided by atropine administration.

▶ [To repeat the authors, ". . . the beta blocking drugs, whilst increasing the protectiveness of surgical anesthesia, may enhance the hazards thereof if not applied with full appreciation of their pharmacology. . . ."—Eds.]

Comparison of Cardiovascular Effects of Halothane, Fluroxene, Ether and Cyclopropane in Man: Resumé. Edmond I. Eger, II, N. Ty Smith, David J. Cullen, Bruce F. Cullen and George A. Gregory[5] examined the cardiovascular effects of halothane, fluroxene, diethyl ether and cyclopropane in fasting, young healthy subjects. Ventilation was controlled before and during halothane and cyclopropane anesthesia. Spontaneous ventilation continued with ether and with 5% alveolar fluroxene. Eight of 11 subjects spontaneously breathed 9% fluroxene. The average $Paco_2$ remained at 35-40 torr in all subjects. In studies with ether, induction was with cyclopropane. Cardiovascular variables were measured in the first 60-90 minutes of anesthesia and after 4 or 5 hours. The subjects were aged 21-30 years.

In the 1st hour of anesthesia, halothane caused the most depression of cardiac output, and cyclopropane caused no depression at light anesthetic levels. Ether stimulated cardiac output at deep levels. Cyclopropane increased arterial pressure without changing cardiac output, with a rise in peripheral resistance at all levels of anesthesia. Right atrial pressure rose with increasing alveolar concentrations of all the anesthetic agents studied except fluroxene. Neither of the ethers affected left ventricular work except for a rise at 12% fluroxene. No anesthetic at light levels altered muscle blood flow, and only halothane consistently reduced it with increasing depth of anesthesia. All the agents increased cutaneous blood flow at light levels. All concentrations except light levels of ether and fluroxene acutely reduced oxygen consumption. Cardiac output rose in late anesthesia at all anesthetic levels, although right atrial pressure fell consistently. Arterial pressures decreased with time at light levels of anesthesia and peripheral resistance decreased. Left ventricular work rose slightly in time with all anesthetics. Stroke work changed little. Muscle blood flow rose greatly with the ethers. Oxygen consumption increased with the time-de-

(5) Anesthesiology 34:25-40, January, 1971.

pendent rise in cardiac output. Base excess values remained statistically unchanged.

Cyclopropane induced anesthesia most rapidly in this study and fluroxene least rapidly. Halothane and cyclopropane permitted intubation without use of neuromuscular blockers. Most subjects given halothane or cyclopropane had ventricular arrhythmias or A-V dissociation or both at some time during anesthesia. Specific patients may deviate from the general patterns observed in these volunteers.

Cardiovascular Effects of Diethyl Ether in Man. Many studies of the cardiovascular effects of ether have failed to relate them to anesthetic partial pressure or to the duration of anesthesia. George A. Gregory, Edmond I. Eger, II, N. Ty Smith, Bruce F. Cullen and David J. Cullen[6] studied the cardiovascular effects of ether in 9 healthy subjects in whom these factors were controlled and also studied the changes in effects that occurred with continued anesthesia. Fasted, unpremedicated subjects breathed pure oxygen for 10-20 minutes and then received cyclopropane-oxygen, followed by diethyl ether instead of cyclopropane. After intubation, 3 and 6% alveolar ether concentrations were administered in the 1st and 5th hours of anesthesia. Nitrous oxide and carbon dioxide were administered at 3-5 hours.

Heart rate increased and cardiac output was little changed in the 1st hour of anesthesia. Stroke volume decreased and right atrial pressure rose slightly. Mean arterial pressure and forearm vascular resistance changed little from waking values at either ether concentration. Oxygen consumption was unchanged. Base excess decreased by 2 mEq./L. Cardiac output and rate increased further in the 5th hour of anesthesia. Right atrial pressures decreased and stroke volumes returned to waking values at both anesthetic concentrations. Mean arterial pressure, total peripheral resistance and forearm vascular resistance decreased and muscle blood flow increased. Oxygen consumption did not change. The circulatory index was significantly increased above the waking value at both 3 and 6% ether concentrations.

Cardiovascular depression did not occur in this study of normal subjects except early in anesthesia at a 6% alveolar ether level. The increased heart rate on deepening of anesthesia may

(6)   Anesthesiology 34:19-24, January, 1971.

be explained by an increase in cervical preganglionic nerve traffic as the end-tidal ether level increased. Total body tissue oxygen and metabolic demands appear to have been met at all times. Recovery of cardiac output may occur more slowly in patients with diseased myocardia, and caution must be used when ether anesthesia is deepened rapidly.

▶ [Excellent resumés of data from unmedicated healthy volunteers without the stimulus of operation!—Eds.]

Vasopressin and Angiotensin on Resistance Vessels of Spleen, Intestine and Liver. Marsha M. Cohen, Daniel S. Sitar, J. Robert McNeill and Clive V. Greenway[7] (Univ. of Manitoba) studied sensitivities of splenic, intestinal and hepatic arterial beds in 36 anesthetized cats of similar body weight during intravenous infusion of vasopressin and angiotensin in a range of doses.

METHOD.—Cats were anesthetized by intraperitoneal injection of sodium pentobarbital, 30 mg./kg. When reflex limb and ear movements returned, an additional 8 mg. pentobarbital was given by cannula in a forelimb cutaneous vein. In one series of cats, splenic arterial flow was recorded with a noncannulating electromagetic flowmeter probe; hepatic arterial flow was recorded in a second series and superior mesenteric flow, in a third series. In each case, a clamp was placed on the artery next to the flow probe, and arterial pressure was recorded distal to this clamp. As systemic arterial pressure increased during drug infusions, the clamp was progressively tightened, and arterial pressure in the vascular bed was maintained constant. Angiotensin and vasopressin were diluted with 0.9% sodium chloride and infused intravenously with a Harvard constant infusion pump. The maximum infusion rate was 0.14 ml. per minute; infusions were continued for 6 minutes, by which time flow was steady at its new level. Conductance was determined from flow and arterial pressure in the vascular bed studied at 1 minute before and at the 5-minute mark during each infusion. Conductance during infusion was expressed as a percentage of that before infusion.

Each cat received vasopressin in a dose series from 0.57 to 57 mU./kg./minute, which covered the range from that causing minimal observable response to that causing arrhythmias. Figure 1 shows dose-response curves, each of which indicates the mean ±S.E. of the responses in 5-7 cats. Vasopressin markedly constricted intestinal and splenic vascular beds; decrease in conductance at each dose level was similar. The hepatic arterial bed dilated during infusions, and the responses in this bed were more variable than in the other 2 vascular beds, as shown by the greater standard errors. Responses to doses above 2.3 mU./kg./minute were significantly different (P<0.01) from

(7)   Am. J. Physiol. 218:1704-1706, June, 1970.

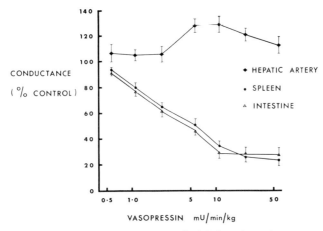

Fig. 1.—Dose-response curves to vasopressin infusions for resistance vessels of hepatic arterial, splenic and intestinal vascular beds. Each curve represents means ± standard error of mean of responses in 5-7 cats. (Courtesy of Cohen, M. M., *et al.:* Am. J. Physiol. 218:1704-1706, June, 1970.)

intestinal and splenic bed responses when analyzed by the un-paired *t*-test.

Each cat received angiotensin in doses from 0.004 to 0.4 μg./ kg./minute, which covered the range from causing minimal ob-servable response to that causing arrhythmias. Figure 2 shows

Fig. 2.—Dose-response curves to angiotensin infusions for resistance vessels of hepatic arterial, splenic and intestinal vascular beds. Each curve represents means ± standard error of mean of responses in 5-7 cats. (Courtesy of Cohen, M. M., *et al.:* Am. J. Physiol. 218:1704-1706, June, 1970.)

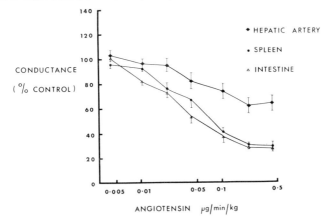

dose-response curves, each of which represents the mean ±S.E. of the responses in 5-7 cats. Whereas angiotensin constricted all 3 vascular beds, responses of the splenic and intestinal beds were similar and greater than those of the hepatic arterial bed. At doses above 0.1 µg./kg./minute responses were significantly different (P<0.05).

Probably there are no fundamental differences between the responses of the spleen and intestinal beds and the responses of the hepatic arterial bed to vasopressin and angiotensin, but in the hepatic arterial bed, vasoconstrictor responses are opposed by a myogenic vasodilatation secondary to the decrease in portal venous flow. The net result is vasodilatation with vasopressin and weak vasoconstriction with angiotensin.

▶ [Does a reflex increase of 30% conductance in the hepatic artery make up for the decreased portal vein flow secondary to marked splanchnic vasoconstriction? This study supports the idea that there is a limited place for vasopressors in clinical practice since the action of the drugs closely simulates the effect of hemorrhage on blood vessels.—Eds.]

Effect of Levodopa on Norepinephrine Stores in Rat Heart. Dopamine, the immediate precursor of L-dopa, exerts a β-adrenergic stimulating effect on the heart and causes renal vasodilation. Large doses of L-dopa are given in parkinsonism and cardiovascular side effects are frequent. Philip L. Liu, Laurence J. Krenis and S. H. Ngai[8] (Columbia Univ.) studied the effect of L-dopa on norepinephrine stores in the rat heart, an organ rich in sympathetic innervation, as well as on brain norepinephrine and dopamine concentrations. Male Sprague-Dawley rats were given 100-200 mg. L-dopa per kg. intraperitoneally or solvent alone and were killed 1-6 hours after injection. Other rats received 200 mg. L-dopa per kg. 30-120 minutes after a tracer dose of norepinephrine-^{3}H was given intravenously.

Brain norepinephrine levels were unchanged in rats given 100 mg. L-dopa per kg., whereas dopamine levels increased at 1 hour. L-Dopa produced a sharp rise in cardiac dopamine concentration, with a peak at 1 hour. At the peak dopamine level, norepinephrine concentration was 55% of the control level, gradually returning to the control level at 4 hours. Specific cardiac norepinephrine activity declined faster in L-dopa-treated rats. There was an almost fourfold rise in norepinephrine turnover in the heart after administration of a large dose of L-dopa. The half-life of specific norepinephrine activity was 4.5 hours in control animals and 1.7 in rats treated with L-dopa.

(8)   Anesthesiology 34:4-8, January, 1971.

The results indicate that dopamine accumulates significantly in the rat heart after L-dopa administration. Dopamine appears to be formed in or transported to adrenergic nerve endings and to displace norepinephrine from its storage site. Normal adrenergic function may be expected during anesthesia when the last dose of L-dopa is given the night before operation. Unexpected cardiovascular complications have not been encountered during anesthesia in parkinsonian patients on L-dopa therapy.

▶ [Accumulation of dopamine and displacement of norepinephrine from peripheral adrenergic stores could explain some of the clinical side effects (arrhythmia and occasional hypertensive effect) seen with L-dopa. Because of the short half-life and rapid turnover rates of components of the peripheral adrenergic system, normal adrenergic function can be expected 6 hours after the last drug dosage. L-Dopa probably does not have to be discontinued for more than 6 hours prior to anesthesia.—Eds.]

Effect of Angiotensin on Myocardial Function was studied by Martin J. Frank, Manouchehr Nadimi, Pablo Casanegra, Paul Stein and Robert Pekaar[9] in the intact anesthetized dog, in order to distinguish between functional changes resulting from changes in initial muscle length and those resulting from an altered force-velocity relationship.

METHOD.—Nine mongrel dogs were anesthetized with intraperitoneal morphine followed by intravenous chloralose or by Dial-urethan. The first time derivative of the ventricular pulse was obtained with use of a resistance-capacitance differentiating circuit. The left ventricular ejection fraction was measured by indicator dilution and left ventricular coronary flow with use of ^{85}Kr-labeled saturated saline. Angiotensin was infused into a peripheral vein in doses of 0.23-0.8 μg. per minute, dosage being varied to raise the aortic diastolic pressure by 3-50 mm. Hg. Force-velocity relations were calculated for each state.

Cardiac output was not significantly changed by angiotensin infusion. The main aortic pressure rose by 22%, and the systemic resistance index by 28%. Left ventricular end-diastolic volume rose by 24%, with a fall in ejection fraction and a rise in end-systolic volume. The mean end-diastolic pressure rose by 35%, but ventricular end-diastolic compliance did not change consistently. Left ventricular coronary flow and myocardial oxygen consumption were unaltered by angiotensin. The coronary resistance index rose by a mean of 27%. A mean decline in contractile state of 24% resulted from failure of the peak rate of pressure rise to increase in proportion with the maximum isovolumetric pressure and fiber length. A significant negative relation was found between percentage change in

(9) Am. J. Physiol. 218: 1267-1272, May, 1970.

stroke work and that in afterload. The ratio of stroke work to fiber length declined to below initial levels.

Angiotensin has a negative inotropic effect on the heart of the intact anesthetized dog. The unchanged myocardial oxygen consumption results from a balance between declining contractility and increasing wall tension. Angiotensin may be dangerous in circumstances where contractility is already compromised.

EFFECTS OF ANESTHETIC AGENTS ON THE CENTRAL NERVOUS SYSTEM

On Dose-Response Curves and Anesthetics. B. E. Waud and D. R. Waud[1] (Harvard Med. School) draw a distinction among graded, quantal and ordered responses. The depth of anesthesia cannot be treated as a graded response, since no natural continuous scale is available. Quantal responses, like waking or sleeping, are all-or-none responses. Anesthetic depth can be managed by a quantal approach if a given end point is considered, such as loss of response to pain, but then the idea of a passage through ordered stages or planes is lost.

Empiric scales such as Guedel's classification or the scale of EEG end points have been introduced to retain the notion of depth as a graded process. Such responses can be called ordered; all that can be said is whether one end point comes before or after another. For convenience, such end points are often plotted at evenly spaced intervals along a scale of ordinates, but conclusions must not be drawn that would change if another spacing were used.

Even with graded responses it is rarely possible to attach any significance to the shape of the dose-response curve. A constant depth of anesthesia can be chosen as an end point and concentrations of agents producing it compared, to provide ratios of potency or "dose ratios." A currently popular index is the end point of just barely responding to a painful stimulus.

The term "concentration-response curves" should be used instead of "dose-response curves;" the term "dose" has meaning only in the sense that a certain volume of distribution is implied, with a given dose leading to a specific concentration at the site of action. Currently, the measurement used is the alveo-

---

(1)   Anesthesiology 33:1-4, July, 1970.

lar concentration reached after a reasonable equilibration period. The combination of this parameter with the end point of marginal response to a painful stimulus provides the minimal alveolar concentration. The minimal alveolar concentration may be useful as a rough measure of potency, but extrapolation to other response levels without direct experimental confirmation is hazardous. If relative potency is to be estimated, it is advisable to make comparisons at several depths of anesthesia in the same group of subjects.

It is not likely that the examination of anesthetic dose-response curves per se will shed much light on mechanisms of action.

▶ [To the vast majority of anesthesiologists, clinical estimation of depth of anesthesia still looks pretty good.—Eds.]

Minimum Alveolar Concentrations in Man on Awakening from Methoxyflurane, Halothane, Ether and Fluroxene Anesthesia: MAC Awake. Robert K. Stoelting, David E. Longnecker and Edmond I. Eger, II[2] measured the alveolar anesthetic concentrations present when patients first opened their eyes on request and those just preventing responses during recovery from methoxyflurane, halothane, ether and fluroxene anesthesia. The minimal alveolar concentration (MAC) on awakening (MAC awake) was defined as the alveolar concentration midway between the values permitting and preventing the response. Volunteers and patients having general anesthesia for elective operations were studied. The volunteers were not premedicated; patients received atropine. Respiration was controlled during the studies. A constant anesthetic level was maintained for. at least 15 minutes to insure equilibration with cerebral partial pressure.

The MAC awake values were 0.081% methoxyflurane, 0.41% halothane, 1.41% ether and 2.20% fluroxene, as determined at constant alveolar concentrations. When alveolar concentrations were allowed to drop spontaneously, awake values were 0.082% methoxyflurane, 0.27% halothane and 1.16% fluroxene. Ratios of MAC awake to MAC with a constant alveolar concentration were 0.52 for methoxyflurane, 0.52 for halothane, 0.67 for ether and 0.60 for fluroxene. Ratios on spontaneous recovery were 0.50 for methoxyflurane, 0.33 for halothane and 0.34 for fluroxene. When the alveolar concentrations fell spontaneously, falsely low MAC awake values were obtained for halothane and

(2)   Anesthesiology 33:5-9, July, 1970.

fluroxene, whereas the value for methoxyflurane was unchanged from that at constant alveolar concentration.

The relative consistency of the ratio of MAC awake to anesthetized MAC, averaging 0.58, permits predictions of MAC awake to be made for other inhalation agents. The predicted MAC awake value for cyclopropane would be about 5.3% and that for nitrous oxide, 59%. Differences between anesthetics in time required for awakening must result only from differences in rates of elimination. This agrees with the clinical impression of slow recovery with highly soluble anesthetics and more rapid recovery with poorly soluble agents.

► [We suspect that MAC awake is likely to prove to be less precise than MAC.—Eds.]

Body Temperature: Possible Ionic Mechanism in Hypothalamus Controlling the Set Point. According to the monoamine theory of thermoregulation, serotonin and norepinephrine are released from the anterior hypothalamus in functional opposition to one another, acting at the same hypothalamic site to active heat-production and heat-loss pathways. This theory, however, does not explain the intrinsic setting of body temperature at about 37 C., noted in most mammals. Perfusion of isotonic saline through the cerebral ventricles of a cat leads to shivering and a rise in temperature, and addition of calcium blocks the hyperthermic response. R. D. Myers and W. L. Veale[3] (Purdue Univ.) propose that the set point for body temperature is localized in the posterior hypothalamus and is maintained by the inherent sodium-calcium ion ratio.

Guide tubes were placed in the rostral and caudal hypothalamus in cats by stereotaxic technic, and body temperature was monitored by a colonic thermistor probe. Bilateral hypothalamic sites were perfused at a rate of 50 μL. per minute for 20-30 minutes. Temperature was unchanged by perfusion with a solution containing 143 mM sodium and 2.6 mM calcium ion. Perfusion with calcium-free solution containing normal or excessive sodium led to shivering and a sharp rise in temperature (Fig. 3), as well as vasoconstriction and piloerection. With calcium in normal or increased amounts but no sodium, the temperature fell sharply, with vasodilation and slight sedation evident. Normal Krebs solution, Krebs solution with doubled ionic constituents and sucrose solution that was isotonic or twice isotonic concentration caused no temperature changes.

---

(3) Science 170:95-97, Oct. 2, 1970.

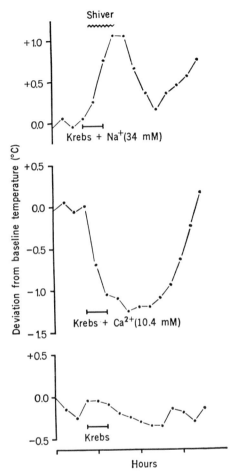

Fig. 3.—Deviation from baseline temperature (degrees C.) in a cat in which the posterior hypothalamus was perfused bilaterally 3 times at 48-hour intervals. Solid bar denotes a 30-minute perfusion with Krebs solution having excess sodium at a concentration of 34 mM. (*top*); excess calcium at a concentration of 10.4 mM. (*center*); and normal values of all salts (*bottom*). Shivering accompanied the sodium perfusion as indicated (*top*). (Courtesy of Myers, R. D., and Veale, W. L.: Science 170: 95-97, Oct. 2, 1970.)

No significant changes occurred with magnesium or potassium ion perfused in two to five times normal physiologic concentrations. The hyperthermic effect of saline was not due to chloride, as seen in studies with a sodium compound having toluene-p-sulfonate as its anion.

These studies showed that the set point for body temperature may be determined in the cat by a balance in sodium and calcium concentrations in the brain stem. A constant ratio between these ions is important. The cellular mechanisms by which ionic balance causes efferent responses in the hypothalamus are not clear. Ions could mobilize intracellular cyclic AMP, ATP and adenylcyclase. An inherent ionic balance within the framework of enzymatic activity may also explain other homeostatic mechanisms involved in functions mediated by the brain stem.

▶ [Many theories of narcosis in the past have invoked changes in intracellular-extracellular calcium ratios as an explanation for general anesthesia. If this were involved in anesthesia, and is now found to affect temperature regulation, it might explain the tendency to hypothermia so commonly seen during anesthesia.—Eds.]

Cerebral Electric Activity during Cyclopropane Anesthesia in Man. Data on visual evoked activity indicate that general anesthetics may block specific afferent activity; however, whether extracranial early evoked waves reflect activity in specific paths is less certain for visual than for somatic potentials. Donald L. Clark, Burton S. Rosner and Charles Beck[4] (Univ. of Pennsylvania) examined somatosensory evoked responses in 16 healthy young men during cyclopropane anesthesia at known $Paco_2$ levels.

METHOD.—Fasting subjects were studied while supine. The ulnar nerve was stimulated for recording the peripheral neurogram. Cerebral evoked responses were recorded from scalp electrodes. Control recordings were obtained with the subject breathing room air. Atropine, 0.6 mg., was given intramuscularly, and anesthesia was induced with cyclopropane, with ventilation controlled by a Bird respirator. Tidal volume was adjusted to produce a minute volume of about 8 L. for normocarbia or up to 20 L. for hypocarbia. Cyclopropane was given in concentrations of 5, 12, 20-25 and 36-43%.

All concentrations of cyclopropane decreased or eliminated both the specific and diffuse components of averaged extracranial evoked somatosensory potentials. Peripheral nerve still responded to percutaneous electric stimuli. As the concentration of cyclopropane was increased from 5 to about 40%, the frontal EEG became larger, slower and more regular. At a 20% cyclopropane concentration, varying the $Paco_2$ from about 20 to 50 torr or more produced EEG changes indicative of increasing depth of anesthesia.

Cyclopropane appeared to affect both lemniscal and extralemniscal sensory pathways. The findings may indicate that

(4)   J. Appl. Physiol. 28:802-807, June, 1970.

early visual potentials recorded extracranially do not originate in the geniculocalcarine system. Alternately, they may represent a pharmacologic difference between the somatic and visual systems.

Effects of Basal Anesthesia on Response of Sympathetic Nervous Activity and Barostatic Reflexes to Subsequent Administration of Halothane were examined by Per Skovsted, Mary L. Price and Henry L. Price[5] (Univ. of Pennsylvania). Halothane, given to the cat, on a background of 50% nitrous oxide anesthesia reduced sympathetic outflow only slightly and did not alter the response to stimulation of the left aortic depressor nerve. Halothane given with chloralose markedly reduced sympathetic activity and abolished the barostatic reflex. Studies were then done on 22 cats initially anesthetized with 4% halothane in oxygen, continuing with 50% nitrous oxide in oxygen. The left cervical sympathetic trunk and left aortic depressor nerve were divided. Six animals were given 3, 2 and 1.5% halothane, followed by chloralose, 40 mg./kg., as 1% solution, nitrous oxide being discontinued. Six received 1.5% halothane without nitrous oxide, and 6 received halothane and then chloralose. In 6 animals, the effect of halothane on the response to baroreceptor nerve stimulation was studied with nitrous oxide or chloralose as basal anesthetic.

Halothane in an end-tidal concentration of 1.2% reduced preganglionic sympathetic activity and abolished barostatic reflexes in cats given chloralose as a basal anesthetic. These effects were not observed when the basal anesthetic consisted of nitrous oxide and gallamine. It is concluded that chloralose can interact with at least one inhalation anesthetic in such a manner that autonomic responses to the latter are profoundly modified.

This study emphasizes the need for caution in attempting to study drug actions in animals given basal anesthetics whose effects remain essentially unknown.

▶ [Many studies of the effects of anesthetic agents require some form of basal anesthesia in order that control measurements may be made. An old favorite has been chloralose, which supposedly had minimal effects on nerve activity. The results described here suggest that chloralose exerts its own neurologic effects, and that we must re-evaluate many studies done in its presence.—Eds.]

Anesthetic Agents and Chemical Sensitivity of Cortical Neurons. J. M. Crawford[6] (Australian Nat'l Univ.) examined the

(5) J. Pharmacol. & Exper. Therap. 175:183-188, October, 1970.
(6) Neuropharmacology 9:31-46, January, 1970.

effects of anesthetics on the sensitivity of cortical neurons to acetylcholine and homocysteic acid as representative excitants and to the depressant γ-aminobutyric acid and compared the effects with changes in spontaneous synaptic firing of the cells.

Studies were done on 45 adult cats prepared under halothane anesthesia. Needles were placed stereotaxically in the pericruciate cortex and various lesions were made. Artificial ventilation was instituted after decerebration, maintaining the end-tidal CO_2 at 3.6-4.2%. Micropipettes were used to record extra-cellular spike potentials from pericruciate neurons. Studies were done using 0.2M homocysteic acid, 0.5 or 1M acetyl-choline, 0.2 or 0.5M γ-aminobutyric acid and either 0.05M 5-hydroxytryptamine or 4M NaCl.

Anesthetics produced similar effects on both spontaneous synaptic firing and responses of given cells to alternate micro-electrophoretic ejection of acetylcholine and excitant amino acids. Barbiturates reduced the chemical sensitivity of cortical neurons in doses well below those necessary for surgical anes-thesia; the duration of depression resembled the persistence of each agent in clinical practice. Subanesthetic doses of urethane were not effective but full anesthetic doses of chloralose mark-edly reduced the chemical sensitivity of the cells for long pe-riods.

Low to moderate concentrations of nitrous oxide, trichlor-ethylene and halothane had little direct effect on neuronal fir-ing. The effects of "anesthetic" levels of nitrous oxide were ob-scured by associated hypoxia but halothane levels exceeding 1.5% depressed cell excitability. Methoxyflurane, 0.2-1.2% did not appreciably alter the chemical sensitivity of neurons, even in full anesthetic levels. None of the agents tested prevented de-pression of the neurons by γ-aminobutyric acid.

General anesthetics appear to nonspecifically reduce the chemical excitability of cortical neurons, possibly by an action on postsynaptic membrane conductance changes. Neurons in various regions of the nervous system differ in their suscepti-bility to particular anesthetics. Only chloralose showed specific antagonism toward the natural transmitters at cortical neurons. More potent analgesic agents had a relatively less depressant effect on the sensitivity of cortical neurons. Analgesia and an-esthesia may result from an action of these compounds at sub-cortical sites.

▶ [The barbiturates appear to act differently in cortical neurons than the inhalation anesthetics, which in clinical concentrations seem to have relatively little effect on the spontaneous activity or chemical sensitivity of these neurons.—Ed.]

LOCAL ANESTHETICS

Mechanism of Convulsions Elicited by Local Anesthetic Agents: I. Local Anesthetic Depression of Electrically Induced Seizures in Man. Jaime A. Wikinski, Jose E. Usubiaga, Raul L. Morales, Alberto Torrieri and Lilia E. Usubiaga[7] (Buenos Aires, Argentina) noted, in studies on the interaction of local anesthetics and succinylcholine, that convulsant doses of procaine and lidocaine made patients completely refractory to electric shock stimulation and prolonged the sleep times.

Study was made of 12 men, aged 20-54, who were to receive electroconvulsive therapy. Controls received thiopental sodium, 4 mg./kg. intravenously, followed by succinylcholine, 0.7 mg./kg. Electric shock was induced by a 60-cps a-c current after fasciculations had subsided. Procaine, in doses of 1-36 mg./kg., was given intravenously in 50% increments after thiopental induction, at a rate of 10 mg./kg./minute. Lidocaine was given in doses of 1-16.5 mg./kg. at a rate of 3 mg./kg./minute.

Both local anesthetics reduced the duration of convulsion in a dose-related manner; lidocaine was more potent than procaine on a mg. for mg. basis. Lidocaine and procaine doses of 11.2 and 24.7 mg./kg., respectively, prevented seizures in half the patients. Larger doses of both agents induced tonic-clonic seizures; afterward electric shock did not induce a seizure in any patient.

The tonic phase of the electrically induced somatic seizure was more vulnerable to local anesthetic depression than the clonic. Recovery was significantly shortened by small doses of the local anesthetics, but larger doses delayed the recovery. Procaine usually produced tachycardia, and both drugs reduced the arterial pressure temporarily. Blood levels of lidocaine were lower than those of procaine and showed a more prolonged delay.

Local anesthetics are antielectroconvulsive and are depressant agents at all dose levels. They probably have a single mechanism of action, though they may influence different receptor sites. Anticonvulsive and convulsive effects of the anesthetics appear to represent depression of different central nerv-

(7) Anesth. & Analg. 49:504-510, May-June, 1970.

ous system structures. Protection from electroconvulsive therapy is most evident at the lower end of the dose scale; greater depression, including convulsions, becomes evident at the higher end.

▶ [Local anesthetics, while causing convulsions at certain dose levels, do so by depressing certain brain centers, not stimulating them. It is somewhat akin to the stimulation via depression caused by alcohol.

This field was an abiding interest of Dr. Jose Usubiaga, who unfortunately died shortly after the article appeared.—Eds.]

Effects of Hepatectomy on Disappearance Rate of Lidocaine from Blood in Man and Dog. Lidocaine has been thought to be primarily metabolized in the liver, with little or no extrahepatic degradation. J. Antonio Aldrete, John Homatas (Univ. of Colorado), R. Nichol Boyes (Worcester, Mass.) and Thomas E. Starzl[8] (Univ. of Colorado) tested this contention in hepatectomized dogs with near-normal cardiodynamics and, during the anhepatic period, in 2 patients undergoing liver transplantation. Five anesthetized mongrel dogs received a 2% solution of lidocaine HCl, 2.5 mg./kg., intravenously, before and after portacaval shunting and total hepatectomy. Two adults having orthotopic liver transplantation were given lidocaine, 2.5 mg./kg., intravenously while anesthetized, as the host liver was being dissected. A second injection was given as host hepatectomy was done a few hours later. The homograft was revascularized 50 minutes after injection of the anesthetic.

Intact dogs had blood lidocaine levels of 0.7 µg./ml. or less at 1 hour, and 0.5 or less 2 hours after injection. Hepatectomized dogs given dilute glucose had 2-hour values above 1.2 µg./ml. When concentrated glucose was given, initial lidocaine levels were 7.9-18.4 µg./ml., and they dropped rapidly to 3-5 µg./ml. Levels remained above 1 µg./ml. at 2 hours. The patients, both with severe hepatic insufficiency, had respective blood lidocaine levels of 6.6 and 5 µg./ml. after injection. One-hour levels were 1.5 and 1.7, and 2-hour levels, 1.1 and 1.4 µg./ml. After revascularization, the level 4 hours after injection was only 0.4 µg./ml. Neither dogs nor patients showed toxic effects from the lidocaine injections.

This study showed that the early phase of lidocaine disappearance was less affected by the anhepatic state than the late phase in both dogs and man. If extrahepatic degradation of lidocaine occurred at all, it must have been at an imperceptible pace.

(8)   Anesth. & Analg. 49:687-690, Sept.-Oct., 1970.

▶ [Caution has been expressed against the use of intravenous regional block with lidocaine in patients with liver disease. This work suggests that other degradation pathways are available.—Eds.]

Nerve Conduction Studies in Regional Intravenous Analgesia Using One Per Cent Lidocaine. Most workers have used 0.5% lidocaine for intravenous regional analgesia, but 1% lidocaine is also safe and effective. C. A. Shanks and J. G. McLeod[9] (Univ. of Sydney) studied the site of action of 1% lidocaine by electrophysiologic technics in 8 healthy men aged 21-48. In 5 subjects, an upper arm cuff was inflated after exsanguination of the limb, and 20 ml. of 1% lidocaine was injected into a hand vein. The median nerve in the forearm and its branches in the hand were studied for the next 30 minutes. In 2 subjects, 10 ml. lidocaine was injected after exsanguination with a cuff 8-10 cm. above the wrist, and in 1 subject exsanguination was not done, but the limb was elevated for 3 minutes before cuff inflation. Control observations were made on the opposite limb with ischemia alone in all subjects.

Pain and tactile sensations were reduced proximal to the injection site about 5 minutes after injection, and full anesthesia was present after 7-15 minutes distal to a strip just below the tourniquet. Forearm muscles were totally paralyzed in 10-25 minutes. With ischemia alone, dysesthesia appeared at about 5 minutes and anesthesia in 15-30; only 1 subject had total paralysis. Anesthesia spread extremely slowly when exsanguination was incomplete. Motor conduction was totally impaired in 25 minutes. When only the wrist and hand were exsanguinated, latency increased earlier and more rapidly with injection of lidocaine. The same was true of sensory conduction. Responses to repetitive stimulation after lidocaine did not differ significantly from those seen with ischemia alone. Peak plasma lidocaine levels in the contralateral arm occurred 1-5 minutes after initial tourniquet release, the maximum value being 4.4 μg./ml.

The site of action of 1% lidocaine in regional intravenous analgesia is the nerve trunks, as well as the peripheral nerve endings. This mode of action may be preferable to the more peripheral effects of 0.5% lidocaine in circumstances that prevent adequate perfusion of the operative site, such as tense fracture hematoma formation.

▶ [The anesthesia seems better with 1% lidocaine, but how much more dangerous is it than 0.5%?—Eds.]

(9) Brit. J. Anaesth. 42:1060-1066, December, 1970.

Plasma Lidocaine Concentrations Following Topical Aerosol Application to the Trachea and Bronchi. D. A. Pelton, M. Daly, P. D. Cooper and A. W. Conn[1] (Univ. of Toronto) examined the effects of avoiding explosive anesthetics for routine clinical practice and of the clinical use of a new endotracheal aerosol with a metering system that can deliver accurate doses of lidocaine. Previously 4% lidocaine was given by spray to the glottic and tracheal regions, and toxic blood levels could readily occur in small infants. Most of the aerosol bomb dispensers examined delivered a dose of lidocaine of about 10 mg., as claimed. A topical dose of 3 mg./kg. was administered to 13 cardiovascular patients with nonshunting lesions. Premedication was with atropine and meperidine plus pentobarbital. Induction was with thiopental, and anesthesia was maintained with halothane and nitrous oxide. Lidocaine was administered after succinylcholine to the larynx and then below the vocal cords. Anesthesia was maintained by controlled ventilation.

The arterial lidocaine level rose to a peak in 2 minutes, followed by a gradual decline. Venous levels reached a peak in 5 minutes and then declined steadily. Maximal arterial and venous blood levels were 2.5 and 3.2 μg./ml., respectively, below the safe level. The rate of absorption probably depends on the state of the mucosa, amount of airway mucus present, rate and depth of respiration, state of the circulation and dose administered. No signs of toxicity occurred with use of the 10% lidocaine spray in this study. This technic is effective and reliable for topical tracheobronchial anesthesia as an adjunct to general anesthesia. The blood concentrations are dose dependent and, in the dosage used, are below toxic levels.

► [Has anyone done a blind study to determine if topical spray before tracheal intubation during general anesthesia is really worthwhile?—Eds.]

Evaluation of Two New Local Anesthetics for Major Conduction Blockade. Recently two agents have been introduced that provide fast, reliable onset of blockade and prolonged blockade. They are the fast-acting carbonated local anesthetics and the long-acting local agent bupivacaine. P. R. Bromage and M. Gertel[2] (McGill Univ.) evaluated these agents for epidural anesthesia and supraclavicular brachial blockade in 320 cases. All the agents studied included 1:200,000 epinephrine. Epidural anesthesia was induced with 2% lidocaine in 65 instances, 2%

(1)   Canad. Anaesth. Soc. J. 17:250-255, May, 1970.
(2)   Ibid., pp. 557-564, November, 1970.

mepivacaine in 25; 0.5% tetracaine in 37, 2% CO_2-lidocaine in 150 and 0.5% bupivacaine in 76. Brachial plexus block was performed by a modification of Kulenkampff's supraclavicular approach. The agent used was 1% lidocaine in 26 instances, 1% mepivacaine in 25, 1% CO_2-lidocaine in 26, 2% CO_2-lidocaine in 26, 0.25% bupivacaine in 28 and 1% CO_2-lidocaine with 0.25% bupivacaine in 10.

In epidural analgesia, orthodox hydrochloride solutions took a considerable time to produce complete blockade. Carbonated lidocaine had the fastest onset of action, with a latency about 30% faster than its hydrochloride counterpart. Bupivacaine acted considerably more slowly. Carbonated lidocaine produced the most intense motor blockade (51.5%) and bupivacaine the least (28.9%). Bupivacaine had the longest duration of action, but the agents were not markedly different in this regard. In brachial plexus block, CO_2-lidocaine solutions showed the shortest duration of action and the least variability and bupivacaine the longest latency and the most variability. Three of 28 patients given bupivacaine had only patchy, incomplete analgesia after 35 minutes. The CO_2 solutions had the shortest duration of action and bupivacaine the longest, with a mean duration of 10¼ hours, providing excellent postoperative analgesia.

These new agents for major conduction blockade each have highly desirable properties. Carbonated solutions are quick acting, powerful and reliable, but their duration of action is rather short. Bupivacaine is slow to take effect and produces less intense blockade, but it is extremely long acting in peripheral nerve blocks. A single drug producing these various desirable effects is still needed; the findings with carbonating ultra-long-acting agents are awaited with interest.

Bupivacaine: Review of 2,077 Cases. Daniel C. Moore, L. Donald Bridenbaugh, Phillip O. Bridenbaugh and Geoffrey T. Tucker[3] (Mason Clinic, Seattle) evaluated bupivacaine in patients having obstetric or surgical procedures or a diagnostic or therapeutic block. The drug was given in concentrations of 0.1, 0.25, 0.5 and 0.75%, with and without epinephrine (1:200,000). The maximum dose was 200 mg. without and 250 mg. with epinephrine. Blood bupivacaine levels were determined by gas chromatography. The 0.1% solution was inadequate for re-

(3)   J.A.M.A. 214:713-718, Oct. 26, 1970.

gional blocks. The other concentrations were tried in 2,077 patients, including 657 having obstetric procedures, 1,334 having surgical procedures and 86 having diagnostic or therapeutic blocks. There were 600 caudal and 57 epidural obstetric procedures. All concentrations over 0.1% produced sensory anesthesia in all regional blocks, but motor block was not profound in all cases with the weaker concentrations.

The lower concentrations were entirely adequate for vaginal deliveries. Muscle relaxation occurred consistently only with 0.75% bupivacaine for major intra-abdominal operations, including cesarean section. The dose ranges for delivery were 8-14 ml. of 0.25% solution and 18-30 ml. of 0.5% solution. Some brachial plexus blocks done with 0.25% solution were incomplete. Onset of block began at 4-10 minutes with the weaker solutions, with maximal anesthesia in 15-30 minutes. With 0.75% solution, onset was at 3-5 minutes and maximum effect was at 8-20 minutes. Duration of anesthesia was several hours but varied considerably, depending on type of block, concentration of drug, and use of epinephrine or not. The mean peak venous blood bupivacaine level in 11 patients having epidural or caudal blocks was 0.64 μg./ml. 15-30 minutes after injection of 125 or 150 mg. Placental transfer of bupivacaine occurred, but newborn depression was not noted. One patient had a total spinal after caudal block. Two patients given intravenous injections had signs of mild cerebral stimulation. Hypotension followed epidural block for surgery in 39.9% of cases, celiac plexus block in 50.3% and caudal block in 7.1%. No anesthesia occurred in 1.1% of attempted blocks. Some patients, especially children, became anxious about a permanent effect since the block lasted so long.

Bupivacaine was highly reliable in this study and provided excellent sensory and motor anesthesia when used appropriately. The complications were those that can result from regional block. Its prolonged action makes bupivacaine useful for peripheral nerve block, epidural block or caudal block for a long surgical or obstetric procedure, to relieve postoperative pain or to produce prolonged vasodilatation in an extremity. Caudal block for rectal procedures and perineorrhaphy is another definite indication.

▶ [An axillary brachial plexus block with 0.25% bupivacaine with 1:200,000 epinephrine resulted in almost 11 hours of anesthesia, a duration unattainable with other drugs available.—Eds.]

AGENTS FOR INDUCTION OF ANESTHESIA

Effect of Intra-Arterial Injections of Barbiturates. Most reports of intra-arterial barbiturate injection have been in conjunction with anesthesia. Dominic Albo, Jr., Larry Cheung, Larry Ruth, Clifford Snyder and Keith Reemtsma[4] (Univ. of Utah) report data on 2 patients who had an intra-arterial secobarbital injection.

CASE 1.—Man, 29, with a 7-year history of barbiturate addiction was seen 48 hours after the self-injection of 100 mg. secobarbital as 10% solution into the radial artery. Severe pain, forearm and hand edema, cyanosis of the finger tips and an absent radial pulse ensued. Intra-arterial papaverine had no effect and sympathetic block was ineffective. An angiogram at 7 days showed occlusion of the midportion of the radial artery and no filling of the volar arch. The thumb and distal index finger were eventually were amputated.

CASE 2.—Woman, 23, was seen 7 hours after injecting 10% secobarbital into the radial artery, with signs similar to those of Case 1. Heparin was infused into the brachial artery to maintain the clotting time at 3 times the control value. Most swelling had subsided after 10 days of therapy and gangrene did not develop. Angiographic changes did not appear at any time in this patient.

Thrombosis eventually develops in all patients with intra-arterial barbiturate injection in which tissue damage occurs. There is little laboratory evidence to support the theory of vasospasm in this condition. Laboratory studies have indicated that heparin therapy and sympathectomy may be useful.

The authors perform arteriography and then place a catheter proximal to the injection site for heparin infusion, to keep the clotting time about 3 times the control value, using a pump and lactated Ringer's solution. Heparin infusion is continued until pain and swelling have subsided, which may require up to 2 weeks of treatment. Concomitant sympathetic block is not advocated but morphine is given to control pain. Gangrenous areas are allowed to demarcate and are treated in the usual manner. Smoking is prohibited. The arm is elevated to enhance resorption of edema fluid.

▶ [A lot more is known about intra-arterial injection of barbiturates than is indicated here. Is the response to intra-arterial secobarbital the same as to intra-arterial thiopental?—Eds.]

Propanidid is discussed by C. M. Conway and D. B. Ellis[5] (London). Propranidid is a non-barbiturate induction agent with a transient action, followed by rapid recovery. In the body,

(4) Am. J. Surg. 120:676-678, November, 1970.
(5) Brit. J. Anaesth. 42:249-254, March, 1970.

it is rapidly metabolized to inert products by esterases, and cumulation does not occur with repeated administration. The main use of propanidid has been to produce transient anesthesia in outpatients. The drug is derived from oil of cloves (eugenol), and clinical solutions contain a solubilizing agent, Cremophor EL, a polyoxyethylated castor oil. Propanidid is available as a 5% solution miscible with water. Propranidid is equipotent with thiopentone in hypnotic effect; a 4 mg./kg. dose of both drugs is needed to induce anesthesia. Serum cholinesterase activity is transiently inhibited by propanidid. The drug is rapidly redistributed to organs with a high blood supply.

Propanidid given intravenously produces loss of consciousness within one arm-brain circulation time, with EEG changes similar to those produced by barbiturates given intravenously. Propanidid-induced sleep is sometimes associated with excitatory phenomena. Vomiting has been reported in up to 28% of the subjects given the drug. Hyperventilation occurs as consciousness is lost, followed by a short period of hypoventilation, periodic breathing or apnea. Most animals show a transient dose-related fall in blood pressure with propanidid. In man, hypotension occurs; falls of over 40 mm. Hg are common with doses exceeding 8 mg./kg. A 4% incidence of local complications has been noted with direct injection of propanidid into a vein, but no local reactions occurred on infusion of the drug. Potentiation of suxamethonium by propanidid may be due to an action of propanidid on the muscle cell membrane.

Rapid, complete recovery follows the use of propanidid for induction intravenously. Patients anesthetized for minor procedures can usually be safely discharged early. The adverse side effects would be most disturbing in elderly or ill patients, especially as the agent is presently given without added oxygen. Despite its advantages the undesirable side effects of propanidid would appear to preclude its wide acceptance.

▶ [Although widely used throughout Britain and Commonwealth nations, on close examination this drug does not measure up to thiopental.—Eds.]

Ketamine as an Induction Agent in Anesthetics is discussed by J. W. Dundee, J. Bovill, J. W. D. Knox, R. S. J. Clarke, G. W. Black, S. H. S. Love, J. Moore, J. Elliott, S. K. Pandit and D. L. Coppel[6] (Belfast). Ketamine, a rapidly acting nonbarbiturate general anesthetic which can be given intravenously or intramuscularly, is especially suitable for children and for

(6)   Lancet 1: 1370-1371, June 27, 1970.

repeat procedures. Over 450 administrations have been documented, most of them in adults. Ketamine produced loss of consciousness before nitrous oxide-oxygen in adults in initial doses of 1-3 mg./kg., except for a few subjects given less than 2 mg./kg. Some hypertonus always occurred, but this rarely interfered with positioning of patients for operation. No patient given 3 mg./kg. required a supplementary induction dose of ketamine. A blood pressure peak occurred in 3-4 minutes, and a systolic rise of over 20 mm. Hg occurred in most of the patients given over 2 mg./kg. Pulse rate changes were minimal. Response to commands was noted on an average of 5.8 minutes after nitrous oxide withdrawal after an induction dose of up to 2 mg./kg. and 8.3 minutes after larger doses. Emergence delirium was dose-related but responded rapidly to small intravenous doses of diazepam. Half of the patients had dreams during recovery, which were usually unpleasant. The optimal adult dose for induction was set at 2 mg./kg.

Some premedicants were found to reduce the undesirable effects of ketamine, but none abolished them completely. The most suitable agents are papaveretum-hyocine and phenoperidine-droperidol. Cardiovascular effects were greater when 2 mg./kg. ketamine was given as induction for major operations, with atropine as the only premedication, but delirium on emergence was much reduced. Ketamine was used in a dose of 8 mg./kg. with 0.6 mg. atropine in about 40 children having minor operations. The children did not respond to peripheral stimuli and were hypotonic. Moderate hypertension lasted 3-4 minutes. Recovery was more prolonged than with rectal or intravenous barbiturates, but the children had full control of their airways. No postoperative delirium was noted.

The term "dissociated" anesthesia is appropriate for ketamine. Adults have a high incidence of undesirable side effects from this agent, and more work is needed to identify the best adjuvant agents and to clarify specific indications for using ketamine.

▶ [Points up the pros and cons well.—Eds.]

Ketamine as Sole Anesthetic in Open Heart Surgery: Preliminary Report. Ketamine has been found to exert strong cardiovascular stimulation, with a rise in both blood pressure components, by a means that is unclear. Guenter Corssen, Rodolfo Allarde, Frederick Brosch and Gertrud Arbenz[7] (Univ.

(7)   Anesth. & Analg. 49:1025-1031, Nov.-Dec., 1970.

of Alabama) used ketamine as the sole anesthetic in operations done to correct heart defects or replace heart valves. Study was made of 11 males and 3 females, aged 4-75 years. Six patients were so ill that survival from operation using conventional anesthesia was doubted. Intravenous ketamine was given in a dose of about 1 mg./lb., with increments of 0.5 mg./lb. at 15-30 minute intervals. During bypass ketamine was injected into the pump. Total dose ranged from 130 to 850 mg., with a mean of 11 supplemental intravenous doses. Mean duration of anesthesia was 6 hours. Tracheal intubation was with use of tubocurarine in most instances. Average duration of bypass was 83 minutes. Moderate hypothermia was induced in all patients.

In none of the 3 deaths was ketamine implicated. The average hospitalization in the other cases was 16 days. Typically anesthesia was unusually smooth and uneventful, with cardiovascular stability maintained. The arterial pressure was characteristically low 10 minutes after the end of bypass. Recently ketamine has been given just before discontinuation of bypass, and pressures afterward have been more nearly normal. Three patients had prolonged disorientation and psychotic behavior.

Ketamine may be a suitable anesthetic for patients having cardiac operations with cardiopulmonary bypass and hypothermia. The drug is a strong cardiovascular stimulant and has antiarrhythmia activity. It is particularly suitable for desperately ill patients who cannot tolerate the further depression of myocardial function that may occur with conventional anesthetics.

▶ [Not convincing at all. Three (of 14 patients) "had prolonged disorientation and psychotic behavior."—Eds.]

Comparison of Diazepam with Thiopental as Induction Agent in Cardiopulmonary Disease. An intravenous agent that maintains cardiopulmonary safety and stability during anesthetic induction has not yet been identified. Richard B. Knapp and Herbert Dubow[8] (Greenwich, Conn.) studied diazepam to determine if it offered any advantages over the commonly administered ultrashort-acting barbiturates, with sodium thiopental being used as the comparison drug. Studies were done in 800 A.S.A. classes III and IV patients over 2 years. Half received intravenous diazepam, and half, thiopental. A dose of 2 mg./kg. body weight of 2.5% thiopental or 0.2 mg./kg. body weight of diazepam was required for loss of the lid reflex. Pre-

(8)   Anesth. & Analg. 49: 722-726, Sept.-Oct., 1970.

medication was with meperidine, hydroxyzine and atropine. Measurements were repeated about 2 minutes after drug injection, just before tracheal intubation or application of a face mask.

The heart rate fell from 80-120 to 60-80 in 20% of both groups of patients. Changes in Pao_2 and $Paco_2$ were not significant. A 15% decrease in tidal and minute volumes occurred with thiopental, and a 10% decrease with diazepam. Cardiac output decreased by over 15% as determined by the dye-dilution technic in 85% of patients given 100-300 mg. thiopental. Fewer than 1% of patients given 5-20 mg. diazepam had a 15% fall in cardiac output. Mean arterial pressure decreased by 15 mm. Hg or more in 270 of 400 patients given thiopental. Of the 400 given diazepam, 350 had no decrease in mean arterial pressure, and 50 had a decrease of less than 10 mm. Hg.

The much greater cardiovascular safety of diazepam compared with the barbiturates warrants further evaluation of its use as an induction agent. Also diazepam may be preferable to the barbiturates as an induction agent in anesthesia for poor-risk patients with cardiopulmonary disease.

► [Drugs come and go and often are predicted to displace the time-honored agents, only to fall by the wayside themselves. However, it begins to look as if diazepam will be around for awhile.—Eds.]

Effects of Diazepam (Valium) on Left Ventricular Function and Systemic Vascular Resistance were studied by Ronald M. Abel, Rudolf N. Staroscik and Robert L. Reis[9] (Nat'l Inst. of Health) in anesthetized adult mongrel dogs. The sinoatrial node was crushed, and the heart was paced at a rate of 170. Total bypass was instituted, and the main pulmonary artery was ligated. A mean aortic pressure of 75-100 mm. Hg was maintained. Isovolumetric left ventricular contractions were provided by an intraventricular balloon. Diazepam was injected in a dose of 0.1 mg./kg., and force-velocity curves were recorded. Length-tension relationships were determined 2, 5, 10 and 30 minutes after diazepam administration. Solvent vehicle alone was injected in some experiments.

Peak left ventricular isovolumetric pressure rose markedly within 2 minutes after diazepam injection. An average increase of 28% was noted at 30 minutes, with an average 23% increase in the peak rate of positive pressure development during left ventricular systole. Force-velocity curves were shifted upward

(9)   J. Pharmacol. & Exper. Therap. 173:364-370, June, 1970.

and to the right after diazepam. The maximum measured contractile element velocity increased, indicating augmentation of the intrinsic contractile state of the myocardium. Length-tension relationships indicated improved cardiac performance after diazepam. The response to a larger injection of 2-3 mg./kg. given 30 minutes after the first injection did not exceed that obtained with the smaller dose. Solvent injection had no consistent effect on ventricular function. Systemic vascular resistance decreased significantly shortly after diazepam injection, but the values at 30 minutes were similar to control values.

With heart rate and mean aortic pressure held constant, diazepam significantly improved left ventricular function. The mechanisms responsible for the positive inotropic effects of diazepam are not evident from the study. They may be related to reflex effects of the drug on the nervous system or to a decrease in coronary vascular resistance with a resultant increased coronary blood flow. A direct or reflex relaxant effect on peripheral vessels is more likely than primary myocardial depression as an explanation of the hypotensive side effects of the drug. Diazepam may have a salutary effect when used as a sedative or tranquilizer in patients with impaired cardiac function.

▶ [Intravenous diazepam has found a place as an agent to induce anesthesia in poor-risk patients. This study lends support to this practice.— Eds.]

Preliminary Clinical Study of CT 1341—Steroid Anesthetic Agent. The recent discovery of CT 1341 has reawakened interest in steroid anesthesia. Donald Campbell, Alex C. Forrester, Donald C. Miller, I Hutton, J. A. Kennedy, T. D. V. Lawrie, A. R. Lorimer and D. McCall[1] (Univ. of Glasgow) conducted three clinical trials in 20 volunteers. A pilot study was done in 8 patients, generally using a dose of 0.1 ml. CT 1341 per kg. given intravenously in 15 seconds. Anesthesia was maintained with 70%-30% nitrous oxide-oxygen, sometimes supplemented with trichloroethylene. Six patients, 3 of each sex, were studied during diagnostic cardiac catheterization, being given 0.1 ml./kg. A more precise dose-body weight relation was sought in 6 unpremedicated patients having minor outpatient operations.

Troublesome muscle movement occurred in 2 subjects in the pilot study. Induction times were 30-80 seconds and recovery times, 15-360 seconds. Most patients were euphoric on recovery.

(1)   Brit. J. Anaesth. 43:14-24, January, 1971.

Tachypnea was common; apnea was not noted. The glottic and laryngeal reflexes were depressed just after induction but returned quickly to normal. All patients exhibited peripheral vasodilatation and a rise in heart rate. A just significant rise in systolic blood pressure occurred; there were no ECG abnormalities. In hemodynamic studies, mean aortic pressure fell before the heart rate increased, and the pressure rose on recovery from anesthesia. Pulmonary artery pressure did not change significantly, and mean cardiac output did not change. Stroke volume fell slightly, and systemic vascular resistance fell in 5 of 6 cases. The mean decrease in Pao_2 was highly significant; the $Paco_2$ did not rise significantly. No nausea or vomiting occurred. More stable anesthesia was obtained with a dose of 0.15 ml./kg.

The steroid CT 1341 appears to be a potent, quick-acting induction agent with a low incidence of undesirable side effects. It is safe and useful for inducing general anesthesia. This new drug seems worthy of further clinical trial.

NARCOTICS, ANTAGONISTS AND SEDATIVES

Use of Fentanyl, Meperidine or Alphaprodine for Neuroleptanesthesia was investigated by Francis F. Foldes, Hans P. Shiffman and Peter P. Kronfeld[2] (Albert Einstein College of Medicine). Droperidol with fentanyl has been widely used with nitrous oxide-oxygen to produce neuroleptanesthesia. Preliminary studies with combinations of droperidol, chlorpromazine, triflupromazine and hydroxyzine and fentanyl indicated that droperidol was preferable. A double-blind study was then undertaken in 527 consecutive surgical patients over age 16 with combinations of droperidol plus fentanyl, meperidine and alphaprodine. Solutions of 2.5 mg. droperidol per ml., 30 μg. fentanyl per ml., 30 mg. meperidine per ml. and 12 mg. alphaprodine per ml. were used, selected on the basis of relative analgesic potencies. Some patients received succinylcholine for tracheal intubation, some received tubocurarine or gallamine as well for relaxation and some were not given neuromuscular blockers. Premedication was with diphenhydramine and scopolamine or atropine. A third of the settling dose of narcotic was given 6-8 minutes after 0.15 mg. droperidol per kg., followed by

(2)   Anesthesiology 33:35-42, July, 1970.

nitrous oxide-oxygen by face mask. Fractional doses of narcotic were then given as needed.

Droperidol moderately increased the pulse rate. Both fentanyl and alphaprodine reduced the pulse, but only the latter significantly. Only alphaprodine significantly reduced blood pressure. Droperidol moderately reduced the respiratory rate. The narcotics reduced the rate by 20-30%. Apnea and ventilatory difficulty were most frequent in patients given alphaprodine. Doses in terms of micrograms per kilogram per minute were greater during short than during longer anesthesias. Consciousness returned most rapidly after fentanyl and least rapidly after meperidine. Postoperative analgesic requirements and nausea were similar in the different narcotic groups. No extrapyramidal excitation or unusual psychotomimetic effects were noted postoperatively. Most patients were well satisfied with the anesthesia.

Fentanyl and meperidine were found to be more suitable than alphaprodine for production or neuroleptanesthesia in conjunction with droperidol. Fentanyl has a lower incidence of apnea than meperidine and permits more rapid recovery of consciousness at the end of anesthesia.

▶ [Well, how about this! Twenty years ago Foldes told us alphaprodine was shorter in duration of action, had less depressant action and led to less nausea!—Eds.]

Parenteral Pentazocine: Effective Analgesia after Orthopedic Surgical Procedures. Pentazocine is a weak narcotic antagonist and has a low abuse potential, even with prolonged use. It can be given by any route. The adverse reactions are usually mild and transient. It is an effective analgesic in many postoperative pain states. David Befeler and Joseph F. Giattini[3] (New York) evaluated pentazocine therapy in 106 males and 104 females, aged 14-91, with pain after orthopedic surgery. Pentazocine was given postoperatively by intramuscular injection in doses of 15-60 mg. every 3-4 hours, depending on need. Concomitant drug therapy was given when indicated to induce euphoria or muscle relaxation. Pain relief was evaluated in the 169 patients who received constant doses.

Of 156 patients given doses of 30-60 mg. pentazocine, 89% had excellent or good pain relief. Of 13 given smaller doses, 85% had excellent or good pain relief. A dose of 30 mg. induced satisfactory analgesia in 91% of 128 patients. Because of dimin-

(3)   Internat. Surg. 54:219-223, September, 1970.

ished pain, oral analgesics later could be used in 39% of the 210 patients.

Due to inadequate euphoria or muscle relaxation, 6 patients were switched to narcotic analgesics given parenterally; 2 of the 6 had had spinal fusions. An ataractic was given with pentazocine for excessive anxiety or extensive muscle dissection to 46 patients. Eight patients (4%) had adverse reactions to pentazocine; these were usually mild and transient. The commonest was dizziness or lightheadedness. Treatment was stopped in 3 patients because of side effects related to pentazocine. Pentazocine was well tolerated by elderly patients; none of 45 patients aged 70-91 had adverse reactions. Most patients stopped taking pentazocine within a week.

Pentazocine given parenterally is a safe, effective analgesic for relieving pain after various orthopedic surgical procedures. The analgesic is especially effective in elderly patients. Little euphoria occurs, and concomitant use of an ataractic may be helpful for patients having excessive anxiety or extensive dissection. Pentazocine should be a major contribution to the management of postoperative pain.

▶ [In the immediate postoperative period, 30-45 mg. pentazocine is well tolerated by adults when injected intravenously.—Eds.]

Premedication in Children: Trial of Intramuscular Droperidol, Droperidol-Phenoperidine, Papaveretum-Hyoscine and Normal Saline. D. R. Davies and A. G. Doughty[4] (Kingston Group, Surrey, England) evaluated several neuroleptanalgesic mixtures as premedication for children undergoing adenotonsillectomy. The goal was to produce analgesia with somnolence and mental detachment but with retention of cooperative ability with a single intramuscular injection. In a double-blind trial, a group of 480 children were given droperidol (0.22 mg./kg.); droperidol (0.22 mg./kg.) with phenoperidine (0.044 mg./kg.); papaveretum (0.314 mg./kg.) with hyoscine (0.006 mg./kg.); or normal saline. Injections were given intramuscularly 90 minutes before induction of anesthesia. Anesthesia was induced with thiopentone and suxamethonium and, after tracheal intubation, maintained with nitrous oxide-oxygen and 0.5% halothane by spontaneous respiration.

Patient demeanor was better with papaveretum-hyoscine than with droperidol alone, and significantly fewer children cried after venipuncture with this medication. There was less

---

(4) Brit. J. Anaesth. 43:65-75, January, 1971.

tendency to reflex hand-withdrawal with papaveretum-hyoscine. Only with droperidol-phenoperidine did behavior improve with increasing patient age. Behavior was most satisfactory in younger patients when papaveretum-hyoscine was given, and this regimen led to the greatest salivary suppression. Respiratory depression was infrequent with all regimens. Postoperative vomiting was most marked with papaveretum-hyoscine. Droperidol suppressed the emetic effect of phenoperidine. The active preparations suppressed crying and screaming after operation. Amnesia was most frequent with papaveretum-hyoscine and droperidol-phenoperidine.

This trial did not reveal a satisfactory new form of premedication as judged by the behavior of children having tonsillectomy. The findings raise the question as to whether routine sedative premedication is necessary. It is difficult to recommend a type short of a basal narcotic that would succeed most often in "difficult" children.

▶ [If more serious efforts were made to make the placebo work, i.e., by doctor visits and establishment of rapport, 70% or more of our premedication needs would be unnecessary.—Eds.]

Comparative Evaluation of Chlorprothixene and Secobarbital for Pediatric Premedication. Chlorprothixene, a thioxanthene derivative with a structure similar to that of chlorpromazine, has been effective in treating psychotic and behavior disorders in adults and children. It rapidly controls psychomotor agitation when injected parenterally. Benjamin Root and James P. Loveland[5] (Mount Sinai Hosp., Cleveland) evaluated chlorprothixene as preoperative medication in over 500 children in good physical condition. The drug was given both parenterally and orally, combined with meperidine or scopolamine or both. Results were compared with those of secobarbital-scopolamine combinations given parenterally, in a previous study, to over 1,600 children. A double-blind study was also carried out, comparing 0.0625 mg. chlorprothixene per lb. plus 0.006 mg. scopolamine per lb. with a "standard" combination of 1 mg. secobarbital per lb. and 0.006 mg. scopolamine per lb. The latter regimen produced moderate or deep hypnosis in 47% of children. A 1.5 mg./lb. dose of secobarbital increased this figure to 63%. Reducing the time before anesthetic induction to less than 45 minutes reduced hypnotic effectiveness substantially. The

(5)   J. Clin. Pharmacol. 11:56-68, Jan.-Feb., 1971.

hypnotic effect was greater in children under age 6½ years than in older children.

A suspension of 0.5 or 1 mg. chlorprothixene per lb. given orally produced minimal hypnotic effects. Addition of 0.67 mg. meperidine per lb. did not potentiate the hypnotic effect of 1 mg. chlorprothixene per lb., and prolonged postoperative drowsiness sometimes occurred. The intramuscular-oral potency ratio was greater than 16:1. Parenterally, 0.0625 mg. chlorprothixene per lb. produced hypnosis comparable to that obtained with 1 mg. secobarbital per lb. It reduced postoperative restlessness without causing marked circulatory disturbances. Addition of meperidine was not helpful. The findings were confirmed in a double-blind study of 242 children. Chlorprothixene moderately delayed postoperative arousal, compared with secobarbital, and slightly reduced the need for postoperative analgesia. There was no change in postoperative vomiting. Circulatory complications were infrequent.

Chlorprothixene definitely has a greater potential for producing circulatory disturbances than secobarbital and it is not recommended for use in premedication.

▶ [Clinical evaluation is necessary, but there is too much to read.—Eds.]

MISCELLANEOUS

Antibacterial Action of Anesthetic Vapors. J. N. Horton, M. Sussman and W. W. Mushin[6] (Royal Infirm., Cardiff, Wales) devised a technic of exposing a known number of bacteria to a given concentration of volatile anesthetic. Escherichia coli were spread on a membrane which was suspended in a gastight jar containing the anesthetic. After exposure to the vapor for a given period, the membrane was removed and placed on nutrient agar. Standard deviations of counts were not more than 7.5% of the mean. A high relative humidity was required for survival of organisms in the absence of other noxious agents. Oxygen did not significantly influence survival of the organisms. Halothane, chloroform, trichloroethylene and methoxyflurane reduced the numbers of surviving organisms. No organisms survived at the highest concentrations of each of these agents. Reduction in survival was proportional to the concentration of anesthetic, but the differences between proportions of survivors at different concentrations were not always significant. Survival was similar with diethyl ether, differences in

(6) Brit. J. Anaesth. 42:483-487, June, 1970.

survival becoming significant at concentrations of 10 and 20%. The proportion of surviving organisms was greater with diethyl ether than with any of the other agents.

Anesthetic vapors in the concentrations commonly produced in anesthetic equipment reduce the viability of E. coli. Killing is complete at higher concentrations. No more than a minimal bactericidal effect is claimed for usual concentrations of anesthetics, and it is not likely that high concentrations will prove effective in sterilizing anesthetic equipment. The antibacterial effect may, however, be at least partly responsible for a lower than expected incidence of postoperative chest infection, especially in view of the disturbed particle-clearing activity of ciliated epithelium. It is planned to test the effect of anesthetic vapors on the common respiratory pathogens.

Preliminary Observations on Effect of Halothane and Oxygen Anesthesia on Immunologic Response in Man. An increasing number of reports describe deleterious effects of anesthetics on reticuloendothelial function. L. J. Humphrey, J. R. Amerson and E. L. Frederickson[7] (Emory Univ.) evaluated immunologic responses in 10 patients with malignancies anesthetized for at least an hour with halothane in oxygen, and in 7 patients with halothane in air. All had been immunized with tetanus toxoid. Generally they had recurrent but not terminal cancer and were having minimal tissue dissection, arterial catheterization or node biopsy. No preoperative medications were given. One patient was studied with each anesthetic regimen. Flows of oxygen and air were 4 and 10 L. per minute, respectively. A Pco_2 near the "apneic threshold" was maintained by assisted ventilation. Intermittent high tidal volumes were used often during anesthesia with halothane in air. Anesthetic depth was as light as possible. Blood was sampled before and 1 and 2 hours after anesthetic induction. In vitro spinner cultures of white cell suspensions were established. Tanned cell hemagglutination and hemolysis in gel were tested.

The mean white cell count fell 16% after halothane in oxygen for 1 hour; 6 of 10 patients had a decrease of over 20%. Less change occurred in patients given halothane in air. Six normal subjects breathing oxygen for 1 hour had a fall in white cell count from 8,980 to 6,617/cu. mm. Differential counts were not altered significantly by halothane or oxygen alone. Viability counts of white cells incubated in spinner culture for 24 hours

(7)   Anesth. & Analg. 49:809-816. Sept.-Oct., 1970.

were similar in all groups. No significant results were obtained in studying the production of antitoxoid antibody by white cells in spinner culture. A decrease in 7S but not 19S antibody-producing cells was noted after halothane and air in 2 patients preimmunized with sheep red cells, on hemolysis in gel tests. Administration of halothane in oxygen reduced both 7S and 19S antibody-producing cells. One of 2 subjects who breathed oxygen for 1 hour showed a significant decrease in 7S antibody-producing cells on Jerne testing, with tanned sheep red cells coated with tetanus toxoid.

The mechanism of the peripheral white cell-lowering effect of halothane in oxygen is not clear. The effect appears to be directed at the entire white cell content.

▶ [Another of the many effects anesthetics produce in addition to analgesia and sleep.—Eds.]

Effect of Anesthesia and Amputation on Tumor and General Immunity of the Mouse. Previous studies in burned animals and patients suggested that stress or anesthetic agents or both are immunosuppressive. L. J. Humphrey, E. L. Frederickson and J. R. Amerson[8] (Emory Univ.) studied the effects of anesthetic agents on immunity in mice. Methylcholanthrene-induced sarcoma was transplanted to the hindleg of female C3h/HeHa mice. Cytotoxic tests were done in spleen or lymph node cell cultures. Anesthesia was with 0.5-0.7% halothane in air. The leg was amputated 2 or 3 weeks after tumor transplantation, after 24 hours of halothane anesthesia or after both. The procedures were repeated after injection of sheep red blood cells in other groups of mice. The effects of oxygen were also studied in mice immune to sheep red blood cells.

Treated mice showed a significantly greater effect on tumor cell growth by spleen and node cells than did controls. Halothane exposure and amputation, alone or together, increased the activity of both spleen and node against tumor cell growth in culture. This was especially apparent in cultures inoculated with spleen cell suspensions. In no instance was tumor cell growth enhanced. Both experimental maneuvers increased antibody-producing spleen cells. Such cells were reduced by exposure to 100% oxygen.

Whether offering a method of immunosuppression in patients anesthetized for kidney transplantation or enhancing immunity during operations on patients with cancer or bacterial in-

(8) J. S. Res. 10:265 270, June, 1970.

fections, the effects of oxygen intoxication and controlled hypoxia in man require further investigation.

► [These studies suggest that immunosuppression from anesthetic agents may be related to the oxygen they are carried in, rather than to the agent itself. Since only one level of halothane was used, this does not rule out a dose-related effect whereby the immune system may be stimulated at light levels, then depressed as the anesthesia is deepened.—Eds.]

Reversible Effect of Inhalation Anesthetic on Lymphocyte Motility. Clinical concentrations of halothane strikingly reduce the motility of certain nonmammalian cells. J. F. Nunn, J. A. Sharp and K. L. Kimball[9] (Univ. of Leeds) studied the behavior of mammalian lymphocytes in tissue culture during exposure to medium equilibrated with halothane vapor. Explants of lung and thymus from newborn mice were grown in TC 199 medium with 10-30% fetal bovine serum.

Two lung lymphocytes became nearly immobile during 30 minutes of halothane exposure; one did not regain mobility after withdrawal of halothane. Macrophages exhibited normal motility during exposure to halothane, and epithelial cells and fibroblasts showed no changes. Velocity of thymic lymphocytes declined significantly during exposure to halothane. About half the cells rapidly regained control velocities during recovery, but the rest remained immobile. Rapid surface "bubbling" was sometimes noted during exposure of both types of cell to halothane. The 2% concentration corresponds to a blood level of about 40 mg./100 ml., the upper clinical limit.

These changes are probably associated with recent observations that halothane reduces the number of circulating lymphocytes and decreases the number of antibody-producing splenic lymphocytes in rats. General anesthetics, besides their well-known properties, may act as rapidly reversible immunosuppressive agents. Microtubule dispersion and depolymerization have been observed with halothane and other inhalation agents, and microtubules have been described in human lymphocytes. The microtubules may be particularly sensitive to inhalation anesthetics. Study of the effects of general anesthetics on different microtubular systems may explain some of their toxic effects and perhaps their mode of action on the central nervous system.

► [A primary effect on lymphocyte morphology and function might well explain the known immunosuppressive capability of inhalation anesthetics. Whether this is caused by microtubule depression is by no means well established.—Eds.]

_____

(9) Nature, London 226:85-86, Apr. 4, 1970.

Genetic and Environmental Influence on Halothane Metabolism in Twins. Halothane biotransformation in man apparently can be affected by environmental factors, but genetic mechanisms also may have a role. Halothane-induced hepatotoxicity may involve sensitization in persons who differ in some way from the general population. H. F. Cascorbi, E. S. Vesell, D. A. Blake and M. Helrich[1] attempted to define the extent of genetic control over halothane biotransformation in twins. Five pairs of identical and 5 pairs of fraternal twins, all in good health, were studied using halothane-14C. Labeled halothane in saline was infused rapidly, and urine was collected at intervals for 24 hours. Urine samples were radioassayed before and after lyophilization.

The cumulative 24-hour urinary excretion of halothane metabolite ranged from 2.7 to 11.4% of the administered dose. The identical twins metabolized considerably more halothane than the fraternal twins. Normalized intrapair differences in

Fig. 4.—Urinary excretion of halothane metabolite in identical (*I*) and fraternal (*N-I*) twins. *DPM*, disintegrations per minute. (Courtesy of Cascorbi, H. F., *et al.*: Clin. Pharmacol. & Therap. 12:50-55, Jan.-Feb., 1971.)

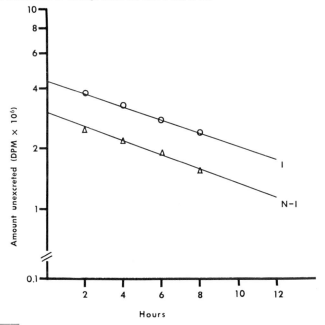

(1) Clin. Pharmacol. & Therap. 12:50-55, Jan.-Feb., 1971.

the percentage of metabolite excreted were appreciably smaller in identical (2.4-17.3%) than in fraternal twins (2.9-70%). Calculations indicated a considerable genetic contribution (88%) to the large individual differences in halothane metabolism observed. Plasma antipyrine half-life was not correlated with the percentage of halothane metabolite excreted or the rate of excretion. A plot of the log amount of unexcreted halothane metabolite against time (Fig. 4) indicated that urinary excretion is a first-order process. The average half-life of urinary excretion was 10.4 hours in identical twins and 9.8 hours in fraternal twins.

Genetic and environmental factors apparently both exert considerable influence on halothane metabolism, but hereditary factors appear to play the greater role. Hereditary factors play an almost exclusive role in the metabolism of phenylbutazone, antipyrine and bishydroxycoumarin, which are metabolized by different enzymes than halothane. Halothane metabolism might be subject to alteration by different types and concentrations of inducing and inhibiting substances in the environment. This would explain the absence of correlation between the metabolism of halothane and that of antipyrine in the subjects.

▶ [After learning only relatively recently that inhalation anesthetics are metabolized, and that their rate of metabolism may be speeded by enzyme stimulation, we now have evidence that their metabolism is also under genetic control. Perhaps we are getting closer to a reason for the toxic effects of anesthetics.—Eds.]

Effect of α-Receptor Blocking Drugs and Disodium Cromoglycate on Histamine Hypersensitivity in Bronchial Asthma was studied by James W. Kerr, M. Govindaraj and K. R. Patel[2] (Glasgow) in 20 patients, aged 13-53 years, with extrinsic-type bronchial asthma. The histamine test was done when the patient had minimal airway obstruction and had not needed an oral bronchodilator drug in the prior 12 hours.

With the patient sitting, baseline levels for vital capacity (VC) and forced expiratory volume in 1 second (FEV_1) in liters were measured. In this time, a normal saline intravenous infusion was set up, and once steady-state readings for VC and FEV_1 were obtained, the infusion was switched to a solution of 50 μg. histamine dihydrochloride in 200 ml. of saline, which was given in 10-15 minutes. The VC and FEV_1 measurements were continued at intervals for 40 minutes thereafter. For the test infusion, the procedure was the same, but just before the histamine

(2)   Brit. M. J. 2:139-141, Apr. 18, 1970.

drip was begun, 7 of 10 patients received 5 mg. phentolamine intravenously into the opposite arm. Three of these 10 received 10 mg. phenoxybenzamine in 150 ml. saline during 2 hours before the histamine drip. The other 10 patients had a histamine control test. Then for 2 weeks they inhaled disodium cromoglycate, three 20-mg. capsules, daily. The histamine test was then repeated after each patient inhaled 40 mg. disodium cromoglycate 30 minutes before the test infusion.

After patients 1-10 received 50 μg. histamine dihydrochloride intravenously, all had a fall in VC and FEV_1, most pronounced at 10 minutes, but considerably returned by 40 minutes (Fig. 5). When these patients received 5 mg. phentolamine or 10 mg. phenoxybenzamine intravenously before histamine infusion, the fall in VC and FEV_1 due to histamine was inhibited (Fig. 5). There was a significant difference in VC and FEV_1 at 5, 10 and 20 minutes, when compared with the control. After patients 11-20 received 50 μg. histamine dihydrochloride intravenously, all had a fall in VC and FEV_1, most pronounced at 20 minutes. When these patients inhaled 40 mg. disodium cromoglycate 30 minutes before histamine infusion, the fall in VC and FEV_1

Fig. 5.—Mean fall in VC (*solid circles*) and FEV_1 (*open triangles*) in 10 subjects after intravenous infusion of 50 μg. histamine dihydrochloride (*broken lines*). This fall in VC and FEV_1 is completely inhibited by prior injection of phentolamine or phenoxybenzamine (*solid lines*). (Courtesy of Kerr, J. W., *et al.*: Brit. M. J. 2: 139-141, Apr. 18, 1970.)

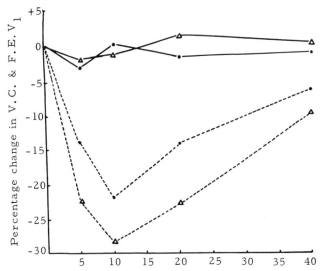

due to histamine was inhibited. There was a significant difference in VC and FEV_1 between 15 and 30 minutes and 10 and 30 minutes, respectively, when compared with the control.

The findings suggest that the bronchial smooth muscle of asthmatics has α-adrenergic receptor sites, and that blockade of these sites with α-receptor antagonists alters the sensitivity of bronchial smooth muscle to histamine. The mechanism by which disodium cromoglycate produces its effect in bronchial asthma remains obscure.

PHYSIOLOGY RELATED TO ANESTHESIA

Norepinephrine Metabolism in Brain Stem of Spontaneously Hypertensive Rats. It has long been thought that catecholamines might play a role in the pathogenesis of hypertension, but elevated levels generally have not been found in relation to hypertension. Yukio Yamori, Walter Lovenberg and Albert Sjoerdsma[3] (Nat'l Inst. of Health) studied catecholamine metabolism in the central nervous system in the spontaneously hypertensive rat, now available as a genetically pure strain and a suitable model of human essential hypertension. Blood pressures were measured without anesthesia by tail plethysmography in male spontaneously hypertensive rats and control rats. Pressures were greatly elevated in the study rats after age 6 weeks. Rats were killed at ages 6, 10 and 20 weeks to examine various parts of the central nervous system for norepinephrine content.

A considerable reduction of norepinephrine was found in the hypothalamus and lower brain stem of study rats. Average concentrations at age 10 weeks were 60-70% of control values. Whole brain norepinephrine levels were also lower. Aromatic L-amino acid decarboxylase activity was reduced in the whole brain stem and the telencephalon. Enzyme activity was not altered in rats with renal or deoxycorticosterone-salt hypertension or in study rats that had been adrenalectomized. No sex differences were noted. Tyrosine hydroxylase activity was not significantly different in the study rats as compared with the controls. Recently, this enzyme activity was reported to be slightly reduced in the mesenteric arteries of spontaneously hypertensive rats (Tarver and Spector, 1970).

---

(3) Science 170:544-546, Oct. 30, 1970.

It appears that catecholamines, while being pressor peripherally, may participate in a central depressor system. The lower levels found in discrete brain areas of spontaneously hypertensive rats suggest a possible relation to the hypertension. The catecholamine precursor L-dopa appears to reduce the blood pressure of spontaneously hypertensive rats treated with peripheral decarboxylase inhibitors. It is concluded that catecholamine mechanisms in the central nervous system may play an important role in blood pressure regulation. Genetic hypertension in the rat and possibly in man may be related to catecholamine deficiency in certain areas of the brain.

▶ [Price has demonstrated the physiologic importance of central mechanisms in mediation of blood pressure changes during anesthesia. Lack of knowledge of the biochemical basis of the central blood pressure regulatory mechanism has impeded further developments. Evidence appears to be accumulating that catecholamine neurotransmitters serve a depressor function centrally. It now remains for a biochemical study to be done on the effects of anesthesia on this system.—Eds.]

Carotid Sinus Origin of Adrenergic Responses Compromising Effectiveness of Artificial Circulatory Support. Timothy S. Harrison, Ramesh C. Chawla, John F. Seaton and Bruce H. Robinson[4] (Ann Arbor, Mich.) examined carotid sinus effects on adrenal medullary secretion.

An adrenal-femoral vein shunt was prepared in healthy mongrel dogs anesthetized with pentobarbital and respired with 98% oxygen. Flow was diverted from one proximal carotid artery to a pulsatile blood pump. Flow from the pump went to both isolated carotid sinuses, to the external carotid arteries and then through a Starling resistance to the femoral vein. Both vagus nerves were divided in the neck. Adrenal blood was sampled after various changes were made in the wave form of the pulses reaching the carotid sinuses. A standard pulse frequency of 100 was used.

Nonpulsatile pressures between 40 and 160 mm. Hg introduced to the carotid sinus had no effect in the adrenomedullary secretion rate of epinephrine. No relation between mean pressure and epinephrine secretion was found when a pulsatile wave form with an amplitude of 40 mm. Hg was used. An inverse logarithmic relation was found between pulse amplitude and epinephrine secretion rate at mean carotid sinus pressures of 60 and 80 mm. Hg (Fig. 6). Markedly aberrant relations were found at low mean carotid sinus pressures of 30 and 40 mm. Hg.

(4) Surgery 68:20-26, July, 1970.

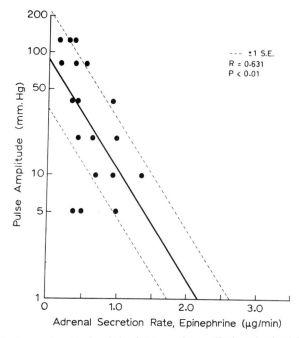

Fig. 6.—Inverse logarithmic relation between pulse amplitude and epinephrine secretion rate is shown at a mean carotid sinus pressure of 80 mm. Hg. Pulse amplitude is plotted logarithmically. (Courtesy of Harrison, T. S., *et al.*: Surgery 68:20-26, July, 1970.)

Hypotension does not stimulate a marked release of catecholamines. Catecholamine secretion increases with low pulse amplitudes at mean arterial pressures of 60 and 80 mm. Hg. These adrenergic responses aid the failing heart but may impair the artificially supported circulation. Adequate safeguarding against the full development of the adrenergic responses can probably be achieved with the use of pulse amplitudes of 50 mm. Hg or more.

▶ [It comes as somewhat of a surprise to learn that hypotension is not associated with a release of catecholamines. However, the authors looked only for epinephrine and only in the adrenal vein. Norepinephrine could be liberated, and at other sites.—Eds.]

Distribution of Ventilation and Perfusion in Lungs of Patients with Airways Obstruction is discussed by F. J. Prime[5] (Inst. of Diseases of the Chest, Brompton, England). Even normal lungs differ regionally in the alveolar ventilation to alve-

(5) Brit. J. Dis. Chest 64:1-4, January, 1970.

olar blood flow (V_A/Q_C) ratio. In the upright subject, this varies from infinity at the lung apexes, where blood flow is absent, to about 0.6 at the bases (West, 1965). Effects of this range of alveolar partial pressures and blood gas contents coincide with a V/Q of about 0.8. In the abnormal lung, ventilation and perfusion in alveoli are altered so that distribution of values for V/Q ratios is usually greatly widened, causing an increased alveolar-arterial oxygen pressure difference, since no amount of overventilation of perfused alveoli can cause the blood flowing through them to take up more than a little oxygen extra to that required to saturate the hemoglobin fully. Thus, final composition of mixed arterial blood will be determined by the contribution of parts of the lung where the V/Q ratio is low. Composition of blood gases from these areas is increasingly like that of mixed venous blood as the V/Q ratio decreases.

In one investigational method, observed alveolar-arterial oxygen partial pressure difference is accounted for by assuming that some mixed venous blood bypasses alveoli and that part of the alveolar ventilation is wasted in unperfused alveoli (Riley and Cournand, 1951). The other approach is that used by Zamel and Kass (1970), which is based on the researches of Briscoe and colleagues and treats the lung as a combination of 2 or more compartments ventilated and perfused together but at different rates. Compartment volumes and their ventilation rates are calculated from intrapulmonary mixing curves obtained when the subject breathes a foreign gas such as helium. One group of alveoli is slowly ventilated, the slow space, and compared with the other, the fast space (Fig. 7). Briscoe (1960) found that in 10 patients with pulmonary emphysema the slow spaces occupied about two thirds of the total alveolar volume and received about half the available blood flow; slow-space ventilation was so low that the V/Q ratio was only one tenth that of the rest of the lung. Briscoe's graph methods have considerably simplified calculations involved in these estimates. The most important of these graphs synthesizes the researches of Briscoe and his co-workers and is shown as Figure 2 in the paper by Zamel and Kass. As a measure of lung inhomogeneity, the value of the complex ratio $(Q_s/Q_t)/(L_s/L_t)$ may be calculated where Q_s, Q_t, L_s and L_t are blood flows (Q) and alveolar volumes (L) of the slow space (s) and the lung as a whole (t). When this equals unity, blood flow is distributed to alve-

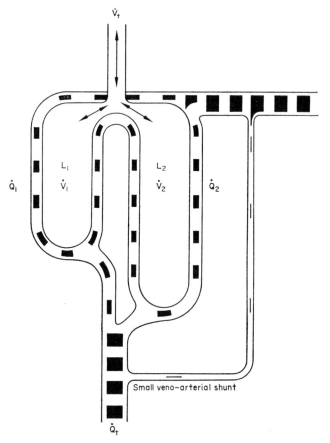

Fig. 7.—At the left, L_1 represents the volume of one group of alveoli. On the right, L_2 is another group of alveoli whose volume is about twice that of L_1. Ventilation of L_2 is only one tenth of that in L_1. Total blood flow (Q_t) is about equally divided between these two groups of alveoli. Distribution of blood is not homogeneous with respect to alveolar volume; in arithmetical terms, Q_1/L_1 is greater than Q_2/L_2. Ventilations of the two compartments are also different. The smaller space has a high ventilation so that here $\dot{V}_1/\dot{Q}_1$ is about 10 times $\dot{V}_2/\dot{Q}_2$. Thus, although L_2 has a lower blood flow per unit volume, it receives more than its share of blood in relation to its ventilation. The diagram may help to show the importance of the slow space in determining mixed arterial blood gas composition; it is modified from Briscoe, W. A.: J. Appl. Physiol. 14:292, 1959. In Briscoe's writings and in the article by Zamel and Kass, L_2 is referred to as the slow space, in reference to its rate of ventilation. (Courtesy of Prime, F. J.: Brit. J. Dis. Chest 64:1-4, January, 1970.)

olar volume evenly throughout fast and slow spaces, and to this extent the lung is homogeneous.

The fact that Zamel and Kass, using the same estimation methods, obtained results different from those of Briscoe and co-workers only increases the interest and importance of the concept on which this work is based.

Overperfusion of Poorly Ventilated Alveoli in Patients with Severe Airways Obstruction. Noe Zamel and Irving Kass[6] (Univ. of Nebraska) studied functional characteristics of slowly ventilated lung space (slow space) in 5 men, aged 40-60, with varying degrees of airway obstruction and pulmonary hyperinflation, hypoxemia and hypercapnia.

METHOD.—Arterial blood was sampled during 5 minutes of expired air collection; oxygen uptake was estimated from the composition of this expired gas, which was measured with a gas chromatograph. Immediately thereafter, functional residual capacity of lungs (Lt) and the volume (Ls) and ventilation of slow space ($\dot{V}_{A,s}$) were estimated by a modification of the open-circuit helium method described by Hickman et al. (1954). The patient first breathed a mixture of 50% helium and 50% oxygen for at least 15 minutes. Then, at the end of a normal expiration, the gas mixture was changed to 100% oxygen. In the next 15 or more minutes, the helium was washed out of the patient's lungs. For the first 10 minutes of this time, the expired gas was collected in a second Douglas bag. During washout, the expired gas was continuously monitored for its helium content until this fell to 0.05%. The recorded output of the helium katharometer was then plotted on log-linear graph paper with helium concentration as ordinate against time as the abscissa; this allowed estimation of the helium fraction in expired gas extrapolated to zero time and the time required for a given fraction to decrease by one half ($T\frac{1}{2}$). The Ls and $\dot{V}_{A,s}$ were then calculated by the formulas of Hickman et al. (1954). The ventilation-perfusion ratio of slow space ($\dot{V}_{A,s}/Qs$) and perfusion of slow space as a fraction of total pulmonary blood perfusion ($Qs/\dot{Q}t$) were calculated with the use of a logarithmic grid (Briscoe et al., 1960). Known parameters on the grid are the ratio of slow-space ventilation to total oxygen uptake ($\dot{V}_{A,s}/\dot{V}o_2$) and arterial oxygen saturation (Sa,o_2) (Fig. 8). Total alveolar ventilation ($\dot{V}_{A,t}$) was calculated by the following formula in which $\dot{V}E$ was total ventilation and f, respiratory frequency per minute (Briscoe et al., 1960): $\dot{V}_{A,t} = \dot{V}E - 0.2$ f. The volume of well-ventilated parts of lungs was computed by subtracting Ls from Lt and alveolar ventilation of these parts, by subtracting $\dot{V}_{A,s}$ from $\dot{V}_{A,t}$. The fractional blood perfusion of well-ventilated parts was the difference between unity and fractional perfusion of slow space. Slow-space determinations were repeated in patients LJF and CME about 15 minutes after inhaling an aerosol containing 0.5% isoprenaline for 1 minute. After treat-

(6) Brit. J. Dis. Chest 64:5-14, January, 1970.

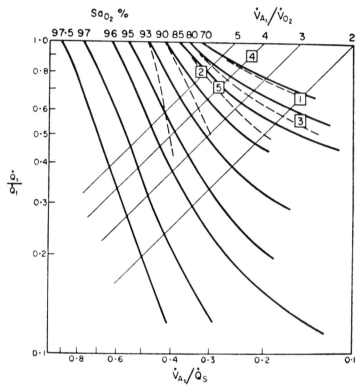

Fig. 8.—Numbers in ascending order refer to patients LJF, CME, ADL, AMK and WH. The ratio of slow space ventilation to oxygen uptake $(\dot{V}A,s/\dot{V}o_2)$ and arterial blood oxygen saturation (Sa,o_2) are known, giving a point on the graph. Perfusion of slow space as a fraction of total perfusion $(\dot{Q}s/\dot{Q}t)$ on the ordinate and ventilation-perfusion ratio of slow space $(\dot{V}A,s/\dot{Q}s)$ on the abscissa are then read from the point. On this reproduction of Figure 4 from Briscoe's article (J. Appl. Physiol. 14:291-298, May, 1959) are marked points obtained from experimental data obtained in the present work. (Courtesy of Zamel, N., and Kass, I.: Brit. J. Dis. Chest 64:5-14, January, 1970.)

ment with antibacterial and bronchodilator drugs, postural drainage and breathing exercises for 9 and 3 weeks, respectively, patients CME and WH were restudied.

Patient LJF had 43% of his lung volume ventilated by 5% of his total alveolar ventilation and perfused by 66% of his total pulmonary blood flow; his $\dot{V}A,s/\dot{Q}s$ ratio was 0.15 and the $\dfrac{\dot{Q}s/\dot{Q}t}{Ls/Lt}$ ratio was 1.5. Patient CME had 79% of lung volume ventilated by 27% of total alveolar ventilation and perfused by

80% of total pulmonary blood flow; $\dot{V}_A,s/\dot{Q}s$ ratio was 0.32 and $\dfrac{\dot{Q}s/\dot{Q}t}{Ls/Lt}$ ratio was 1.0. Patient ADL had 57% of volume ventilated by 15% of total alveolar ventilation and perfused by 56% of total pulmonary blood flow; $\dot{V}_A,s/\dot{Q}s$ was 0.15 and $\dfrac{\dot{Q}s/\dot{Q}t}{Ls/Lt}$ ratio was 1.0. Patient AMK had 50% of volume ventilated by 13% of total alveolar ventilation and perfused by 90% of total pulmonary blood flow; $\dot{V}_A,s/\dot{Q}s$ ratio was 0.22 and $\dfrac{\dot{Q}s/\dot{Q}t}{Ls/Lt}$ ratio was 1.8. Patient WH had 42% of volume ventilated by 17% of total alveolar ventilation and perfused by 72% of total pulmonary blood flow; $\dot{V}_A,s/\dot{Q}s$ ratio was 0.28 and $\dfrac{\dot{Q}s/\dot{Q}t}{Ls/Lt}$ ratio was 1.7. Isoprenaline inhalation failed to alter slow-space values in patients LJF and CME. In patient CME, there were no significant differences in slow-space characteristics at the time of restudy; in patient WH, fractional ventilation and perfusion ratios of slow space were further decreased, but still the $\dfrac{\dot{Q}s/\dot{Q}t}{Ls/Lt}$ ratio was greater than unity (1.34).

The $\dot{V}_A,s/\dot{Q}s$ ratios in these 5 patients were similar to those in the 10 studied by Briscoe *et al.* (1960), yet 7 of the latter had $\dfrac{\dot{Q}s/\dot{Q}t}{Ls/Lt}$ ratios under 1.0. That 1 (AMK) of the 5 patients died and the other 4 failed to improve suggests that a $\dfrac{\dot{Q}s/\dot{Q}t}{Ls/Lt}$ value of 1.0 or over indicates a poor prognosis.

▶ [Anesthesiologists, despite their expertise in the practical management of ventilation, do not necessarily have the experience or training to care for many pulmonary cripples. It is incumbent upon those who insist in self-adulation that they are also the Intensivist and the Pulmonary Superstar that they read and assimilate data such as these.—Eds.]

Constant Positive-Pressure Breathing and Cardiorespiratory Function. Evidence indicates that constant positive-pressure breathing (CPPB) may raise the arterial oxygen tension to higher levels than intermittent positive-pressure breathing (IPPB). Current methods of CPPB include adjusting airflow resistance in expiration to produce a positive end-expiratory pressure and breathing without expiratory resistance but with an end-expiratory plateau of positive pressure. Frank J. Colgan,

Robert E. Barrow and Gary L. Fanning[7] (Univ. of Rochester) evaluated the cardiovascular responses of 10 dogs to periods of spontaneous respiration, IPPB and the two methods of CPPB. Anesthesia was induced with thiopental and maintained with 1% halothane. Cardiac output was measured by the dye-dilution technic, and intrapulmonary volume changes using a capacitance respirometer. Measurements were repeated after 15 minutes of IPPB, CPPB with end-expired pressures of 5 and 10 cm. of water and CPPB-5 with expiratory resistance.

There was no significant change in cardiac output, functional residual capacity or true shunting after a change from spontaneous respiration to IPPB during oxygen inhalation. The cardiac index fell significantly with CPPB-5, and the functional residual capacity rose 18%. With CPPB-10, the functional residual capacity rose to 38% above control level, and the cardiac index was further reduced. Addition of expiratory resistance did not alter the cardiac index significantly. The cardiac index was significantly lower with expiratory resistance at an end-expired pressure of 5 cm. water. Lung deflation was prolonged, increasing the mean airway pressure. The mean total shunt was significantly reduced during CPPB-5 but not further reduced by CPPB-10 or with expiratory resistance. The true shunt measured during oxygen inhalation decreased significantly with increases in mean airway pressure, falling from 14.5% on spontaneous respiration to a low of 8.8% with CPPB-10. No significant changes in alveolar-arterial Do_2 were evident. Pulmonary oxygen content differences were unchanged, but systemic oxygen content differences changed in accordance with changes in mean airway pressure.

The changes seen with positive-pressure respiration in this study suggest a reduction in atelectasis or vascular shunting, rather than a more equitable distribution of ventilation relative to perfusion. Assessment of the effects of CPPB on intrapulmonary shunting requires knowledge of the systemic effect of CPPB. In lieu of measuring cardiac output, this can be done most easily by simultaneous measurements on arterial and mixed venous blood.

▶ [The severe reduction in right heart filling from elevation in end-expiratory pressures often feared in anesthesia practice is not as common as predicted.—Eds.]

Effects of Age and Body Position on "Airway Closure" in Man. Impairment of ventilation to dependent lung zones in

(7)   Anesthesiology 34:145-151, February, 1971.

various positions has been attributed to airway closure, or trapping, in these zones. Pulmonary flow to the lower lung zones is less seriously impaired at low lung volumes, with resultant impaired gas exchange. P. Leblanc, F. Ruff and J. Milic-Emili[8] (McGill Univ.) used the radioxenon technic to measure the "closing volume" in 80 normal seated subjects aged 18-82. Forty were also examined while supine. None of the 74 males and 6 females studied had a history of chronic cardiorespiratory disease, and all had normal body weights. Lung volumes were measured by the helium dilution technic or by volume body plethysmography. Closing volume was measured by the ^{133}Xe bolus method.

The ratios of both functional residual capacity and residual volume to total lung capacity increased with age, the change being more marked for residual volume. In seated subjects the ratio of closing volume to total lung capacity increased about linearly with age, the average annual change being 0.57% of total lung capacity. Smokers tended to have slightly higher closing volumes than nonsmokers. Closing volume was lower than functional residual capacity in young subjects, but the former increased at a greater rate with age and in elderly subjects was greater than functional residual capacity. In supine subjects the closing volume changed by an average of 0.56% of vital capacity per year of age. The critical age at which the closing volume exceeded the expiratory reserve volume was considerably lower in the supine than in the sitting position, the respective critical ages being 44 and about 65 years.

"Closing volume" increases with advancing age. Arterial oxygen tension and oxygen saturation are often measured in blood sampled from supine subjects and the values compared with normal standards that are usually obtained from seated subjects. Such comparisons may not be valid, since the supine position per se may have a considerable effect on the arterial blood gas composition.

▶ [It's an old story—you can't compare apples and pears!—Eds.]

Nonlinear Model for Uptake and Distribution of Halothane in Man is described by Michael N. Ashman (Columbia Univ.), William B. Blesser (Brooklyn, N. Y.) and Robert M. Epstein[9] (Columbia Univ.). Nonlinearities introduce mathematical complexity which can be formidable, but work with models that in-

(8)   J. Appl. Physiol. 28:448-451, April, 1970.
(9)   Anesthesiology 33:419-429, October. 1970.

corporate them is required to obtain evidence of their importance. A nonlinear model would permit the more detailed study of some anesthetic effects that may be large, as under conditions of hemorrhagic shock or poor cardiac reserve. Changes in cardiac output can affect halothane uptake. A first step in obtaining a more exact description of halothane uptake could be to include this cardiovascular nonlinearity in system equations. Such a model was used to develop a program for inducing halothane anesthesia in man. Body tissues are divided into five compartments according to circulatory and solubility criteria, and the perfusion of each compartment is assumed to be evenly distributed, without shunting or diffusion barriers. A set of differential equations has been derived describing the rate of change of compartmental partial pressures as a function of inflow minus outflow of anesthetic agent.

An analog computer simulation of halothane uptake and distribution in man provided partial pressures in each tissue compartment in response to a constant inspired partial pressure of 1% atmospheric. A theoretic derivation of the inspired partial pressure necessary to achieve instantaneously a constant anesthetic depth was included. Using a nonrebreathing anesthesia circuit, with a maximal inspired partial pressure of 4% atmospheric, the program developed achieves a partial pressure of 0.75% atmospheric in the well-perfused tissues in 6 minutes without overshoot and will maintain this partial pressure indefinitely. The difference between this model and a linear one having fixed cardiac output was found to be insignificant for the first 5 minutes. Nonlinearity elevated the partial pressures in well-perfused tissues and the lung by 6% after 1 hour of anesthesia, with an inspired partial pressure of 1% atmospheric.

The nonlinearity in this study was due to a uniformly distributed reduction of cardiac output as anesthetic partial pressure in the viscera increased. The construction of more realistic models depends on inclusion of respiratory as well as more detailed circulatory effects of anesthesia in the mathematical description of the system.

▶ [Sounds like the disparity between West Point classic war strategy and the realities of Vietnam warfare, but see Eger and Halsey's editorial in the same issue of *Anesthesiology*.—Eds.]

Influence of Anesthesia on Regional Distribution of Perfusion and Ventilation in the Lung. The substantial increase in the difference between alveolar and arterial Po_2 that follows induction of anesthesia remains unexplained. Usually, some increase in measured venous admixture occurs. G. H. Hulands, R. Greene, L. D. Iliff and J. F. Nunn[1] (Royal Postgrad. Med. School, London) measured the effect of anesthesia with paralysis and artificial ventilation on the distribution of ventilation and pulmonary blood flow, using radioxenon, in 4 patients, aged 27-51 years, who were free from cardiovascular and pulmonary disease.

METHOD.—Scans were performed in supine patients just before and during anesthesia. Premedication was with morphine and atropine. Anesthesia was induced with thiopentone and maintained with 0.75% halothane in oxygen. Intubation was facilitated with suxamethonium, and full muscle paralysis was assured with tubocurarine. Ventilation was continued manually with an end-expiratory Pco_2 maintained close to 5%. The lungs were inflated passively before scans were obtained.

Distribution of lung volume was unchanged by anesthesia, and the lung geometry of individual patients was faithfully preserved. Distribution of ventilation per unit lung volume slightly favored the dependent parts of the lungs. One patient showed a significant change toward greater uniformity after induction of anesthesia. All patients showed preferential perfusion of the lower parts of the lungs, which received about double the perfusion of the upper parts. Three patients had less uniform distribution after induction, accentuating the preferential perfusion of dependent areas. There was no evidence of failure of perfusion of the uppermost parts of the lungs. Ventilation-perfusion ratios were higher in the uppermost parts of the lungs before anesthesia. Three patients showed greater nonuniformity after anesthesia, 2 primarily because of altered distribution of blood flow and 1 primarily because of altered distribution of ventilation. One patient showed no change.

In this study, ventilation-perfusion inequality alone was insufficient to explain the alveolar-arterial Po_2 difference usually noted during anesthesia. Pulmonary arteriovenous shunting remains a possible explanation; this is supported by the constancy of the calculated venous admixture found at different levels of inspired oxygen. If shunting is the cause of the increased alveolar-arterial Po_2 difference, its pathway remains obscure. Shunting through collapsed lung has not been proved.

Ventilation-Perfusion Ratio during Intermittent Positive-Pressure Ventilation: Importance of No-Flow Interval during

(1) Clin. Sc. 38:451-460, April, 1970.

Insufflation. Model studies have shown that an uneven distribution of respiratory air referable to a difference in flow resistance between lung compartments can be improved if a no-flow interval is inserted between the end of insufflation and the start of expiration. Dog studies have given similar results. Søren Lyager[2] (Univ. of Aarhus) studied the influence of a no-flow interval after the end of insufflation on the ventilation-perfusion ratio in normal dogs. Physiologic dead space, venous shunt and alveoloarterial oxygen pressure gradient were assessed in dogs ventilated with and without a no-flow interval. Fourteen dogs were anesthetized with thiomebumal sodium, 15-30 mg./kg., given intravenously. The animals were provided with an endotracheal tube whose cuff was inflated. During the experiment, the dogs were completely paralyzed with gallamonium iodide, 40-60 mg. given intravenously. Animals were ventilated by an Engström respirator with air at a constant tidal volume of 15-20 ml./kg. The ratio of insufflation and expiration times was 1:2; insufflation plus the no-flow interval extended over 1 second at a respiratory rate of 20. Volume acceleration was carried out in some studies, with and without a no-flow interval.

Physiologic dead space fell significantly when a no-flow interval was used. The dead space did not depend on whether insufflation occurred with or without volume acceleration. Volume acceleration resulted in a great increase in tracheal pressure and a higher intrathoracic mean pressure. Both cardiac output and venous admixture were reduced with a long no-flow interval, and/or if a certain pressure rise was obtained during insufflation. A long no-flow interval led to a significant fall in CO_2 pressures. The respiratory exchange ratio and oxygen uptake were independent of the respiratory pattern. Compliance was a little greater when a no-flow interval was used.

Dogs in this study exhibited an increased ventilation-perfusion ratio when a no-flow interval was inserted between the end of insufflation and the start of expiration. The cause is assumed to be a redistribution of both ventilation and perfusion. When a no-flow interval is used, the ratio between ventilation and perfusion becomes more even, though not ideal.

Age as a Factor in Distribution of Lower Airway Conductance and Pathologic Anatomy of Obstructive Lung Disease. Chronic obstructive lung diseases, except for asthma, are strik-

(2) Acta anaesth. scandinav. 14:211-232, 1970.

ingly separated by age. The airways beyond the 12th to 15th generation contribute little to total airways resistance in the adult lung, and severe disease may affect them without being clinically apparent. J. C. Hogg, J. Williams, J. B. Richardson, P. T. Macklem and W. M. Thurlbeck[3] studied the effects of lung growth on distribution of airway conductance in the normal lung and observed disturbances in the pattern present in obstructive airway disease. Study was made of 16 normal and 5 abnormal lungs obtained from the autopsy services of the Royal Victoria Hospital, Montreal, Quebec, and the Montreal Children's Hospital.

Central airway conductance per gram was relatively constant at all ages in normal lungs, whereas peripheral conductance per gram increased greatly at about age 5 years. The number of generations of airways changed little from birth to the 7th decade. The estimated number of airways smaller than the catheter tip showed no change with age. The lung grows by adding alveoli rapidly in the first few years of life, their linear dimensions remaining relatively constant during this time. It is likely that a true reduction in conductance was found in a case of bronchiolitis in a child aged 3 months, with a reduced number of airways peripheral to the catheter tip. A child aged $6\frac{1}{2}$ years had a reduced peripheral conductance value but a normal number of peripheral airways; inflammatory infiltrate thickened the walls of nearly all of the small airways. Findings were similar in the lungs of a woman aged 63 who had no previous history of respiratory symptoms but had a marked infiltrate in the walls of small airways. Central airway conductance was reduced in 2 of 3 children who died of fibrocystic disease; peripheral airway conductance was markedly reduced in all 3 cases. Widespread mucus plugging of small airways was noted, with an actual reduction in the number of peripheral airways counted in at least 2 of the 3 cases. Findings were similar in 1 case of bronchiectasis in an adult.

Acute lower respiratory tract inflammation probably involves both bronchi and bronchioles at all ages. This results in serious illness in young children, with normally low bronchiolar conductance but is manifested only as acute bronchitis in adults, in whom peripheral airway conductance is large. Atelectasis occurs with chronic inflammation of the lower airways when the collateral paths are poorly developed, but in older

(3) New England J. Med. 282:1283-1287, June 4, 1970.

patients with well-developed collateral channels, atelectasis is prevented, although collateral ventilation of obstructed units may erode and destroy the alveolar walls and produce emphysema.

Dead Space during Anesthesia: Effect of Added Oxygen. The physiologic dead space and dead space-tidal volume ratio are known to increase when anesthesia is induced and to increase further when ventilation is controlled. The increase in dead space has been attributed to a maldistribution of inspired gas and to a drop in pulmonary artery pressure. Another possibility is an increase in stratified ventilation-perfusion inequality at the alveolar level, possibly due to abolition of homeostatic mechanisms by a direct anesthetic effect on pulmonary vessels or through an increase in alveolar oxygen tension. M. K. Sykes and W. E. I. Finlay[4] (London) studied the effects of an increase in inspired oxygen concentration on physiologic dead space during anesthesia with controlled ventilation. Studies were done on 14 patients having open heart surgical procedures for aortic or mitral valve replacement. Measurements were made 30-60 minutes after induction of anesthesia and repeated 45-75 minutes after bypass, generally with the pleura closed.

Patients were premedicated with rectal quinalbarbitone, followed by pethidine and promethazine. Anesthesia was induced with thiopentone and d-tubocurarine and maintained with nitrous oxide, oxygen and pethidine. Gamma-hydroxybutyrate was given 30 minutes before study to maintain unconsciousness during 100% oxygen administration. An Engström ventilator was used to produce a Pao_2 close to 100 mm. Hg. An end-expiratory pressure of 5 or 10 cm. water was produced. Measurements were made on about 25% oxygen with the chest open, about an hour after anesthetic induction, and again on 100% oxygen after 10-15 minutes. The lungs were inflated three times to 30 cm. water before each reading. The inspired oxygen tension was 165.1 mm. Hg before and 179.0 mm. Hg after perfusion for satisfactory Pao_2. The mean Pao_2 levels were 89.5 mm. Hg before and 90.1 mm. Hg after perfusion, respectively. Physiologic dead space increased significantly with a change to 100% oxygen before perfusion, but the dead space-tidal volume ratio did not change significantly. With perfusion, the ratio increased significantly on 100% oxygen. The ratio decreased

(4)   Anaesthesia 26:22-27, January, 1971.

significantly after bypass on both oxygen concentrations, and CO_2 output increased significantly at this time.

All patients showing a significant rise in dead space-tidal volume in the postperfusion period also showed a rise before perfusion, suggesting an individual rather than a general response. The rise in dead space occurring in a proportion of patients with 100% oxygen inhalation is mainly in the alveolar compartment. It may contribute to the increase in dead space noted during anesthesia.

▶ [As the authors say, "The mean increase is, however, relatively small and the statistical significance of the results is borderline."—Eds.]

Gas Exchange Abnormalities in Mild Bronchitis and Asymptomatic Asthma. Patients with minimal bronchitis or asymptomatic asthma may show frequency dependence of compliance and ventilation-perfusion abnormalities despite relatively normal lung function, attributed to obstruction in some peripheral airways. Gerald Levine, E. Housley, P. MacLeod and Peter T. Macklem[5] (Montreal, Que.) studied gas exchange at rest and during upright bicycle exercise in 8 patients with minimal chronic bronchitis, 7 asthmatic patients without symptoms but with histories of episodic bronchospasm and 11 control subjects with an average age of 50. Most asthmatic patients were taking corticosteroids and bronchodilators at the time of the study. Dynamic compliance and pulmonary resistance were measured; gas exchange was measured on the same day as the dynamic compliance study in most patients.

Residual volume was increased in the bronchitic patients. The asthmatic patients had mildly abnormal lung volumes and flow rates. All patients had normal or minimally increased pulmonary resistance. All showed frequency dependence of compliance, defined as a fall of over 20% in compliance from the lowest to the highest breathing frequency. The alveolar-arterial oxygen tension difference, well above control levels at rest, improved on exercise in 5 and worsened in 2 patients with bronchitis; it improved in 4 asthmatic patients. The ratio of physiologic dead space to tidal volume was elevated at rest in both groups and changed little on exercise in all but 1 bronchitic patient. The asthmatic group showed a greater trend toward normality in this respect.

Residual volume was the only consistently abnormal routine

(5)   New England J. Med. 282:1277-1282, June 4, 1970.

lung function in the bronchitic subjects in this study. Patients with mild chronic bronchitis and asymptomatic asthma have abnormal gas exchange despite relatively normal routine lung function test results and airway resistance. This confirms the view that abnormal ventilation distribution and gas exchange becomes evident before other abnormalities of lung function appear.

The Lung's "Quiet Zone" is discussed by Jere Mead.[6] Earlier work indicated that the small bronchi must contribute importantly to gas flow resistance in airways. Weibel's recent measurements indicate that the increase in cross-sections at successive levels of branching is so rapid that resistance per unit length should be less rather than more in the smaller airways. Direct measurements of airway resistance have confirmed this; about 90% of the resistance of the tracheobronchial tree was found in airways greater than 1 mm. in internal diameter. Substantial changes in the cross-sectional area of small airways would then be expected to have only a small, perhaps undetectable, influence on total airway resistance, and hence on ventilatory function. Patency of small airways, however, has a major influence on distribution of lung distention, and thus on lung distensibility. Abnormal distensibility has been found in patients with mild bronchitis, with the abnormality magnified on more rapid breathing. Apparently abnormal distribution secondary to small airway disease impairs gas exchange during spontaneous breathing, but the embarrassment is not great.

Small airways contribute importantly to total airway resistance in the early years of life, with an abrupt change to an adult distribution at about the age when alveolar proliferation is complete. The small airways in adult lungs can be considered a "silent zone" within the lungs, obstruction within them causing little change in tests designed to detect it until the obstruction is far advanced. In young children the same zone may be far from quiet. The age of the patient may be of crucial importance in determining whether lower airway inflammation affecting the entire length of the tracheobronchial tree is manifested clinically as bronchitis or bronchiolitis.

Effect of Hyperventilation on Size and Shape of Alveoli. It has been suggested that hyperventilation reduces effective pulmonary surfactant and lung compliance, and this should be

(6)   New England J. Med. 282:1318-1319, June 4, 1970.

reflected in a change in the size and shape of alveoli but not of alveolar ducts. J. B. Forrest[7] (Glasgow) conducted a morphometric study of alveoli and alveolar ducts after a period of hyperventilation in anesthetized guinea pigs. The animals were artificially ventilated and rapidly frozen at the instant of cessation of ventilation at a selected point on the respiratory cycle. Guinea pigs were anesthetized with pentobarbital and ventilated for two breaths or for 5, 10 or 15 minutes at a rate of 32 strokes per minute. The negative ventilation pressure ranged from -30 to -40 cm. water, with positive pressure of 3 cm. water. Ventilation was stopped at low lung volume or at 30 or 60% inflation or full inflation.

The mean alveolar volumetric fraction of control lungs was significantly higher at midinflation than at low or high inflation. Hyperventilation reduced the fraction at all degrees of lung inflation, especially at midinflation (50% reduction after 15 minutes). Alveolar duct volumetric fractions did not differ with inflation or ventilation. Hyperventilation reduced total alveolar volume, especially at midinflation. Control lungs showed a greater increase in total alveolar volume when inflated from low than from high lung volume. Hyperventilation reduced this effect. Total alveolar surface area was reduced with progressive hyperventilation, being less than the predicted control value after 15 minutes. The alveolar shape coefficient (surface-to-volume ratio) tended to decrease as the lung was inflated and with hyperventilation.

Hyperventilation reduces the amount of effective pulmonary surfactant, requiring higher pressures to inflate the alveoli. Repeated overinflation of the lungs, as in mechanical ventilation, promotes alveolar atelectasis and transudation of alveolar capillary fluid into the interstitial space. This results in impaired gaseous diffusion and a tendency to complete alveolar collapse at the end of expirations. This may contribute to postoperative atelectasis and hypoxia, especially when respiration is already impaired from other causes such as pain or "heavy" sedation.

Diffusion Hypoxia Following Nitrous Oxide Anesthesia. Recently, Frumin and Edelist (1969) have cast doubt on the clinical significance of diffusion hypoxia, arguing that patients without significant cardiorespiratory disease do not become hypoxic when switched from 79% N_2O-21% oxygen to room air, if

(7)   Brit. J. Anaesth. 42:810-817, October, 1970.

respiratory irregularities or obstruction do not occur. Gary L. Fanning and Frank J. Colgan[8] (Univ. of Rochester) re-examined the problem of diffusion hypoxia, using simultaneous measurements of alveolar and arterial oxygen tensions during N_2O washout. Three healthy dogs were anesthetized with thiopental and, after tracheal intubation, breathed spontaneously. Mixtures of N_2O-oxygen were admitted in ratios of 4:2 or 6:2, and, after at least 30 minutes of equilibration with a given mixture and attainment of a stable P_{AO_2}, room air was suddenly breathed as the P_{AO_2} was continuously monitored. Four adult patients undergoing major surgical procedures were studied after anesthesia with thiopental and maintenance with N_2O-oxygen mixture and curare or halothane, with ventilation controlled. Radial arterial blood was sampled during washout.

Both Pa_{O_2} and P_{AO_2} were higher during N_2O-oxygen breathing than on room air and provided arterial oxygen saturations greater than 97%. Both values were significantly below values obtained 10-15 minutes later, 2-3 minutes after the switch to room air. The mean P_{AO_2} was 159 torr before washout, 83 torr at the lowest point during washout and 102 torr at equilibration with room air. The corresponding mean values for Pa_{O_2} were 112, 56 and 75 torr. The mean saturation values were 97.6, 83.7 and 94.3%, respectively. All the patients showed dilution of alveolar oxygen and a reduction in Pa_{O_2} in the first several minutes of N_2O washout, and 3 of the 4 patients became hypoxic. All these 3 patients had major intra-abdominal operations.

A given patient may initially be quite safe with a Pa_{O_2} of 60 torr during N_2O washout, but an untoward airway problem results in a rapid fall in Sa_{O_2} as the Pa_{O_2} drops below 60 torr. Supernormal oxygen concentrations must be available in the alveoli during washout to preclude hypoxemia. All patients should receive high inspired oxygen concentrations in the early washout period following N_2O anesthesia, forestalling the development of severe hypoxia should some unforeseen airway problem occur.

▶ [This has been an overworked hypothesis, anyway. All patients should be spontaneously breathing room air before transport from operating room to recovery room. If not, they must be transported with respiration assisted with oxygen.—Eds.]

Airway Closure and Lung Volumes in Surgical Positions. Closure of small airways in dependent lung zones of normal subjects has been described. Closure is thought to occur when

(8) Anesth. & Analg. 50:86-91, Jan.-Feb., 1971.

the net forces acting on small airways are such as to induce their collapse. The functional consequence is impaired ventilation to affected lung regions, with a reduction in ventilation-perfusion ratios and adverse pulmonary gas exchange. Trapped gas is sometimes absorbed, producing atelectasis and further impairing gas exchange. Douglas B. Craig, W. M. Wahba and Hillary Don[9] (McGill Univ.) studied the effects of several surgical positions on airway closure and lung volumes. Studies were done on 10 normal males, aged 28-53 years, in the seated, supine, supine with 15-degree head-down and lithotomy plus 15-degree head-down positions. Lung volumes were measured and airway closure determined by a modified single-breath nitrogen technic.

All lung volumes except vital capacity decreased significantly with the change from sitting to supine. With addition of the 15-degree head-down position, total lung capacity and functional residual capacity changed significantly. Further addition of the lithotomy position did not significantly alter any parameter. Airway closure involved increasing lung volumes with increasing age. In the seated position, the age at which the closing volume exceeded functional residual capacity was 49 years. The age decreased to 36 years in the supine position, 35.5 years with the head-down position and 32 years with the combined lithotomy and head-down position.

Pulmonary gas exchange is likely to be impaired in subjects in whom airway closure occurs within the tidal volume range. Airway closure appears to have important effects on gas exchange, and the role of posture provides significant added implications for the anesthetic and perioperative periods. Body position importantly affects the critical relation between closing volume and functional residual capacity and, thus, the functional results of airway closure.

▶ [Too bad they didn't look at the prone and the lateral kidney positions. How important is the change if respiration is controlled or assisted?—Eds.]

Properties of Alveolar Cells and Tissues That Strengthen Alveolar Defenses are discussed by Sergei P. Sorokin[1] (Harvard Med. School). Some of the properties of alveolar cells that contribute to their defensive capacity against inhaled agents are held in common with cells of other regions, and some are unique to alveolar cells. Many of the general defensive measures of a region are enacted in its connective tissue and

(9) Canad. Anaesth. Soc. J. 18:92-99, January, 1971.
(1) Arch. Int. Med. 126:450-463, September, 1970.

concern its plasma cells, mast cells and macrophages. The alveolar surface is specialized toward facilitating diffusion between the external and internal environments but the alveolar wall is organized along the same lines as other exposed surfaces. The alveolar epithelium is inhomogeneous, consisting principally of attenuated squamous alveolar cells and pleomorphic great alveolar cells. Defenses include mucociliary mechanisms and others present higher up in the respiratory tract, those arising from physical properties of the alveoli and the alveolar microcirculation, the phagocytic activity of alveolar macrophages, and those contributed by the epithelium.

The connective tissue may contribute significantly to alveolar defense through maintaining alveolar differentiation. The alveolar macrophages are the predominant defensive cells. These cells resemble great alveolar cells histochemically more closely than any other component of the alveolar wall. The defensive capacity of alveolar macrophages resides mainly in their ability to digest harmful objects. The alveolar epithelium is a barrier to macromolecules and a surface suitable for phagocytic action. It is also a possible source of bacteriostatic or other salutary agents. Secretory activity is carried out mainly by the great alveolar cells, which are distributed fairly uniformly over the alveolar surface. Secreted materials may include some with detergent or hydrolytic actions associated with bacteriostasis or others useful in promoting phagocytosis.

Effect of Acute Hypoxia on Vascular Responsiveness in Man. —I. Responsiveness to lower body negative pressure and ice on the forehead.—Donald D. Heistad and Robert C. Wheeler[2] (US Army Res. Inst. of Environmental Medicine) studied the effect of hypoxia on vascular responsiveness to lower body negative pressure and to ice on the forehead in 12 healthy men, aged 19-24.

METHOD.—An airtight box enclosed the lower part of the supine subject's body to iliac-crest level. Blood pressure was determined by auscultation every 30 seconds. In measuring forearm blood flow by water plethysmograph, a pneumatic cuff placed around the upper arm was periodically inflated above venous pressure for 8-12 seconds; arm volume change was measured as hydrostatic pressure change. In 8 of 12 subjects, blood flow to the hand was measured on the same arm. The subject breathed room air, 12% oxygen (in nitrogen) and 10% oxygen for 16 minutes with 10-minute rests between gases. After a gas was breathed for 5 minutes, control measurements were taken for 3 minutes before response to reflex vaso-

(2)　J. Clin. Invest. 49:1252-1265, June, 1970.

constrictor stimuli was studied. Pressure within the box was reduced to 40 mm. Hg below atmospheric pressure and maintained for 1.5 minutes. Lower body negative pressure was applied twice while breathing each gas mixture, separated by a 1.5-minute rest period. After a 2-minute rest, the subject had ice to the forehead for 1 minute. Blood flow to forearm and hand was calculated from the rate of volume increase during venous occlusion. Forearm vascular resistance was derived by dividing mean arterial pressure by forearm blood flow, and mean arterial pressure was derived by adding one third of the pulse pressure to the diastolic pressure.

The subjects' mean arterial pressure and forearm vascular resistance were not significantly different as they breathed air, 12% oxygen or 10% oxygen. In 8, mean blood flow to the hand decreased during hypoxia; the decrease was statistically significant during 10% oxygen administration. During lower body negative pressure, mean arterial pressure increased minimally during air breathing and fell during oxygen breathing; increase in forearm vascular resistance was significantly greater during normoxia than during either level of hypoxia. During ice on the forehead, increase in mean arterial pressure was similar during air and oxygen breathing; increase in forearm vascular resistance during air breathing was significantly reduced during hypoxia.

II. Responses to norepinephrine and angiotensin.—The authors studied the effect of hypoxia on vascular response to norepinephrine and angiotensin during 24 experiments in 15 men.

METHOD.—In 12 subjects, a cannula was passed about 2 inches into the brachial artery and connected to a pressure transducer and syringe for drug infusions. Forearm and hand blood were measured as before. After control measurements were made, the supine subject received the drug by Harvard constant infusion pump at 75 mμg. per minute for 3 minutes and then at 150 mμg. per minute for 3 minutes. Each subject received norepinephrine while breathing air, 12% oxygen and 10% oxygen and angiotensin while breathing air and 10% oxygen. The Po_2, Pco_2 and pH were determined in blood samples obtained after breathing each gas for 6 minutes. In measuring calf blood flow by water plethysmograph in 12 subjects, a pneumatic cuff placed around the thigh was periodically inflated for 10-15 seconds to pressures sufficient to produce venous occlusion. Blood pressure was determined by auscultation. The subject received norepinephrine, 3 and 6 μg. per minute, into the basilic vein as he breathed each gas mixture.

Average arterial blood Po_2 fell from 90 mm. Hg during air breathing to 41 mm. Hg during 12% oxygen and 35 mm. Hg during 10% oxygen breathing. Accompanying the decrease in Po_2 during hypoxia, Pco_2 fell and pH rose. Norepinephrine and angiotensin doses were insufficient to cause detectable changes in blood pressure or heart rate. Reduction in blood flow to the forearm during drug administration was significantly less during hypoxia than during normoxia. Resting mean arterial pressure was not significantly different during air and oxygen breathing during norepinephrine. Blood pressure increase in response to norepinephrine was significantly less during hypoxia than during normoxia. Resting calf vascular resistance was not significantly changed by hypoxia; increase in resistance during norepinephrine administration was not significantly different during normoxia and hypoxia.

III. Effect of hypoxia and hypocapnia.—The authors assessed responses to lower body negative pressure and to ice on the forehead in 12 men during normoxia and normocapnia while breathing air; hypoxia and hypocapnia while breathing 12% oxygen; hypoxia and normocapnia while breathing 10.5% oxygen with carbon dioxide replacement; and normoxia and hypocapnia during hyperventilation while breathing room air.

METHOD.—During hypoxia and normocapnia, end-tidal carbon dioxide was measured directly by an infrared carbon dioxide analyzer with continuous sampling at the mouthpiece; carbon dioxide was added to inspired 10.5% oxygen at flow rates sufficient to maintain end-tidal carbon dioxide at values similar to those obtained while breathing air. In normoxia and hypocapnia, the subject adjusted his respiration to maintain end-tidal carbon dioxide similar to the level achieved while breathing 12% oxygen. Alveolar samples were obtained after breathing each gas mixture for 6-14 minutes and analyzed for Po_2 and Pco_2. Forearm and hand blood flows were measured by water plethysmographs, and blood pressure was determined by auscultation. Expiratory minute volume was collected and measured.

Alveolar Pco_2 during 12% oxygen breathing was the same as in hyperventilation during air breathing; Pco_2 was similar during air breathing and breathing of 10.5% oxygen with carbon dioxide replacement. The alveolar Po_2 was reduced to similar levels during breathing of 12% oxygen and 10.5% oxygen with carbon dioxide replacement. Mean arterial pressure and forearm vascular resistance were not significantly altered by hypoxia or hypocapnia. Hand blood flow was significantly greater during air breathing than during hypoxia or hypocapnia. Lower body negative pressure caused a similar fall in mean arterial pressure during hypoxia with and without carbon dioxide replacement and a neglible fall during hyperventilation hypocapnia. Increase in forearm vascular resistance in response to lower body negative pressure was decreased during hypoxia with and without carbon dioxide replacement. Increase in mean arterial pressure during ice on the forehead was not significantly altered during hypoxia or hypocapnia. The increase in forearm vascular resistance, which occurs with ice on the forehead while breathing air, was markedly reduced during hypoxia, with and without carbon dioxide replacement, and by hyperventilation hypocapnia.

These experiments suggest that hypoxia levels which do not consistently alter resting vascular resistance and arterial pressure still markedly decrease vasoconstrictor responsiveness.

▶ [Clinical situations where hypoxemia is of this degree are generally accompanied by metabolic acidosis, which further obtunds vascular reactivity.—Eds.]

Screening Tests of Pulmonary Function are reviewed by J. H. Comroe, Jr., and J. A. Nadel[3] (Univ. of California). Ideally, pulmonary function screening tests should be done with inexpensive, easy-to-use portable apparatus; be error free; pinpoint the function abnormality and provide quantitative data.

The simplest tests measure vital capacity and maximal expiratory flow rate. For both, the patient inspires maximally, but in the former the patient exhales slowly and in the latter, rapidly and forcefully. The maximal volume exhaled slowly is vital capacity and that exhaled rapidly is usually quantified as the volume exhaled in the first second, expressed as a percentage of vital capacity (forced expired volume in 1 second/vital capacity). These screening tests properly belong in the physician's office. Vital capacity may be decreased in both restrictive and obstructive pulmonary disease, but the patient with the former can exhale rapidly and the one with the latter cannot. If the test is repeated after the patient inhales 0.5% isoproterenol, obstruction due to smooth muscle contraction in the airways is partly or wholly reversed but that due to destructive or organic disease is not.

A rapid, single-breath screening test of pulmonary diffusing capacity helps detect obstructive disorders of pulmonary circulation. The patient inhales a low, nontoxic concentration of carbon monoxide, holds his breath for 10 seconds and then exhales. The test measures the transfer of carbon monoxide molecules across alveolar capillary membranes and their combination with hemoglobin in red blood cells in pulmonary

(3)   New England J. Med. 282: 1249-1253, May 28, 1970.

capillaries; the test is useful in detecting infiltrative lung disease, pulmonary vascular disease and disease associated with loss of alveolar-capillary surface area. Although the test requires a skilled operator and costly equipment, it provides an easy and safe way to measure diffusing capacity repeatedly. The present authors believe that the previously described screening tests should be used in the differential diagnosis of all patients with dyspnea.

Screening tests are also used to detect the presence, location and extent of regional lung disease. In the single-breath oxygen test, nitrogen concentration in expired gas is measured by an electric analyzer after the patient inhales oxygen. Abnormal results show that some lung regions are filling and emptying unevenly. Except in the case of asthmatic-type obstruction, the data cannot tell what or where the abnormality is. Large lesions are reasonably well located by the single-breath xenon (^{133}Xe) test. As the patient inhales gas containing ^{133}Xe, an external stationary detector records count distribution from both lungs during breath-holding at end inspiration and during ^{133}Xe clearance by normal breathing. Exposure to radiation is like that during a chest x-ray. The test gives information on gas distribution to different lung areas and on the ventilation rates of these regions. Although material and apparatus are costly, the test gives specific information quickly. A method in which powdered tantalum is insufflated provides excellent bronchograms without interfering with pulmonary function and seemingly without producing local or systemic toxicity; this method may become applicable as a screening test (Nadel et al., 1968). Poorly perfused lung areas can be located by intravenously injected macroaggregates of radioactive iodinated serum albumin (Wagner et al., 1964); aggregates, larger in diameter than small arterioles or capillaries, are carried by flowing pulmonary blood and lodged in previously patent arterioles or capillaries. An external detector maps the perfused areas. The test can be redone after 24 hours, since the body removes the particles rapidly.

The patient about to have a lobe or lung removed should have complete pulmonary function tests. Those about to have extrathoracic operations should have screening tests to uncover unsuspected pulmonary abnormalities or to determine quantitatively a known or suspected functional defect. Effective preoperative treatment of airway obstruction reduces the frequency of postoperative complications. Patients to have Ethiodol injections should have pulmonary diffusing capacity measured.

To detect hypoventilation, an infrared carbon dioxide analyzer is used; it continuously samples and analyzes inspired and expired gas just beyond the patient's lips. If breathing is not rapid and lungs are normal, end-expired Pco_2, alveolar gas Pco_2 and arterial blood Pco_2 are about equal. An end-expired Pco_2 of over 44 mm. Hg shows hypoventilation (in relation to the patient's metabolic rate). An inexpensive chemical gas analyzer, as described by Hackney and Collier (1965), can be used to measure Pco_2 in expired gas; with this value, arterial Pco_2 can be estimated. Analyzer use takes about as much time and skill as do simple spirometric studies. Direct measurement of Po_2, Pco_2 and pH of arterial blood is necessary in hospital recovery rooms, intensive coronary and respiratory care units and medical wards for optimal management of patients with hypoxemia and respiratory failure. Pulmonary function tests also allow the physician to try his therapeutic recommendations on the patient and determine which is most beneficial or to follow the course of pulmonary disease for which no therapy is specific or effective.

Airway resistance can be measured quantitatively by the body plethysmograph as the patient with airway obstruction sits in a small closed chamber and breathes through a flowmeter. The test gives a value for lung volume at which resistance was measured. The test has been used for evaluating large populations and effects of air pollution and industrial exposures. By mounting any of the previously mentioned apparatus into mobile units, an investigator can study whole populations far removed from a major medical center or a pulmonary function laboratory.

▶ [With more frequent use of such methods preoperatively, we now can identify patients at risk from pulmonary pathophysiology in sufficient time to get them into optimal condition before operation. Preoperative studies may also form a baseline of information from which conclusions can be drawn when the postoperative course is unsatisfactory.—Eds.]

Pulmonary Function in Thoracic Scoliosis: Before and after Corrective Surgery. Hugh D. Westgate[4] (Univ. of Minnesota) compared thoracic spinal curvature and lung function parameters before and at intervals up to 5 years after correction of thoracic scoliosis by the Harrington rod technic. Study was made of 74 patients with scoliosis, with or without kyphosis,

(4)   Minnesota Med. 53:839-847, August, 1970.

seen since 1961. Most were aged 13-22 years. Scoliosis was secondary to poliomyelitis in 37 patients and congenital in 13; in 24 it was considered idiopathic. Spinal fusion was produced with bank bone or iliac crest bone after placement of the Harrington rods.

Minute volume and alveolar minute ventilation were normal before and after operation. Cough was normal except in patients having tracheotomy preoperatively. The average spinal curvature was 87 degrees before and 53 degrees 2 years after operation; it remained the same 5 years postoperatively. Vital capacity was significantly related negatively to the degree of curvature only in the idiopathic group, and it was positively correlated with maximum breathing capacity. These parameters were not related to changes in angulation after operation. Maximum breathing capacity decreased from 55 to 51% of predicted a year after operation but increased from 61 to 64% in the idiopathic group. Arterial oxygen saturation correlated negatively with curvature in the idiopathic group. It improved significantly 2 years after operation. Fifteen patients required tracheotomy, 12 of them electively, including 7 with postpoliomyelitic scoliosis. Two poliomyelitis patients and 1 with congenital scoliosis required tracheotomy and assisted ventilation postoperatively.

The Harrington method of correcting thoracic scoliosis did not improve average vital capacity or maximum breathing capacity in this series, but it did improve the over-all ventilation-perfusion ratio. Overenthusiastic correction of the curve is to be avoided in patients with postpoliomyelitic scoliosis, but treatment should be started as soon as a curve is observed. Idiopathic scoliosis should be treated when there is any sudden increase in curvature or as early as possible if the curve is progressing slowly, since in this group the vital capacity decreases proportional to the increase in spinal curvature. Treatment should aim primarily at restoration or preservation of function, not anatomic perfection alone.

▶ [In effect, this study shows little improvement in pulmonary mechanics in kyphoscoliotic patients after vigorous corrective surgery. Nonetheless, individual patients did have better blood gas values postoperatively, and the need for preoperative baseline blood gas values is obvious if one is to follow these patients postoperatively.—Eds.]

Effect of Hypothermia on Respiratory Response to Carbon Dioxide. Gerald Edelist[5] (Univ. of Toronto) noted low $Paco_2$

(5) Canad. Anaesth. Soc. J. 17:551-556, November, 1970.

levels in the postoperative period in patients having hypothermia during operation for cerebral aneurysm. In the present study, 5 dogs were anesthetized with halothane and nitrous oxide and had their tracheas intubated. When the end-tidal halothane level and end-tidal Pco_2 were stable, resting minute ventilation was estimated as arterial blood was sampled, and the end-tidal Pco_2 was then raised. The dog was then cooled about 10 C. by surface ice application, and responses to normal and raised CO_2 levels were again determined. Measurements were repeated after the halothane concentration was raised to about double that needed to prevent movement in response to tail clamp at normothermia.

With a 10-degree drop in temperature, the minimum alveolar concentration of halothane fell 49%, from 0.84 to 0.43, a highly significant change. Resting ventilation did not change significantly, but the resting $Paco_2$ was significantly lower, 23.4 compared with 34.6 torr. At ventilation of 10 L. per minute, the $Paco_2$ was 41.5 torr at normothermia and 32 torr at hypothermia. There was a considerable shift to the left of the CO_2 response curve during hypothermia, exhibited by each dog studied. The mean slope of the curves was not significantly decreased, and changes in slope were inconsistent. In the 3 dogs cooled while the anesthetic level was kept at the normothermic minimum alveolar concentration, the slope was profoundly depressed, due to deepening of anesthesia rather than to any effect of the hypothermia itself.

The mechanism by which the threshold of the respiratory center is lowered by hypothermia remains obscure. Generally, any increased afferent input into the center from the periphery will shift the CO_2 response curve to the left. The primary effect of hypothermia on the respiratory response to CO_2 in dogs is a shift of the response curve to the left, with no significant change in slope. Not considering that anesthesia deepens during hypothermia for the same anesthetic concentration, the slope of the response curve is markedly depressed. This may account for the clinical impression held by some that hypothermia depresses ventilation.

Clinical Interpretation of Arterial Oxygen Measurements is discussed by Richard W. Hyde[6] (Univ. of Rochester). Identification of the physiologic cause of arterial hypoxia can help in diagnosis and management of the patient with cardiopulmonary

---

(6)   M. Clin. North America 54:617-629, May, 1970.

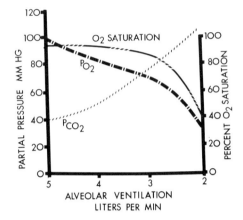

Fig. 9.—Effect of fall in alveolar ventilation (hypoventilation) on O_2 saturation, Po_2 and Pco_2 of arterial blood. Note that Pco_2 shows an almost linear rise in value with decreasing levels of ventilation. Arterial Po_2 shows about a reciprocal fall. The O_2 saturation does not decrease appreciably until ventilation falls to about three fifths of normal value. This alinearity is the result of the curved shape of the O_2 dissociation curve for blood. Data for this figure were calculated from the alveolar air equation, using a constant CO_2 production of 220 ml. STPD (standard temperature and pressure, dry) per minute and a respiratory quotient of 0.85. Alveolar and arterial Po_2 were considered to be equal and no unevenness of ventilation or perfusion was assumed to be present. (Courtesy of Hyde, R. W.: M. Clin. North America 54:617-629, May, 1970.)

disease. The Pao_2 is considered low if less than about 75 mm. Hg during air breathing at sea level. The corresponding arterial blood oxygen saturation is about 95%. The four basic mechanisms of arterial hypoxia are hypoventilation (Fig. 9), uneven matching of pulmonary ventilation to perfusion, impaired diffusion of oxygen from the alveolus to the pulmonary capillary blood and right-to-left shunts.

During breathing of 100% oxygen, the Po_2 of blood leaving the ventilated alveoli rises to a high, predictable level; thus a lesser amount of oxygen in arterial blood is attributable to venous blood bypassing the pulmonary capillaries. Such measurements can distinguish hypoxia due to right-to-left shunting from that due to other mechanisms. Underventilation or uneven distribution of ventilation to perfusion is usually accompanied by arterial hypoxemia during air breathing, with a rise to near normal when oxygen is breathed. Also, hypoxemia due to impaired diffusion usually disappears during pure oxygen breathing. The blood gas changes associated with the various abnormalities causing hypoxemia are shown in the table.

From these measurements, formulas have been derived for

SUMMARY OF ABNORMALITIES IN BLOOD GASES SEEN IN THE FOUR
BASIC PHYSIOLOGIC ABNORMALITIES CAUSING ARTERIAL HYPOXIA

PHYSIOLOGIC DEFECT	ARTERIAL P_{CO_2}*	ARTERIAL P_{O_2} BREATHING AIR†	ARTERIAL P_{O_2} BREATHING 100% O_2‡
Hypoventilation	High	Low	Normal
Uneven ventilation to perfusion	Normal	Low	Normal
Impairment of pulmonary diffusion	Normal or low	Low	Normal
Right-to-left shunt	Normal	Low	Low

*Normal range for arterial P_{CO_2} is 35-46 mm. Hg.
†Lower limit of normal for arterial P_{O_2} is about 75 mm. Hg.
‡This value should be greater than 550 mm. Hg in normal subjects.

calculating the size of right-to-left shunts. Small shunts (5-15%) may be found in patients with emphysema, pulmonary fibrosis, congestive heart failure, obesity or hepatic cirrhosis. The measured shunt in healthy subjects or patients with no apparent lung disease should be less than 6-8%.

Abnormal shunting of blood around ventilated alveoli is present in a hypoxic patient if ventilation with 100% oxygen for 15 minutes does not raise the Pa_{O_2} to 500 mm. Hg or higher. Conditions such as atelectasis and pneumonia must be excluded before an intracardiac shunt or other abnormal communication can be diagnosed. Patients with a normal Pa_{CO_2} and arterial hypoxia during air breathing who have a Pa_{O_2} greater than 500 mm. Hg during breathing of 100% oxygen have hypoxia secondary to uneven matching of ventilation to pulmonary perfusion or the "alveolar-capillary block" syndrome.

▶ [A worthwhile review for teaching purposes.—Eds.]

O_2 **Exchange across Spleen during Asphyxia.** Splenic contraction can increase the blood oxygen content in hypoxia by increasing the number of circulating red cells. In complete asphyxia, the spleen could also serve as an oxygen source through a slower decrease in splenic tissue P_{O_2} than in Pa_{O_2} during asphyxia, since the mass of red cells in the spleen is large and its oxygen storage capacity is high. Splenic venous oxygen tension would then exceed arterial oxygen tension during asphyxia, reversing the usual oxygen tension gradient. Neil S. Cherniack, Norman H. Edelman and Alfred P. Fishman[7] (Univ. of Pennsylvania) compared the oxygen balance of the intact and denervated spleen of the dog during asphyxia. A flowmeter was placed in the splenic vein of 16 anesthetized mongrel dogs and another in the splenic artery. About one third of the splenic mass was excluded from the circulation by the surgical procedures. Both phasic and mean flows were recorded. Flow was recorded after the respiratory pump was stopped in 8 dogs. Splenic contraction was induced in 5 animals by the injection into the splenic artery of 2 ml. of 1:1000 epinephrine. Splenic pulp pressure rose to 40-60 mm. Hg in 60 seconds with contraction, and venous outflow exceeded arterial inflow. Denervation delayed the onset of contraction and reduced the rise in pulp pressure. Added bilateral adrenalectomy abolished splenic contraction during asphyxia.

In the first 3 minutes of asphyxia, the intact contracting spleen added 24.2 ml. of oxygen to the venous blood. After a minute of asphyxia, splenic venous blood had a higher oxygen tension and content than did arterial blood. Even the noncontracting spleen contributed an average of 15 ml. of oxygen to venous blood during 3 minutes of asphyxia.

The spleen acts as a source of oxygen during acute hypoxia both by contracting, with an increase in red cells, and by releasing red cells richer in oxygen than those entering the spleen. The spleen may be a significant oxygen source during asphyxia even in species, such as man, where splenic contraction is feeble. The spleen may also serve as a site of CO_2 storage, but this is probably a less important function in emergency situations, since there are many sites of CO_2 storage in the body, especially muscle.

► [An interesting phenomenon, which must be remembered by those doing experimental studies in dogs. It is probably of little significance to the clinician.—Eds.]

Affinity of Hemoglobin for Oxygen: Its Control and In Vivo Significance were investigated by Leonard D. Miller, Frank A. Oski, Joseph F. Diaco, Harvey J. Sugerman, A. J. Gottlieb, Douglas Davidson and Maria Delivoria-Papadopoulos[8] (Philadelphia).

The red blood cell can no longer be considered a passive carrier of hemoglobin; it responds actively to the oxygen requirements of tissues. The position of the adult's oxyhemoglobin dissociation curve is largely controlled by the interaction

(7) Am. J. Physiol. 219:1585-1589, December, 1970.
(8) Surgery 68:187-195, July, 1970.

of hemoglobin with organic phosphates within the red blood cell, 70-80% of which is composed of 2,3-diphosphoglycerate, a normal glycolytic intermediate of the Embden-Meyerhoff cycle within the red blood cell. The curve shifts to the right with higher 2,3-diphosphoglycerate levels, with a decreased affinity of hemoglobin for oxygen. A maladaptive "left shift" occurs, however, in patients in septic shock, those given large volumes of stored blood and infants with infection or respiratory distress syndrome, or both, despite their need for increased oxygen transport.

Serial measurements of 2,3-diphosphogylcerate were made in 11 patients admitted to the hospital in septic shock. The 2,3-diphosphoglycerate level correlated well with the position of the oxyhemoglobin equilibrium curve, and it also mirrored the patient's general clinical state, being lower with a poor state. Most of the patients had signs of a "hyperdynamic state" at some time, with inadequate oxygen consumption and an elevated cardiac index. A steadily decreasing oxygen consumption often provided a clue to unresolved sepsis (Fig. 10). Presumably, one can shift only so far "to the left" before the capillary-tissue cell oxygen gradient drops to an inadequate degree, in terms of tissue requirements, i.e., a critical Po_2 is reached. This critical Po_2, defined as the Po_2 below which organ deterioration occurs, probably varies in different organs and may depend on an organ's functional state and its ability to increase local flow. Other physiologic parameters of impaired function such as arteriovenous oxygen content difference and decreasing oxygen consumption correlated well with the 2,3-diphosphoglycerate levels.

Determinations of 2,3-diphosphoglycerate made on banked blood before it was administered to patients showed that 2,3-diphosphoglycerate had fallen to 50% of control values after 3 days of storage, to 25% after 6 days and to 5% after 10 days. In these patients 2,3-diphosphoglycerate levels correlated appropriately with the storage time of the blood transfused, and low values correlated with dropping central venous Po_2 values, despite marked variations in blood pressure and peripheral blood flow. Addition of inosine, pyruvate and phosphate to stored blood restored normal 2,3-diphosphoglycerate levels.

Studies done in 28 premature infants showed a marked "left shift" of the oxygen equilibrium curve compared with normal adults. A fraction of 2,3-diphosphoglycerate can inter-

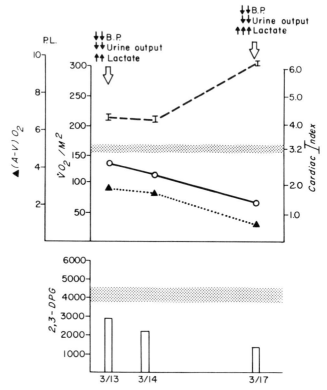

Fig. 10.—The "hyperdynamic state." In uncontrolled sepsis, oxygen consumption continues to fall, and clinical signs of peripheral perfusion deteriorate, despite a high and rising cardiac index. The 2,3-diphosphoglycerate concentration falls as clinical status worsens. Efforts to compensate, in terms of flow, in this patient were still insufficient to salvage his life. (Courtesy of Miller, L. D., *et al.:* Surgery 68:187-195, July, 1970.)

act with the lesser amount of adult hemoglobin present in the newborn's red blood cells. Added oxygen could be provided without added myocardial stress by replacing fetal red blood cells with fresh adult red blood cells in sick infants. Above a venous Po_2 of about 15 mm. Hg, the "right-shifted" child is better oxygenated than a "left-shifted" one at the same hemoglobin level. The absolute hemoglobin level is less important than how the hemoglobin is functioning in terms of delivery of oxygen to the tissues.

Regulatory Mechanisms of Hemoglobin Oxygen Affinity in Acidosis and Alkalosis. Hemoglobin oxygen affinity has been found to be reduced by 2,3-diphosphoglycerate (2,3-DPG), present in high concentrations in red cells, and diabetic acidosis is associated with a low red cell 2,3-DPG level. A. J. Bellingham, J. C. Detter and C. Lenfant[9] (Univ. of Washington) studied the effects of acidosis and alkalosis on the oxygen dissociation curve in normal man.

Acidosis was induced in 4 healthy subjects by giving acetazolamide intravenously and acetazolamide and ammonium chloride orally. Acidosis was then corrected, and alkalosis was induced with sodium bicarbonate. Measurements were made on arterialized blood with a hemoglobin oxygen saturation of 80% or greater. Hemoglobin affinity for oxygen was determined by the mixing technic. Results were expressed as the partial pres-

Fig. 11.—Changes in plasma pH, red cell 2,3-DPG, P50 (7.4) and in vivo hemoglobin oxygen affinity ($P50$ (in vivo)) occurring in 4 subjects during a week of acidosis followed by a week of alkalosis. Each subject is represented by a different symbol. Note the changing time scale. (Courtesy of Bellingham, A. J., et al.: J. Clin. Invest. 50:700-706, March, 1971.)

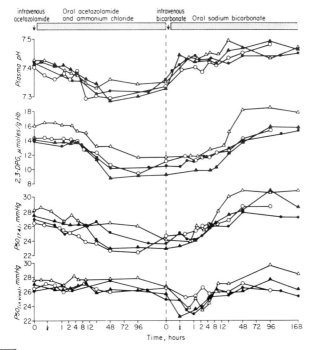

(9) J. Clin. Invest. 50:700-706, March, 1971.

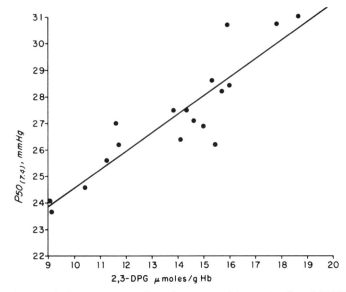

Fig. 12.—The P50(7.4), corrected to a base excess of 0, as a function of 2,3-DPG in samples obtained for control and last phase of both acidosis and alkalosis. The regression line, P50(7.4) = 0.694 DPG + 17.63, is shown (r = 0.9, P < 0.001). (Courtesy of Bellingham, A. J., et al.: J. Clin. Invest. 50:700-706, March, 1971.)

sure of oxygen at half saturation at pH 7.4 and 37 C. ($P50_{(7.4)}$). Red cell organic phosphate content was assessed by extraction and fractionation.

The mean plasma pH fell to 7.332 in acidosis and rose to 7.45 in alkalosis. The mean control red cell 2,3-DPG level was 14.5 μM./Gm. hemoglobin, falling to 10.4 at the end of acidosis and rising to 16.2 μM. in alkalosis (Fig. 11). The hemoglobin oxygen affinity at pH 7.4 fell from 27.2 to 24.1 mm. Hg with acidosis and rose to 29.2 mm. Hg at the end of alkalosis. The in vivo affinity did not change significantly in acidosis, but fell transiently in alkalosis. The mean corpuscular hemoglobin concentration fell rapidly early in acidosis but then returned to normal. It rose in alkalosis and then was normalized. Plasma Pco_2 and base excess were reduced in acidosis and elevated in alkalosis. Red cell ATP, blood urea nitrogen and plasma sodium levels did not change significantly.

The observed changes in hemoglobin oxygen affinity at pH 7.4 are attributed to changes in red cell volume, through alterations in both intracellular hemoglobin concentration and 2,3-

DPG concentration. The observations are illustrated in Figure 12. About 35% of the change in hemoglobin oxygen affinity resulting from an alteration in red cell 2,3-DPG is explained by the effect of 2,3-DPG on the red cell pH.

▶ [The clinical significance of the 2,3-diphosphoglycerate level in red blood cells is becoming apparent. Not only is its lack an important factor in causing tissue hypoxia in the patient in shock but it also could be of importance in the surgical patient who has had massive transfusion with old blood. In the discussion that followed this article, it was pointed out that the 2,3-diphosphoglycerate changes very little in blood stored at −85 C. for as long as 37 months. Perhaps we will soon be in a position to treat old blood with inosine, pyruvate and phosphate or with 2,3-diphosphoglycerate. —Eds.]

Effects of Diethyl Ether Anesthesia and Surgery on Carbohydrate and Fat Metabolism in Man. Tsutomu Oyama and T. Takazawa[1] (Hirosaki Univ., Japan) studied the effects of ether anesthesia alone on carbohydrate and fat metabolism and compared them with the effects of surgery superimposed on anesthesia. Studies were done on 20 males, aged 22-56 years, who underwent elective operations; none had hepatorenal or endocrine disease or had had steroid therapy. Pentobarbital, meperidine and atropine were given before induction with nitrous oxide-oxygen. Plane 1-2 anesthesia was maintained after intubation; tubocurarine was used for muscle relaxation. Respiration was assisted intermittently. Anesthesia lasted at least 45 minutes in each case. Ether was added from a Copper Kettle vaporizer. Blood was sampled 10 minutes before and 15, 30 and 45 minutes after induction, 5-10, 30 and 60 minutes after the start of operation, and again when the patient awakened in the recovery room. Plasma cortisol was measured using ^{3}H-corticosterone.

Plasma growth hormone was significantly elevated at 3.2 mμg./ml. after 30 minutes of ether anesthesia, and a further rise to 3.9 mμg. was noted at 45 minutes. The peak value, 10.2 mμg./ml., was found an hour after the start of operation. Plasma insulin fell to 25.6 μU./ml. an hour after the start of operation, a significant fall from the control level of 37.7 μU./ml. The blood glucose an hour after the start of operation was 155 mg./100 ml., compared with a control level of 85 mg. Free fatty acids did not change significantly. Plasma cortisol rose from 15.2 μg./ml. in the control period to 27.5 μg./ml. an hour after the start of surgery; the recovery room level was 31.0 μg./ml.

Plasma growth hormone increased significantly with surgery

(1) Canad. Anaesth. Soc. J. 18:51-59, January, 1971.

and ether anesthesia in this study. Plasma insulin showed a relative decrease. Fatty acids did not change significantly. Plasma cortisol increased stepwise significantly during anesthesia and surgery. The growth hormone, insulin and cortisol changes appear to play a role in the rise in blood glucose noted during ether anesthesia and operation in man.

► [The failure of a rise in plasma insulin in the face of an elevated blood sugar probably represents the inhibitory effect of elevated plasma catecholamine levels on the insulin-secreting mechanism.—Eds.]

CEREBRAL CIRCULATION

Cerebrovascular Response to Acute Hypocapnic and Eucapnic Hypoxia in Normal Man. Little information is available on the separate, possibly antagonistic effects on the cerebral vasculature of the hypocapnia often associated with exposure to acute hypoxia. William Shapiro, Albert J. Wasserman, James P. Baker and John L. Patterson, Jr.[2] examined cerebral blood flow and related blood constituents in healthy subjects after induction of various degrees of acute hypoxia. A total of 28 studies was done in 13 healthy men, aged 25-40 years, in the postabsorptive resting state. Arterial and jugular venous bulb blood was sampled after serial 5-minute inhalations of air, 18, 16, 14, 12 and 10% oxygen and 10% oxygen with carbon dioxide added to restore the end-tidal carbon dioxide level as closely as possible to the control level. In 12 studies an 8-minute period of 10% oxygen inhalation was given. In 10 studies subjects breathed air, 18, 14, 9.5, 10.4 and 9.5% oxygen for 10-minute periods, with carbon dioxide added during inhalation of 18 and 14% oxygen and the first 9.5% oxygen period. Subjects hyperventilated during the second period of 9.5% oxygen inhalation.

Significant increases in cerebral blood flow followed inhalation of 12 and 10% oxygen, although cerebrovascular resistance was reduced after less marked hypoxemia. Addition of carbon dioxide resulted in a further rise in flow and drop in resistance. The estimated total oxygen delivery to the brain was significantly increased with 10% oxygen, with and without added carbon dioxide. Jugular venous oxygen tensions decreased less than the Pao_2. With prolonged 10% oxygen inhalation, maximal cerebral flow occurred in about 6 or 7 minutes. Time and

---

(2)   J. Clin. Invest. 49: 2362-2368, December, 1970.

$Paco_2$ were significant correlates of cerebral flow during 10% oxygen inhalation. When eucapnia was maintained, cerebral flow increased significantly after slight reductions in inspired oxygen concentration. Hyperventilation during 9.5% oxygen inhalation significantly decreased the $Paco_2$, with no material change in Po_2, compared with previous inhalation of 10.4% oxygen without added carbon dioxide. The cerebral flow-Pao_2 curve during eucapnic hypoxemia showed a steeper flow response with decreasing arterial oxygen tension than did the curve during graded hypoxemia without maintenance of normal arterial CO_2 levels.

Mild to moderate hypocapnia may blunt or abolish the vasodilatory stimulus of fairly severe hypoxia. The findings indicate the powerful cerebrovascular constrictor effects of modest reductions in carbon dioxide tension counterbalances the vasodilating influence of hypoxia represented by Pao_2 reductions to about 40 mm. Hg. The effects of hypoxia on control of the cerebral circulation must be analyzed in terms of the effects of any associated changes in carbon dioxide tension.

▶ [When we deliberately hyperventilate patients to hypocapnic levels, we must be especially careful that we maintain normal oxygen tensions. This will particularly apply to the patient with cerebrovascular disease.—Eds.]

Clinical Methods of Reducing Intracranial Pressure: Role of Cerebral Circulation. Henry A. Shenkin and William F. Bouzarth[3] (Episcopal Hosp., Philadelphia) review differing effects on cerebral blood flow produced by various methods of lowering intracranial pressure.

Since respiratory alkalosis reduces cerebral circulation, hyperventilation is an attractive way to control intracranial pressure in the operative approach to vascular brain lesions but not in the patient with impaired cerebral vasculature, due to the risk of causing total occlusion of a damaged vessel, leading to focal, irreversible cerebral ischemia. Cerebral hypoxia induced by hyperventilation seems relatively mild and reversible when maintained 60-90 minutes, but whether more prolonged respiratory alkalosis causes irreversible damage has not been fully explored. Gotoh *et al.* (1961) suggest that the intracellular pH of smooth muscle fibers of cerebral arteries regulates their size. Carbon dioxide diffuses freely through the endothelial membrane but hydrogen and bicarbonate ions (HCO_3) do not, so intravascular carbon dioxide and extravascular HCO_3 determine

(3) New England J. Med. 282:1465-1471, June 25, 1970.

the pH around and within the smooth muscle of vessels. In severely contused areas, the acidotic tissue and dilated vessels increase intracranial pressure by increasing blood volume. Observers have suggested that at some point of tissue acidosis, autoregulation is lost and vasoparalysis occurs. Hyperventilation could be a means of reducing tissue acidosis, maintaining vessel reactivity and lowering intracranial pressure with the possibility of better cerebral perfusion.

Hypertonic solutions of glucose, urea and mannitol effectively produce an osmotic gradient between brain water and plasma for quick reduction of the former. Osmotic agents also increase cerebral circulation by 21-47%, at least during infusion and shortly thereafter (Goluboff et al., 1964). Whereas use of these agents seems to be a poor way to control intracranial pressure in patients with vascular brain lesions, their use should be the method of choice for reducing such pressure in older people with impaired cerebral circulation. The present authors' recent treatment of 7 patients with acute cerebral infarction by rapid infusion (within 20 minutes) of 500 ml. of 20% mannitol solution gave encouraging results, presumably because over-all increase in cerebral blood flow improved collateral circulation and simultaneous hyperosmolar action reduced edema about the infarcted area.

Controlled hypotension during operation is expedited by use of ganglionic blocking agents. Brain relaxation, noted in the early application of this method (Mazzia et al., 1956), must result from a fall in transmural pressures since systemic hypotension is accompanied by increased size of the cerebrovascular bed (Finnerty et al., 1954) and, therefore, increased cerebral blood volume. Drake (1968) dissected and obliterated vertebral-basilar aneurysms at a systolic pressure of 40-45 mm. Hg; only 1 of 33 patients did not tolerate this procedure, although hypotension of over 1 hour was used in some. The present authors use a maximum of 20 minutes of hypotension at a systolic pressure of 60 mm. Hg and combine it only with spinal drainage to facilitate exposure. Hyperventilation should be used cautiously with hypotension, since both tend to reduce cerebral blood flow and the critical value for hypotension may occur at a higher level in the presence of respiratory alkalosis.

In 3 patients under hypothermia, Stone et al. (1956) found distinctly reduced cerebral blood flow when body temperature was 28-29 C., especially if shivering was prevented. Arterial blood pressure was well maintained, but cerebrovascular resistance rose despite a Pco_2 rise; a hematocrit, and presumably blood viscosity, increase accounted for at least some of the increased resistance. Adams *et al.* (1957) noted that cerebral blood flow at hypothermic levels did not drop if systemic blood pressure was maintained. The present authors' experience with 10 patients with acute, severe craniocerebral trauma, who had immediate hypothermia and subsequent arteriography, may be of interest in that 7 had subdural hemorrhages, a much higher proportion than in a similar group not treated with hypothermia. The present authors believe that maintenance of normothermia is the best policy in treating patients with intracranial injury.

Shenkin and Gutterman (1969) found that patients who had craniotomy for brain tumor and were treated with pharmacologic doses of dexamethasone had increased urinary output and excretion of sodium and chloride, which inhibited the usual expansion of the extracellular fluid space. This suggests that the beneficial effect of corticosteroids in reducing brain edema is through this dehydrating mechanism.

Christensen *et al.* (1967), directly measuring cerebral blood flow in normal adults, concluded that halothane was a cerebral vasodilator and also noted potentiation of this vasodilatation with hypotension or hypercapnia in patients with cerebrovascular disease. Wollman *et al.* (1965) confirmed Søndergård's observation (1961) that nitrous oxide had no effect on cerebral blood flow at normal arterial Pco_2, but cerebral oxygen uptake decreased 23%; when mean arterial Pco_2 was decreased to 18 mm. Hg, cerebral blood flow was halved, but the cerebral metabolic rate for oxygen did not change. Since properly given thiopental sodium has no effect on cerebrospinal fluid pressure or cerebral blood flow despite marked reduction in cerebral metabolism, it is useful for inducing general anesthesia and inserting the endotracheal tube. Anesthesia can be maintained by nitrous oxide and oxygen inhalation supplemented with intravenously given thiopental and *d*-tubocurarine without causing brain swelling.

► [The authors, neurosurgeons, favor nitrous oxide-thiopental-curare anesthesia for patients with elevated intracranial pressure. They do so on rather shaky grounds and don't even consider the merits of controlled vs. assisted respiration, tracheal analgesia to prevent coughing and other important facets of this choice of anesthesia. The authors misquote their own article (ref. 49) and say subdural hemorrhage occurred in 7 of 10 hypothermic patients, whereas their original article stated 10 of 14 patients. Nonethe-

less, this is a useful review article and offers a 60-reference bibliography.
—Eds.]

Influence of Anesthesia and of Arterial Hypocapnia on Regional Blood Flow in Normal Human Cerebral Hemisphere.
I. M. S. Wilkinson and Doreen R. G. Browne[4] (Nat'l Hosp. for Nervous Diseases, London) studied regional patterns of cerebral perfusion during the unconscious state produced by a specific anesthetic regime and the patterns present during anesthesia at low arterial CO_2 tensions. The patients studied were undergoing diagnostic arteriography for a suspected intracranial lesion. Arteriograms were normal, and there were no abnormal signs referable to the cerebral hemisphere. Six anesthetized patients were studied at a $Paco_2$ of 45 mm. Hg and 6 others at a level of about 30 mm. Hg. After premedication with droperidol and phenoperidine, sleep was induced with methohexitone, and suxamethonium was given for tracheal intubation. Tubocurarine was subsequently given for control of ventilation by a Beaver ventilator. Incremental doses of phenoperidine were given during the procedure. Regional cerebral flow was estimated using radioxenon injected into the internal carotid artery, 45-90 minutes after anesthetic induction.

Grey and white matter perfusion values in the normocapnic group were 77.3 and 20.8 ml./100 Gm./minute, respectively. Patients showed considerable variation in mean hemispheric values for perfusion of grey matter. The mean grey and white matter perfusion values in the hypocapnic group were 45.6 and 15.1 ml., significantly different from those in normacapnic patients. Normocapnic patients had temporary grey matter perfusion 14-21% below the mean hemispheric value. Frontoparietal perfusion was 14-17% higher than the mean value. Grey matter perfusion was relatively homogeneous in hypocapnic patients. White matter perfusion was relatively high in the internal capsule region in normocapnic patients, and low in the frontal region. Findings in hypocapnic patients were similar. Perfusion in the internal capsule region was 19-20% above that of the rest of the hemisphere in both groups of patients.

Grey matter perfusion is not homogeneous through the "normal" cerebral hemisphere in anesthetized patients, except under hypocapnic conditions. White matter perfusion is relatively great in the internal capsule region in both normocapnic and hypocapnic patients under anesthesia with nitrous oxide sup-

---

(4)   Brit. J. Anaesth. 42:472-482, June, 1970.

plemented by neuroleptanalgesia. Grey matter perfusion is insignificantly lower in anesthetized than in conscious patients. White matter perfusion is very similar in anesthetized and conscious patients.

▶ [Significant changes in cerebral blood flow could not be observed between conscious and anesthetized subjects and between white and gray matter. Hypocapnia did lower cerebral flow, more so in gray than in white matter.—Eds.]

PREOPERATIVE JUDGMENTS

Preoperative Laboratory Screening before Administration of General Anesthesia in Office. Roger A. Meyer[5] (Bellingham, Wash.) surveyed the results of routine blood and urine screening in healthy patients before general anesthesia was given them in the office. Patients requiring oral surgical procedures who were ASA class I or II risks were considered. A complete blood count and routine urinalysis were carried out. Study was made of 758 good-risk females and 591 males seen in 1968-69, all with normal histories and physical findings. Blood or urine abnormalities were found in 158 subjects (11.7%). Undiagnosed medical conditions that directly contraindicated general anesthesia in the office were found in 24 subjects (1.8%). Eleven of these had severe anemia, 10 had diabetes, 2 had leukemia and 1 had infectious mononucleosis.

The incidence of anemia in this series, with a hemoglobin below 12 Gm., was 6%. In 11 instances, the hemoglobin was less than 10 Gm. Two patients with severe anemia had occult bleeding peptic ulcers; the others had iron deficiency anemia. The incidence of previously undiagnosed diabetes mellitus was 0.7%. Pulmonary fibrosis was found in a patient employed in a fiber glass factory who had a highly elevated eosinophil count. Although they do not directly contraindicate general anesthesia, urinary tract infections are best treated in their asymptomatic early stages.

Routine screening of blood and urine is recommended as part of oral surgery practice in all patients scheduled for general anesthesia in the office.

▶ [Amen!!—Eds.]

Evaluation of Peridural Anesthesia in Outpatient Culdoscopy was done by Turhan S. Dogu and Jerry A. Dorsch[6]

(5) J. Oral Surg. 28:332-334, May, 1970.
(6) Am. J. Obst. & Gynec. 108:468-470, Oct. 1, 1970.

(Univ. of Pittsburgh) in 91 women, aged 20-41, seen in 1967-69. All patients but 1 were ASA status 1. Premedication was with a narcotic, belladonna, barbiturate, phenothiazine or a combination thereof; stable patients were not given premedication. Most blocks were done by anesthesia residents. Lumbar epidural block was performed in 66 cases; a continuous technic was used in 1 case. There were 23 single caudal injections and 1 continuous caudal injection.

Eighteen patients required supplemental analgesia. Two patients had a drop in blood pressure of 25% or more; 1 received a vasopressor. Dural puncture occurred in 2 cases, shivering in 3 and nausea in 1. One patient lost consciousness briefly. One rectal perforation occurred without further complication.

Nine of 80 patients questioned after several months reported having had undue discomfort during the procedure. Five had had supplementary analgesia inhalationally or intravenously. Fifteen patients (18.7%) reported having discomfort during administration of the block. Multiple attempts to enter the epidural space were necessary in 5 of these cases. Discomfort postoperatively was reported by 38.7% of the 80 patients; the commonest type was chest or shoulder pain. Most patients preferred epidural to general anesthesia.

The value of epidural anesthesia for culdoscopy has been demonstrated. Peridural anesthesia is readily accepted by patients. If an anesthesiologist sees the patient and performs the peridural block, a high success rate and a low incidence of complications may be expected.

► [Seems like a long run for a short slide!—Eds.]

Ventricular Function Following Acute Alcohol Administration: A Strain Gauge Analysis of Depressed Ventricular Dynamics. An examination of ventricular dynamics must consider the load the ventricle works against and the contractility or inotropic state of the ventricle. Walter H. Newman and Joseph F. Valicenti, Jr.[7] (Univ. of South Carolina) used strain gauge methods to continuously monitor changes in these parameters in 12 mongrel dogs anesthetized with pentobarbital and ventilated with air.

Walton-Brodie, isotonic and Hefner-type strain gauge arches were placed before 6 of the animals were given 25-minute infusions of alcohol, 2 Gm./kg., 40% in saline, and pentobarbital (30 mg./kg.). Six others were given two successive alcohol infu-

---

(7)   Am. Heart J. 81:61-68, January, 1971.

sions. When a steady state was reached, ouabain, 0.025 mg./kg., was injected by slow infusion, supplemented by doses of 0.005 mg./kg. until digitalization was evident.

Contractile force was depressed by alcohol infusion, and mural force was elevated; ventricular circumference was increased, as indicated by the change in muscle segment length. Aortic pressure was essentially unchanged. The parameters did not become normal in 1 hour. The mean blood alcohol level 5 minutes after the initial alcohol infusion was 273 mg./100 ml. Initial responses to pentobarbital infusion were similar, but aortic pressure fell near the end of the infusion, with shortening of the muscle segment and a reduction of the previously increasing mural force. Infusion of ouabain was followed by a return of all parameters toward control levels in all experiments. There was a highly significant correlation between measured mural force and the load on the ventricle as calculated from intraventricular pressures.

The ventricle depressed by alcohol or pentobarbital operates under an increased load. Compensation is through the limited Frank-Starling mechanism. Ouabain reversed the depression. The findings indicate the precarious state of ventricular function at moderate blood alcohol levels and may explain the lability of acutely intoxicated patients to hemodynamic stress. Further sudden stress, such as acute blood loss, might place cardiac function on the descending limb of the Starling curve. ► [This suggests that halothane should not be used on the acute alcoholic, or, if given and cardiovascular collapse ensues, ouabain might be of help.—Eds.]

Changes in Plasma and Extracellular Fluid Volumes in Patients with Essential Hypertension during Long-Term Treatment with Hydrochlorothiazide. It is not yet clear whether the antihypertensive effect of thiazides can be explained by a reduction in plasma and extracellular fluid volumes. During short-term treatment, the thiazides reduce fluid volumes of the body, whereas long-term effects have not been thoroughly studied. Arne Leth[8] (Copenhagen, Denmark) studied the effects of hydrochlorothiazide on plasma and extracellular fluid volumes during the long-term treatment of essential hypertension. Studies were done in 13 patients without signs of congestive heart failure or clinical edema. Previous treatment had been stopped at least a month before the study. Plasma volume was

(8)   Circulation 42:479-485, September, 1970.

measured with the use of Evans blue dye, and extracellular fluid volume with $^{82}Br^-$. The patients received 50-100 mg. hydrochlorothiazide daily, the mean dose being 86 mg., and measurements were repeated after 1, 2, 4 and 6 months of treatment. Six patients were dropped from the study after variable periods.

The results are shown in Figure 13. Average plasma volume was invariable reduced and significantly so after 1, 2 and 4 months. Extracellular fluid volume was also reduced, but the change was significant only after 1 and 2 months of treatment. Mean blood pressure was reduced significantly in all the patients, the average reduction being 13 mm. Hg at 1 month and 26 mm. Hg at 6 months. A definite correlation between reduction in pressure and that in plasma volume was apparent only after 2 months of treatmnt. Hemoglobin and hematocrit values both increased during treatment. The average rise in hemoglobin value was significant at 1 and 2 months, and that in hematocrit value at 2 months. Body weight decreased by an average of 1.2 kg. during treatment, but many patients had

Fig. 13.—The effect of hydrochlorothiazide on plasma volume after 1, 2, 4 and 6 months of treatment. The horizontal lines of the columns represent the average values and the whole column indicates 2 S.D. (Courtesy of Leth, A.: Circulation 42:479-485, September, 1970.)

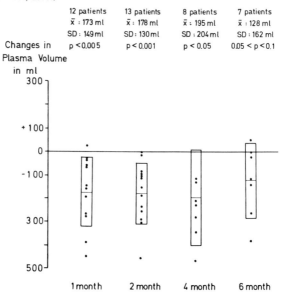

voluntarily reduced their weight. Weight loss was not related to the reduction in extracellular fluid volume.

Several facts support the view that thiazides exert a continued volume-depleting effect during long-term treatment. The volume depletion produced initially by thiazide therapy is maintained, although at a lower level. This is probably important in the long-term effect of thiazide therapy on blood pressure.

▶ [It is probably also important in our preoperative assessment of volemia in a patient receiving such drug therapy.—Eds.]

Studies of Anesthesia in Relation to Hypertension: I. Cardiovascular Responses of Treated and Untreated Patients. Opinion is divided as to whether it is necessary or wise to stop antihypertensive therapy before anesthesia. C. Prys-Roberts, R. Meloche and P. Foëx[9] (Univ. of Oxford), with the technical assistance of A. Ryder, studied the cardiovascular responses of hypertensive patients to anesthesia and operation.

Study was made of 7 elderly normotensive patients, 7 elderly hypertensive patients not on antihypertensive drug therapy and 15 patients, most of them elderly, treated with various antihypertensive agents. Nine treated hypertensive patients had full hemodynamic studies. Observations were made during steady-state anesthesia before and after operation and in the postoperative period. Anesthesia was induced with thiopentone and maintained with 1% halothane in 70% nitrous oxide-30% oxygen. Suxamethonium was given for relaxation.

Mean arterial pressures were significantly higher before anesthesia in both hypertensive groups than they were in the normotensive group. Five untreated and 3 treated hypertensive patients who had high arterial pressures before anesthesia had severe reductions in pressure, associated with ECG evidence of myocardial ischemia, during anesthesia. Other treated hypertensives, whose arterial pressures were well controlled, behaved similarly to normotensive patients during anesthesia. Cardiac output fell about 30% in all three groups. Reductions in arterial pressure were largely due to decrease in initially high systemic vascular resistance. Baroreflex control of the heart rate was significantly depressed in hypertensive patients both before and during anesthesia. No specific cardiovascular response could be related to any particular form of drug therapy.

(9) Brit. J. Anaesth. 43:122-137, February, 1971.

Untreated high arterial pressure constitutes a serious risk to patients undergoing anesthesia and operation. The withdrawal of antihypertensive therapy before anesthesia is potentially dangerous, and therapy should be considered for otherwise symptom-free patients before anesthesia and operation. Premedication of elderly patients is a matter for individual consideration. The lowest possible dose of thiopentone should be used to induce anesthesia, and other induction agents may be preferable. Further studies are needed on the effects of artificial ventilation on hypertensive patients. The ventilatory and circulatory depressant effects of halothane should be carefully weighed against the possible benefits of using this agent.

▶ [We've had a full swing of the pendulum on this one—from stop the drug well ahead of the anesthesia to keep the patient on the drug. But this article says, ". . . should not be withdrawn without a compelling reason." What could the reason be?—Eds.]

Lung Diffusing Capacity: Normal Values in Male Smokers and Nonsmokers Using Breath-Holding Technic. The influence of smoking on pulmonary diffusing capacity is still debated. Dan B. Teculescu and Dan C. Stănescu[1] (Bucharest) used the breath-holding technic with a mixture of 1.5% helium and 0.2% carbon monoxide in air to determine lung diffusing capacity in healthy smoking and nonsmoking men. About three fourths of the subjects were employees of a transport company, with average physical activity levels. Chest x-rays were normal and there were no respiratory complaints and no history of exposure to respiratory irritants. Vital capacity and forced expiratory volume were normal. The 42 smokers and 47 nonsmokers examined were aged 19-67. Only cigarette smokers were included; average consumption was 17.4 cigarettes daily for an average of 20.9 years. Mean number of pack-years smoked was 19.3.

Permeability of the alveolar membrane decreased with age and was lower in smokers than in nonsmokers at each age level. The difference of mean values for smokers and nonsmokers was highly significant. The predictability was slightly weaker for smokers. The intra-age group variability was greater in older subjects.

Prediction equations were developed for pulmonary diffusing capacity and "permeability" for smokers and nonsmokers. The accuracy of prediction of diffusing capacity compared favorably with that obtained in other studies. The effects of aging

---

(1) Scandinav. J. Resp. Dis. 51:137-149, 1970.

on lung permeability appear to differ in different persons. ▶ [And so the data accumulate.—Eds.]

Abnormal Distribution of Pulmonary Blood Flow in Aortic Valve Disease: Relation between Pulmonary Function and Chest Radiograph. Patients with aortic valve disease who complain of breathlessness cannot reduce their wasted ventilatory volume-tidal volume ratio normally on exertion. This abnormality, unrelated to a reduced tidal volume, suggests abnormal perfusion in some lung areas. Lucy S. Goodenday, George Simon, Hazel Craig and Lola Dalby[2] (Univ. of London) examined 17 patients with aortic valve disease of varying severity. Lung function was studied before and after aortic valve replacement in 3 patients. There was no evidence of noncardiac lung disease in these patients. Wasted ventilatory volume and tidal volume were determined at rest and on cycle exercise at a low work load. The wasted ventilatory volume-tidal volume ratio was considered abnormal if it did not decrease on exertion or if the exercising value was over 40%.

There was agreement between the chest radiographic and pulmonary function evidence of over-all maldistribution of pulmonary blood flow in 14 of 20 studies. One of the other patients had bilateral pleural effusions, and another had a borderline exercise ventilatory ratio. Even including these patients, agreement between the observations was significant.

The abnormal distribution of flow in patients with aortic valve disease is less simple than a mechanical model would imply. There are areas of patchy interstitial edema throughout the lung, which may have blood flow reduced proportionately more than ventilation. Some correlation was found in the present patients between an abnormally high ratio of wasted ventilatory volume to tidal volume on exertion and an abnormal diversion of blood from the lung bases to the upper lobes on chest radiographic examination. This suggests that such a mechanism of blood diversion is one cause of the abnormal ventilation-perfusion relations found in pulmonary venous hypertension.

Unusual Problems in Airway Management: II. Influence of Temporomandibular Joint, Mandible and Associated Structures on Endotracheal Intubation is discussed by Charles Block and Verne L. Brechner[3] (Univ. of California, Los Angeles). Anoma-

(2) Brit. Heart J. 32:406-408, May, 1970.
(3) Anesth. & Analg. 50:114-123, Jan.-Feb., 1971.

lies that arise in the temporomandibular joint, the mandible and associated structures may preclude successful tracheal intubation. Kowledge of such anomalies may forewarn the anesthesiologist of necessary precautions to be taken or modifications for proper placement of an endotracheal tube. All candidates for intubation should be carefully evaluated in terms of the functional integrity of the temporomandibular joint and the range of mandibular motion. The oral cavity should be examined for abnormalities of anatomy or dentition or other changes that may influence laryngoscopy or intubation.

In the Pierre Robin syndrome, the mandible is small and receded, and cleft palate and micrognathia are present. The tongue may be sutured to the lip or chin or a mechanical airway used. Lateral, downward placement of the face may also aid in maintaining airway patency. Tracheostomy is not favored. The mandible is usually hypoplastic in the Treacher Collins syndrome. In unilateral facial agenesis, there is macrostomia and failure of formation of the mandibular ramus and condyle. The mandible is shortened in progressive hemifacial atrophy, and secondary temporomandibular joint involvement is not uncommon. Mandibular hypoplasia may also occur in oculoauriculovertebral dysplasia, orodigitofacial dysostosis and progeria. The temporomandibular joint may be involved in rheumatoid arthritis and other polyarthritic conditions, as well as in degenerative joint disease. Regional infection may limit mandibular opening. Trismus may be a result of masticator space infections, practically always of dental origin. Blind nasotracheal intubation with the patient awake may be indicated in such cases. Laryngeal edema may occur in lateral pharyngeal space infections, and tracheostomy is indicated in this circumstance. A patent airway must be assured in cases of Ludwig's angina before general anesthesia is induced; tracheostomy is the simplest measure. Blind nasotracheal intubation is preferred in cases of temporomandibular joint ankylosis. The tongue may be involved by rhabdomyoma or carcinoma, or in reactive edema.

Nasotracheal intubation is popular in reducing and stabilizing mandibular fractures. Often an endotracheal tube is left in place for several hours after the surgical correction of deformities of the mandible. When the laryngoscopy is difficult, the head may be extended but the neck should be flexed.

► [The article has excellent pictures of the Pierre Robin and Treacher

Collins syndrome facies. Those who have anesthetized such patients know that intubation of the trachea can be impossible.—Eds.]

Paraplegia: Problems Confronting the Anesthesiologist are discussed by John Desmond[4] (Toronto Gen'l Hosp.). Information was gleaned from replies to questionnaires sent to 3,186 paraplegics in 1967-68, 2,253 of which were returned. The ratio of males to females was 4.5:1. Work and automobile accidents accounted for over half the injuries. In the paraplegic the part of the spinal cord distal to the lesion recovers after initial shock, and its reflex function becomes highly excitable. Reflexes largely lose their local response, reactions being massive rather than specific. Paroxysmal hypertension is followed by bradycardia. Heart block and ventricular ectopic beats can also result from vagal hyperactivity. Afferent impulses from the aortic arch and carotid sinus are relayed in the vasomotor center, resulting in vasodilation above and sweating and piloerection below the level of the lesion.

Patients tend to adjust well mentally to paraplegia. Burning pains of the trunk and legs are frequent. The patients tend to have a low pain threshold. Autonomic hyperreflexia develops in some but not all patients with injuries above the T7 level. Too little anesthesia evokes a hypertensive crisis and too much is not tolerated. The blood pressure often falls precipitously during anesthetic induction but then rises when operation is begun and must be lowered by deepening anesthesia or giving a ganglion-blocking agent. It is probably best to block the afferent visceral pathways, but spinal anesthesia carries risks in paraplegic patients. Oral hexamethonium has been suggested. The ECG must be monitored whenever general anesthesia is given. Artificial cough is produced by manual pressure on the abdomen in expiration. The danger of aspiration is always present. The anesthetist should check the genitourinary status carefully. Enemas are dangerous in paraplegics. Anemia is frequent and may require transfusions, since oral iron preparations lead to constipation. The quadriplegic is essentially poikilothermic below the site of the lesion. Pathologic fractures may result from even apparently normal movements. Pressure sores should be guarded against, especially in pregnancy. Premature labor is a great hazard. Toxemia would be expected to be common, but this has not been the case.

▶ [We are not sure the author's concern about using spinal anesthesia in these patients is justified.—Eds.]

(4) Canad. Anaesth. Soc. J. 17:435-451, September, 1970.

Neurologic Disorders Seen in the Uremic Patient are discussed by H. Richard Tyler[5] (Harvard Med. School). Patients in renal failure may exhibit a wide variety of signs and symptoms of nervous system dysfunction. Difficulty in concentration and failure to complete complex tasks are early signs of uremic encephalopathy. Some patients have a marked tendency to mental fatigue; there are often striking swings between states of confusion and mental lucidity. Stupor and coma eventually occur.

Hypertonus is often associated with decorticate postures. Restoration of electrolyte levels to normal does not always produce immediate clinical improvement. Myoclonus and asterixis may occur in uremic patients, with a lapse of electromyographic activity. Seizures are not common except when patients become acidotic and water intoxicated; they are usually generalized with tonic and clonic phases. A few patients have photosensitive seizures. The routine EEG is not of much practical use; it is not definitively related to any specific electrolyte change.

The pathogenesis of these encephalopathic syndromes has not been elucidated. Generally they are more related to the rate of ion changes than to the nature of the changes. There may be a membrane defect or defects in the sodium-potassium ion pump. No definite gross neuropathology has been described.

"Uremic amaurosis" is noted rarely. Hypertensive patients may have isolated cranial nerve lesions. Muscle weakness is fairly common; it is primarily proximal and limb muscle wasting is not unusual. Mildly decompensated uremic patients may have muscle cramps.

Hemodialysis may be associated with an intracranial bleeding tendency and other hemorrhagic complications. Patients may acquire fungous meningitis or brain abscess after transplantation and transplant patients have a high incidence of reticuloendothelial tumors. Chronic paralytic neuropathy may complicate long-standing renal failure.

Both burning-feet and restless-leg syndromes may be observed. Rarely polyneuritis is fulminant. Slowing of motor and sensory nerve conduction is common in uremic patients. Cerebrospinal fluid examination is usually noncontributory. Some patients given immunosuppressive and steroid therapy have an

(5)   Arch. Int. Med. 126:781-786, November, 1970.

increased incidence of cytomegalic inclusion body disease. Pontine myelinolysis has been noted in uremia.

▶ [This suggests that regional anesthesia might be unwise in these patients; on the other hand, uremic patients are often slow in regaining their preanesthetic state after general anesthesia.—Eds.]

Anesthesia for the Asthmatic Patient. Martin I. Gold[6] (Univ. of Maryland) points out that vital capacity is reduced during an asthmatic attack, and residual volume and frictional resistance increase, with a reduction in compliance. The Pao_2 gradually decreases and the dead space-tidal volume ratio increases. Oxygen uptake and CO_2 production increase, as does the cardiac output, probably in relation to increased work of breathing. Pulmonary arterial pressures increases, and the oxygen-diffusing capacity on exericse decreases. Regional abnormalities of pulmonary blood flow exist. Physiologic changes may occur even in asthmatics who are asymptomatic between attacks.

All asthmatics should have vital capacity estimated before operation. Severe asthmatics should have a trial of isoproterenol, with or without intermittent positive-pressure breathing. Psychotherapy is important in preparing such patients. Anemia and obesity should be corrected preoperatively. Pentobarbital is a good sedative for sleep the night before operation. An antihistamine may be useful. Steroids have been recommended for preventing respiratory complications during and after anesthesia. Oxybarbiturates are useful as induction agents. Halothane was the preferred general anesthetic in two large series. When bronchoconstriction occurs during anesthesia, an asthmatic attack must be distinguished from too light anesthesia. A higher oxygen concentration should be given, and positive-pressure ventilation may be helpful. Humidity should be increased in the recovery room. Pharyngeal and tracheal suction may be necessary at this point. Long-term mechanical ventilation should be considered only when the asthmatic fails to respond to other treatment and is working extremely hard without improvement or if the $Paco_2$ rises significantly above the control level. The essence of intermittent positive-pressure breathing therapy is correct timing. Blood gases must be monitored regardless of the flow rate or pressure used.

Tracheal intubation has the advantage of maintaining airway adequacy but the disadvantage of possibly initiating an attack

(6) Anesth. & Analg. 49:881-888, Nov.-Dec., 1970.

of bronchospasm in the asthmatic patient. The skill and experience of the anesthesiologist are more important than the agent or technic used.

▶ [We would agree that the skill and experience of the anesthesiologist are more important than the agent or technic used in anesthetizing the asthmatic.—Eds.]

ANESTHETIC TECHNICS

Diazepam and Local Analgesia for Lumbar Air Encephalography. Lumbar air encephalography can be very distressing when done under local analgesia, and general anesthesia may lead to hypotension in the sitting position. Narcotics, butyrophenone drugs and phenothiazine drugs all have serious potential disadvantages. J. C. Edwards and G. D. Flowerdew[7] (London, England) evaluated intravenous diazepam as an adjuvant to local analgesia for lumbar air encephalography. All patients who were not comatose and who were not children were considered for the study. Diazepam was given intravenously in a dose of 1 mg./7 kg. body weight as a 0.1% aqueous solution, and encephalography was begun 8 minutes later, after 3 minutes in the sitting position. The pulse and blood pressure were recorded every 5 minutes during the procedure and for 2 hours afterward. If the patients needed further sedation, diazepam was injected in increments of 0.5 mg./7 kg. of body weight. The goal was a drowsy, relaxed state. Study was made of 26 patients aged 16-70 years. Encephalography was completed with diazepam and local analgesia in 25 cases; 1 patient with a very scarred back required general anesthesia.

The mean duration of the procedure was 107 minutes, and the mean amount of air injected, 38.5 ml. The total dose of diazepam ranged from 9 to 54 mg. The mean period between increments was 22 minutes. Usually two or three increments sufficed for shorter studies. The total dose was related to the length of the procedure and to body weight. Three of the 4 patients who became disoriented and agitated during the procedure were demented. No significant pulse or blood pressure changes occurred. All patients had headache within 24 hours after the procedure, and 7 vomited during this period. Seventeen of 23 patients did not recall the procedure at all. Radiographers found the procedure more difficult than when pa-

(7) Brit. J. Anaesth. 42:999-1004, November, 1970.

tients were fully anesthetized, but the radiographs obtained were satisfactory.

Diazepam can be used as an adjuvant to local analgesia for lumbar air encephalography in adults. Severe dementia appears to be a contraindication to use of the technic.

▶ [Not a very enthusiastic report.—Eds.]

Anesthesia Suitable for Prolonged Bronchoscopic Examination. Topical anesthesia for bronchoscopy is unpleasant for most patients. A general anesthetic technic permitting a lengthy examination is required. E. C. Attwood, W. Brooks and W. J. H. Leckie[8] (Hereford, England) describe a technic of combined general and topical anesthesia permitting spontaneous ventilation that proved extremely satisfactory in over 200 clinical cases and did not cause serious complications.

Blood gases were measured in 19 patients having diagnostic bronchoscopy who had satisfactory peripheral circulation. Capillary blood was taken by finger prick from about the time the bronchoscope was introduced until the examination was completed. Anesthesia was induced with thiopentone 30 minutes after atropine, and gallamine was given, usually 60 mg. The larynx was sprayed with 4% lignocaine solution. The lungs of apneic patients were ventilated with oxygen through a Magill circuit, after which the respiratory tract was sprayed with local anesthetic. All patients then breathed 2-4% halothane in oxygen at a flow rate of 5 L. per minute. Recently, patients breathed oxygen through the side tube of the bronchoscope during the examination; incremental doses of thiopentone were not required. Neostigmine was given after atropine at the end of examination.

All subjects were satisfactorily anesthetized and, in all cases but 1, prolonged examination was possible. The mean time of bronchoscopy was 11.8 minutes. The mean resting Pao_2 was 62.2 mm. Hg. Two patients had a brief fall in Pao_2 to below 40 mm. Hg before oxygen was given during the examination. Subsequently only one value under 75 mm. Hg was obtained. Only 1 patient acquired serious hypoventilation, with the $Paco_2$ 135 mm. Hg and the Pao_2 40 mm. Hg. The $Paco_2$ tended to drop whether air or oxygen was breathed during bronchoscopy. The mean recovery time was 7 minutes and the range, $1\frac{1}{2}$-19 minutes.

This technic, involving spontaneous ventilation, proved satisfactory for bronchoscopy. Dangerous hypoxemia did not occur when oxygen was administered during the examination.

New and Simple Method for Ventilating Patients Undergoing Bronchoscopy. Technics of assisting or controlling ventilation in anesthetized patients for bronchoscopy have varied widely over the years. E. Carden, W. G. Trapp and J: Oulton[9] (Univ. of British Columbia) describe a method of ventilation that utilizes the bronchoscopic sidearm only for attachment. A length of high-pressure oxygen hose with a male bayonet connector is used, with an adjustable one-stage reducing valve, an ARO Corporation Blow Gun, and a length of soft rubber tubing. The bayonet connector is plugged into the hospital oxygen pipeline and the hose attached to the inlet of the valve. A further length of pressure hose connects the valve outlet to the input of the blow gun, the output of which is connected to the bronchoscopic sidearm with the rubber hose. Pressure is exerted intermittently on the blow gun button after the reducing valve is set.

Six patients premedicated with meperidine and atropine were studied. The reducing valve was adjusted to give a peak bronchoscope pressure of 45 cm. water. A sleep dose of thiopental was given, followed by succinylcholine and ventilation with oxygen by mask for introduction of the bronchoscope. Ventilation was continued by the sidearm alone. Additional thiopental was given as needed. Small variations in extent and duration of blow gun button depression occurred. A rate of about 15 cycles per minute was used. An airway pressure of 45 cm. water is very unlikely to occur in the lungs themselves. Flow rates were adequate, and delivered oxygen concentrations were never below 98%. The button was depressed just enough to give the desired flow rate as judged by observing chest expansion. Study of CO_2 levels indicated adequate ventilation; oxygen levels were always above 250 mm. Hg. The endoscopists had no complaints and were impressed by the clear field of vision and the freedom from misting of the lenses due to dry gas flow.

▶ [This requires great cooperation between surgeon and anesthesiologist.—Eds.]

Intravenous Lidocaine: Adjunct to General Anesthesia for Endoscopy. Louis S. Blancato, Alfred T. C. Peng and Delia Alonsabe[1] (St. Luke's Hosp. Center, New York) have used

(9) Anesthesiology 33: 454-458, October, 1970.
(1) New York J. Med. 70: 1659-1660, June 15, 1970.

intravenous and topical lidocaine as a supplement to general anesthesia in 214 procedures performed on 210 patients since 1966. Review was also made of 156 endoscopies performed under conventional apneic or recovery anesthesia. The 136 male and 74 female study patients were aged 3-85 years. Premedication was with atropine and meperidine. Thiopental or halothane was used for induction, and anesthesia was maintained with 1-2% halothane with oxygen in a semiclosed system. Patients were given lidocaine, 4-4.6 mg./kg., intravenously in 3 minutes, 5 minutes after induction. The larynx and trachea were sprayed with 2% lidocaine before the bronchoscope was inserted. Halothane-oxygen was insufflated via the sidearm of the bronchoscope or via a nasal catheter when a laryngoscope was used. Increments of 25% of the initial lidocaine dose were given at 5-10 minute intervals as needed. The maximal dose given was less than 600 mg. Anesthesia lasted 20-57 minutes and endoscopy, 2-30 minutes. Respiration was spontaneous throughout the procedure.

Anesthetic results were good in 79.9% of cases, fair in 15.9% and poor in 4.2%. In the control group, results were good in 28.8% of cases, fair in 34% and poor in 37.2%. Fewer than 20% of older study patients developed hypotension and momentary apnea. Two patients developed laryngospasm. Recovery in the lidocaine group was remarkably uneventful; straining, buckling and paroxysmal coughing with cyanosis were not observed.

Good anesthesia was obtained in a large majority of patients having endoscopy using lidocaine in this series. There was no serious morbidity, and no deaths occurred. The patient breathes spontaneously throughout the procedure, and the surgeon is not hurried. The vital signs are stable. The recovery period is quiet.

▶ [Six hundred milligrams of lidocaine, plus meperidine, plus atropine, plus thiopental, plus halothane add up to a good deal of myocardial depression.—Eds.]

Mediastinoscopy. J. Keith Ross, John R. Mikhail, R. A. B. Drury, R. D. Levis and D. N. Mitchell[2] (London) report the findings at mediastinoscopy in 124 patients. General anesthesia was induced with thiopentone and suxamethonium. A spray of 4% lignocaine was topically applied to the vocal cords and trachea, and a 2% water-soluble lignocaine gel was applied to

(2) Thorax 25:312-316, May, 1970.

the oral cuffed tube or bronchoscope. Anesthesia was maintained with 0.5-1% halothane, nitrous oxide and oxygen; a semi-open circuit was used. Gallamine was used as a relaxant. The paratracheal lymph nodes were located using a laryngoscope inserted into a suprasternal incision. Bronchial biopsy forceps were used to biopsy the nodes. Mobile nodes were sometimes removed whole. Serious bleeding never occurred. Drainage was not used.

The right pleura was entered in two examinations; neither patient had pneumothorax postoperatively. The final diagnosis was sarcoidosis in 102 cases. A lymph node was found in 93 of these, and 86 showed histologic changes compatible with sarcoidosis; tissue other than lymph node tissue was obtained in 8 cases. One patient with a pulsatile swelling did not undergo biopsy. Fifteen patients were found to have tuberculous infection causing mediastinal lymph node enlargement. Seven others had malignant disease.

Mediastinal node biopsy is valuable for investigating chest lesions of undetermined cause.

▶ [A "minor" surgical procedure with "major" potential for complications.—Eds.]

Simultaneous Evaluation of Cardiorespiratory and Analgesic Effects of Intravenous Analgesia in Combination with Local Anesthesia. Gaither B. Everett and Gerald D. Allen[3] (Univ. of Washington) attempted to establish intravenous analgesia for dentistry on a sound physiologic basis by controlled studies of cardiovascular and respiratory response and correlation of analgesia levels with the physiologic status of the patient as required.

METHOD.—Nine men, aged 21-38 years, without disease were unpremedicated and seated in a dental chair. After control measurements were made, 30 mg. alphaprodine, 25 mg. hydroxyzine and 0.4 mg. scopolamine were injected intravenously in 2-3 minutes. Measurements were made at 5 and 15 minutes. Immediately thereafter, 10 mg. methohexital was given intravenously and followed within 3 minutes by unilateral mandibular nerve block with 2% lidocaine with 1:100,000 epinephrine. Measurements were again made at 5 and 15 minutes and 10 mg. methohexital was again given intravenously.

Mean arterial pressure declined steadily throughout the study period, with significant depression 5 minutes after each dose of methohexital. Central venous pressure did not change significantly. Cardiac output rose significantly five minutes af-

(3) J.A.D.A. 81:926-931, October, 1970.

ter injection of the drug combination, but fell after the second methohexital injection to about 21% below control level at 45 minutes. Total peripheral resistance dropped significantly until after the second methohexital injection, when a rapid rise occurred. Heart rate rose after the drug combination and then fell progressively, reaching 30% below control level at 45 minutes. Stroke volume and stroke work rose significantly after the block. The Pao_2 was significantly decreased 5 minutes after the drug combination, but then rose to near control values; and $Paco_2$ rose significantly and remained elevated. Most subjects had no memory of the procedures 5 minutes after the block.

Cardiovascular depression might have been less profound in these studies had atropine been used. Intravenous analgesia can relieve the patient's anxiety, but physiologic parameters are altered significantly. The technic is not innocuous. Minimal physiologic disturbance is assured only when regional anesthesia is complete and intravenous drugs are used only to alleviate apprehension.

▶ [Presumably this technic is intended for outpatients. If so, alphaprodine, hydroxyzine, scopolamine, methohexital and 2% lidocaine is a hazardous combination.—Eds.]

Cardiovascular Changes during Dental Anesthesia and Sedation. W. Ryder[4] (Newcastle upon Tyne, England) studied the effects of intravenous anesthetic technics, now widely used in dentistry, on the physiology of healthy dental outpatients. Three groups of patients were studied: group I—114 patients having extractions with intermittent intravenous methohexitone; group II—patients having conservative dental procedures with intermittent intravenous methohexitone (abandoned after 12 sessions as potentially too dangerous); and group III—20 patients having conservative dentistry or periodontal operations with a single injection of diazepam and local analgesia, who were monitored on 51 occasions. All patients had functionally normal cardiovascular systems. Sedative levels of consciousness were maintained for conservative operations with methohexitone. The ECG was monitored continuously in all patients. Blood pressure was monitored in most patients given methohexitone for conservative procedures and in all those given diazepam.

In group I, the age range was 2-60 years, with 65% of the patients under age 12. In group III the age range was 11-46

(4) D. Pract. 21:89-93, November, 1970.

years. In group I, the initial dose was 1-1.5 mg./kg., with increments of one third to one quarter of this; the dose range was 30-220 mg. In group II, the mean dose was 484 mg. In group III, dose range was 7.5-25 mg., the mean dose being 17 mg.

Mean duration of anesthesia was $3\frac{1}{2}$ minutes in group I, 67 minutes in group II and 43 minutes in group III. Most group I and group II patients had transient slight falls in blood pressure on induction, followed by rises of 25-76 mm. Hg. Only 5 group III patients had a rise in pressure; the mean fall in 46 instances was 35 mm. Hg. The heart rhythm was regular in all instances. Pulse rates rose significantly in groups I and II but generally fell in group III patients. Large falls in pulse tended to be from initially high levels.

Indications must be carefully considered in deciding whether to use anesthesia or sedation in dentistry. The various technics should be used only to make the impossible possible, not the possible easy.

▶ [There is choice anesthetic philosophy here!—Eds.]

Superior Laryngeal Nerve Block is described by E. H. Shultz, F. K. Chin and J. D. Williams[5] (Torrance, Calif.). Superior laryngeal nerve block is extremely helpful in performing laryngography, transglottic bronchography, laryngoscopy, bronchoscopy and esophagoscopy. The technic is effective and is easy to administer, and patient discomfort is mild. Less time is needed for the examination.

A no. 22 needle is placed 1 cm. anterior to the superior cornu of the thyroid cartilage and advanced to the thyrohyoid membrane, where about 2-3 ml. of 1 or 2% lidocaine is introduced after aspiration. The procedure is repeated on the other side. The technic blocks the internal branch of the superior laryngeal nerve as it pierces the thyrohyoid membrane. This nerve supplies sensory fibers to the endolarynx, aryepiglottic folds and the posterior epiglottic surface, as well as the parasympathetic secretomotor fibers. The anesthetic takes effect in 5 minutes. The injection of 2-4 ml. transtracheally through the cricothyroid membrane or between any two proximal tracheal rings also provides subglottic anesthesia, further guarding against irritation when contrast material or a tube reaches this region.

No complications occurred in over 500 superior laryngeal blocks administered during 3 years. Distortion of the superior

(5) Radiology 97:94, October, 1970.

piriform sinus from accidental submucosal injection was not observed.

▶ [Five hundred successful cases is impressive.—Eds.]

Safe Management of Child with Contracted Neck: New Method. Many children with thermal injuries are left with severely contracted necks and may be troubled by daily airway obstruction. Aggravation with anesthesia may result in a crisis in such children. Roy D. Wilson, Christa Knapp, D. L. Traber and Barbara Evans[6] (Galveston, Tex.) reviewed 38 burn patients seen in 21 months with moderate to severe neck contraction. The mean age was 7.5 years, and the range, 21 months to 15 years. Ten patients were operated on in the acute phase of burn injury. Eighteen children had anesthesia induced with 1% methohexital, 0.75 mg./kg., after premedication with scopolamine and hydroxyzine, and were then given halothane in a closed system by face mask, followed by a laryngeal spray of 2-4% lidocaine and, in 1-2 minutes, nasotracheal intubation of the larynx. Five patients received ketamine, 8 mg./kg., after scopolamine. Fifteen others received ketamine followed by closed-system anesthesia with tracheal intubation using combined ketamine-halothane anesthesia. Two patients received nitrous oxide-oxygen following tracheal intubation, with repeated doses of ketamine.

One patient in the methohexital-halothane group became seriously obstructed on three occasions. Laryngeal difficulties did not occur in the ketamine-halothane group, even in patients with the most severely contracted necks. No problems occurred with ketamine alone, but, with this technic, the airway is not accessible to the anesthesiologist, and carbon dioxide is retained under the drapes placed over the airway. Two patients with a history of difficult tracheostomies were managed in this way, however, with good results.

Management of the contracted neck is made much easier by ketamine. Various problems of airway obstruction may be managed with facility by using this agent.

▶ [But don't count on ketamine being trouble free when you are not there anticipating trouble.—Eds.]

Roentgenographic Analysis of Positions of Catheters in the Epidural Space. In epidural anesthesia it is desirable to place the catheter tip opposite a predetermined segment, so that the

---

(6) South. M. J. 63:1420-1425, December, 1970.

zone of blockade can be restricted to a minimum; the catheter should be inserted at the nearest possible spinal level. Manno-suke Muneyuki, Kimei Shirai and Akira Inamoto[7] (Kyoto Univ.) determined how far catheter tips were threaded into the lumbar or thoracic epidural space in 151 patients scheduled for abdominal operations. Most were adults in good condition aged 20-60 years. Epidural puncture was done with the patient in the lateral flexed position, using a modified Tuohy needle with a Huber point and the loss-of-resistance test. A median approach was generally used, but a paramedian approach was taken in the thoracic region when necessary. The catheter was not advanced further when excessive force was felt to be re-quired. Soft polyethylene catheters 0.50 and 0.91 mm. in in-ternal diameters and hard polyvinyl catheters of similar diam-eters were used to enter the lumbar epidural space in 100 pa-tients. Polyethylene catheters were used to enter the thoracic epidural space. X-rays were obtained after 0.2 ml. Myodil was injected through the catheter.

The catheter was kinked or curled in 35% of patients having a soft 0.50-mm. catheter placed, in 75% of those having a soft 0.91-mm. catheter placed and in 56% of those having a hard catheter placed in the lumbar epidural space. In the thoracic group, catheters were curled in 31% of cases. Only the differ-ence between the two sizes of soft lumbar catheter was signifi-cant. The probability that the catheter tip was located three segments beyond the intervertebral space of insertion was about 50% in the thoracic group and only about 0.5% in the lumbar group. There were significant differences between the two regions for both length of catheter directly inserted and distance of the catheter tip from the puncture site.

The cause of the differences found in this study between thoracic and lumbar epidural catheterization is unclear, but they may be due to different angles of insertion of the needle. In the thoracic region the catheter is thrust through the needle parallel to the epidural canal; in the lumbar region it impinges on the dura or other structures at a right angle, with little chance of passing further cephalad.

▶ [It is surprising that the smallest catheter curled the least. The lesson is apparent—advance the catheter no more than 2-3 cm. beyond the needle tip.—Eds.]

Simultaneous Systemic and Hepatic Hemodynamic Measure-ments during High Spinal Anesthesia in Normal Man. William

(7) Anesthesiology 33:19-24, July, 1970.

F. Kennedy, Jr., Gaither B. Everett, Leonard A. Cobb and Gerald D. Allen[8] (Univ. of Washington) studied the simultaneous systemic hemodynamic and hepatic blood flow changes occurring with high spinal anesthesia in 10 males, aged 20-35 years, without cardiovascular or liver disease. Subjects fasted for at least 12 hours and received no premedication. Hepatic volume was measured with albumin-[131]I. A spinal anesthetic to the T5 sensory level was produced with 42-49 mg. of 5% lidocaine in 7.5% dextrose. Measurements were repeated when the sensory level was stable and then at 30-minute intervals until cutaneous analgesia disappeared.

The mean arterial pressure and total peripheral resistance decreased by a maximum of 17%. Cardiac output and heart rate rose a little initially, then fell below control levels. Stroke volume and central venous pressure fell slightly, then rose to just above control levels. The Pao_2 was reduced throughout anesthesia but not significantly. Estimated hepatic plasma flow dropped a maximum of 22% at 30 minutes and then gradually returned to control level. The hematocrit did not change significantly. Splanchnic vascular resistance rose for the 1st hour, then fell to just below control level at the end of anesthesia. The extraction ratio remained at 71% for 30 minutes, then fell significantly. At 90 minutes, when anesthetic effects had disappeared, the ratio was 24% below control level.

The systemic cardiovascular effects of high spinal anesthesia were similar to those noted previously. The decrease in extraction ratio in the latter part of anesthesia might have been due to dye saturation of the Kupffer cells or endothelial cells in the hepatic sinusoids. The reduction in hepatic blood flow was associated with a significant reduction in arterial pressure, but unmeasured factors may have contributed to the flow reduction. Splanchnic vascular resistance and cardiac output were not significantly altered during high spinal anesthesia.

Caudal Anesthesia in Children and Spread of 1% Lignocaine: A Statistical Study is reported by O. Schulte-Steinberg (Starnberg, Germany) and V. W. Rahlfs[9] (Munich, Germany). A combination of light general anesthesia and regional blockade is useful in small children and infants, but the dose of local analgesic must be guarded closely. Study was made of 52 children, aged 7-598 weeks, who were to have lower abdominal or geni-

(8) Anesth. & Analg. 49:1016-1024, Nov.-Dec., 1970.
(9) Brit. J. Anaesth. 42:1093-1099, December, 1970.

tourinary operations. Anesthesia was induced with nitrous ox-
ide-oxygen-halothane in a partial rebreathing system. The sacral epidural space was then injected with 1% lignocaine with
1:100,000 epinephrine in a dose of 0.1 ml. per dermatome to be
blocked per year of age. The dose never exceeded 6 mg./kg.
The injection was made at a rate of about 1 ml. per second. The
halothane concentration was reduced from 1.5 to 1 or 0.5%
about 10 minutes later and then maintained at a level just sufficient to prevent movement. Much lower concentrations were
required than for unblocked patients.

On multiple regression analysis of the relation of dose requirements to age, weight and height, the highest correlation
was found with age, followed by weight and then height, but
the relation to height was still highly significant. Age alone
was sufficient for establishing an optimal model for prediction.
Dose requirements increased linearly with age. A regression
equation could be used to determine dose requirements in clinical practice. This method permits a more precise estimate of
dose requirements for infants and young children than was
previously available.

▶ [As a study of the spread of lidocaine in the epidural space, this is interesting. As a technic for surgical procedures in children it seems cumber-
some.—Eds.]

**Review of Complications of Spinal Anesthesia with Experi-
ences in Canadian Teaching Hospitals from 1959 to 1969** is reported by A. B. Noble and J. G. Murray[1] (Univ. of Toronto).
Modern methods of controlling spinal anesthesia are effective,
and serious complications will not occur in experienced hands.
The most common cause of total spinal anesthesia today is
probably the inadvertent intraspinal injection of a large volume
of local anesthetic solution during attempted epidural anesthesia. A survey of 27 Canadian university-affiliated hospitals revealed a total of 78,746 spinal anesthetics given in the past 10
years. No deaths were attributable to spinal anesthesia in this
series. Anesthesia contributed to cardiac arrest in three instances. There were no serious permanent complications. There
were 2 cases of neuropathy affecting lumbar segments, and 1
of abducens paralysis; all these patients recovered within 3
months. Anesthetists appeared to be becoming more selective
in using spinal anesthesia; in most cases, it is now used for procedures below the umbilicus.

(1)   Canad. Anaesth. Soc. J. 18:5-17, January, 1971.

The most important morbid effect of spinal anesthesia is postspinal headache, due to altered cerebrospinal fluid dynamics. Control or avoidance of leakage through the dura has markedly reduced the incidence of this complication. One effective method is to inject a small amount of blood into the epidural space to plug the dural hole. Spinal anesthesia is a rare cause of disk injury. The most important serious complication is chronic adhesive arachnoiditis. The cauda equina region is involved most often. Aseptic meningitis is a result of reversible meningeal irritation. Utmost care is necessary in sterilizing needles and syringes. Septic meningitis is a rare and preventable complication. Conditions that may simulate complications of spinal anesthesia include unrelated neurologic manifestations, hysterical paralysis and porphyria. Electromyography is an important differential measure. In a true complication of spinal anesthesia, denervation will not be noted until 3 weeks after anesthesia, and fibrillatory potentials will be restricted to the paraspinal muscles, pelvic girdle and muscles of the lower extremities.

The mortality and morbidity rates from spinal anesthesia have been definitely reduced to the point where the hazards are no greater than with any other anesthetic technic.

▶ [As the authors imply, there are many situations where spinal anesthesia is the technic of choice.—Eds.]

Plasma Levels of Cortisol in Man during Spinal Anesthesia and Surgery. Spinal anesthesia has been considered not to be usually associated with significant increases in plasma cortisol levels. Tsutomu Oyama and A. Matsuki[2] (Hirosaki Univ.) studied the effect of spinal anesthesia on plasma cortisol in 40 surgical patients. All 47 patients, aged 16-62 years, studied had operations except the 7 who served as controls. Blood loss over 500 ml. was replaced by transfusion. No patient was premedicated. Hyperbaric spinal anesthesia was performed with spinal puncture at L3-4 or L4-5, using 200 mg. of a short-acting anesthetic, quatacain (Tanacaine), diluted to 3% in 10% glucose in 20 patients and 3% lidocaine in the 20 others. The average doses of quatacain and lidocaine were each 2.6 ml., and mean durations of anesthesia were 113 and 114 minutes, respectively. Respective mean analgesic levels were T7 and T8. Plasma free cortisol was determined by spectrofluorometry 10 minutes af-

(2) Canad. Anaesth. Soc. J. 17:234-241, May, 1970.

ter the start of anesthesia, 15 minutes after the incision and $3\frac{1}{2}$ hours after the start of spinal anesthesia.

Controls had a mean initial plasma cortisol level of 8.9 μg./ 100 ml., rising to a peak of 9.4 μg./100 ml. 30 minutes later. The quatacain group had a significant rise to 17.9 μg./100 ml. at 15 minutes; the level $3\frac{1}{2}$ hours after the start of spinal anesthesia was 16.3. The lidocaine patients had a significant rise in plasma cortisol to 18.5 μg./100 ml. 15 minutes after the incision.

Study patients had relatively high cortisol levels just before spinal anesthesia, attributed to emotional stress in the absence of preanesthetic medication. Spinal anesthesia alone had no significant effect on cortisol levels, but the levels rose significantly when operation was begun. Most of the patients had minor operations. Spinal anesthesia, even to an adequate level, does not appear necessarily to block adrenocortical activity. It is therefore not always the technic of choice for patients with hyperadrenocortical function.

▶ [There should be more correlation between operation performed, level of anesthesia, comfort of patient during operation and preoperative condition.—Eds.]

Adrenal Function during Long-Term Anesthesia in Man was studied by Klaus von Werder, Wendell C. Stevens, Thomas H. Cromwell, Edmond I. Eger, II, Satoshi Hane and Peter H. Forsham[3] (Univ. of California). Of 12 healthy unmedicated men, aged 21-30, 5 had anesthesia induced with 40-80% nitrous oxide and then were given halothane; their tracheas were intubated without relaxants. Blood glucose levels were kept constant by slow infusion of 5% glucose. The alveolar halothane level was adjusted to 0.5% in 70% nitrous oxide, and the concentration was raised to 1 and then 1.5% at 15-minute intervals. Concentrations were again varied after $3\frac{1}{2}$ hours of maintenance on 1% alveolar halothane. Nitrous oxide was omitted in 7 subjects given 1 or 1.6% halothane; these subjects were challenged with increasing CO_2 concentrations before and during anesthesia. One received 1 mg., and 1, 4 mg. hydrocortisone succinate per hour of anesthesia.

The first 5 subjects had a rise in plasma 11-hydroxycorticosteroids (11-OHCS) proportional to the length and degree of the excitement stage of anesthesia. The mean rise was 25.7 μg./ 100 ml. A rise to a peak of 32.9 μg. occurred 4-5$\frac{1}{2}$ hours after the start of anesthesia; this was not correlated with changes in

(3)   Proc. Soc. Exper. Biol. & Med. 135:854-858, December, 1970.

halothane concentration. No significant excitement occurred in the group given halothane alone and there was no rise in plasma 11-OHCS; instead, a drop to 3.1 μg./100 ml. occurred. There was a rise to a peak of 30.8 μg. after 2-4½ hours of anesthesia. Challenge with CO_2 did not increase the plasma 11-OHCS level in the waking state or during anesthesia. No fall in plasma 11-OHCS occurred in the subject given 4 mg. hydrocortisone succinate, but a late rise occurred.

Short-term general anesthesia with nitrous oxide-halothane may increase blood cortisol levels significantly before the start of operation in unmedicated patients. The rise is proportional to the duration of the excitement phase during anesthetic induction. Induction in itself does not activate the hypothalamic-pituitary-adrenal axis. The cause of the late rise in plasma 11-OHCS noted during long-term anesthesia is not clear. The early suppression of the axis with inhibition of corticotropin secretion can be overcome by the stress of operation. Catecholamine secretion is not altered by halothane anesthesia.

ANESTHETIC EQUIPMENT

Isocapnic Ventilation during Surgical Operations: Description of Equipment and First Results is presented by Michael Keeri-Szanto[4] (Univ. of Western Ontario). Precise respiratory homeostasis during anesthesia is preferable to reliance on the recuperative powers of the patient or on well-intentioned overcompensation. Thorough mixing of the contents of the entire ventilation system, with "hyperventilation" of the patient, eliminates CO_2 gradients within the system but does not alter the escape concentration at which equilibrium is attained.

A pedestal Boyle anesthesia machine was modified by replacing the soda lime canisters, directional valves and double breathing tubes with a Bird Mark II respirator with its supermuffler, double-walled breathing bag and automatic overflow valve. The valve was placed at the mouth of the patient. A large aneroid manometer was also supplied. For induction, patients were ventilated by manual compression of the bag. Gas flow was then reduced and the escape valve was opened so that the inflowing and escaping gas volumes balanced. The flow of nitrous

(4)   Anesth. & Analg. 49:406-412, May-June, 1970.

oxide-oxygen fresh gas was $3 + 1.5$ L. per minute. If needed, the compliance of the patient was adapted or respirator settings were altered during operation. Fresh gas flow was reduced to $1 + 1$ L. per minute at the end of operation with resetting of the overflow valve. The apparatus may be used, though less efficiently, for anesthesia under mask or for endotracheal anesthesia with spontaneous respirations.

This technic has been used in over a thousand major operations, including neurosurgical procedures and open chest operations. Arterial expired gas analyses showed a relatively small CO_2 gradient. The technic has the advantages of compact, inexpensive equipment, independent regulation of oxygenation and CO_2 blowoff, and increased precision in maintaining a given level of anesthesia by eliminating the complicating factor of changing CO_2 homeostasis. Independent regulation of oxygen homeostasis, as with isocapnic ventilaton, would greatly simplify prolonged artificial ventilation. However, the apparatus must have safety features added before it can be used where supervision is not as close as that in the operating room.

▶ [It would be great to get rid of double breathing tubes, carbon dioxide absorbing canisters and valves. An article worth reading.—Eds.]

Intermittently Closed Anesthesia Circuit. In controlled respiration the semiclosed anesthetic circuit counters the aim of lung inflation, some gas being vented through the valve on compression of the bag. There is no precise way of adjusting the valve. Henning Ruben[5] (Finsen Inst., Copenhagen) describes a circuit providing better control of respiratory minute volume, with less untoward effect on pressure conditions within the chest. The circuit, an intermittently closed one, can be improvised from generally available components. It is closed during inflation and open to the atmosphere during expiration. An intermitter incorporating a small bellows is included in the system to force the pop-off valve into a closed position with each bag compression. There is also a check valve to minimize initial air loss through the pop-off valve. There is a magnet in the intermitter to counteract blocking of the valve from a high fresh-gas flow; a flow exceeding 10 L. per minute can be used without unintended blocking. A button is provided to deblock the valve should it be blocked by improper handling of the bag.

This circuit has been used for over 2 years for major and minor operations. Insufflated respiratory volume is defined by

---

(5)   Acta anaesth. scandinav. 14:71-75, 1970.

compression of the bag. Changes in air resistance and lung-chest compliance can be evaluated from the feeling of the bag during compression. Resistance in the expiratory valve can be set at a minimum, with a resultant reduced influence on mean intrathoracic pressure. The intermitter can be used to convert a standard anesthetic circuit to an intermittently closed circuit.

▶ [We were about to order one until we again tried the "Georgia Valve," available in the United States, and thought it totally acceptable.—Eds.]

New Concept for Continuous Monitoring of Anesthetic Gases: II. Halothane—Comparison of Various Vaporizers' Outputs. Recently a new anesthetic gas analyzer was introduced, using the property of the dielectric constant of the gas being measured. M. Bluth, E. J. Gelb and S. N. Steen[6] (Jamaica, N. Y.) compared the accuracy and reproducibility of the analyzer, the Model H-10, with the performance of an analyzer in common use over a wide range of halothane concentrations. Both analyzers were calibrated for halothane, using a cylinder containing 5.3% v/v halothane in 52.5% nitrous oxide and 42.2% oxygen. The analyzers were then exposed to 10.5% halothane in 48.3% nitrous oxide and 41.2% oxygen and to 2.0% halothane in 45% nitrous oxide and 53.0% oxygen. Outputs of a Fluomatic vaporizer and a Fluotec Mark II vaporizer were monitored, at a total flow of 3 L. per minute. The Fluotec was also monitored at flows of 6 and 8 L. per minute. Output concentrations of 0.5, 1.0 and 2.0% were then delivered at total flows of 0.5-13.0 L. per minute. Output of a Vernitrol vaporizer was monitored at total flows of 4 and 6 L. per minute, using an equiproportional mixture of nitrous oxide and nitrogen.

Results with the LB-1 analyzer were not linear at the higher halothane concentrations, whereas those with the H-10 were linear to 10.5%. Fluotec readings were acceptable at flows of 6 and 8 L. per minute but higher than anticipated at over 2% at 3 L. per minute. The Fluomatic readings exceeded acceptable values. When total flows varied at constant vaporizer dial settings, small concentrations at low flows differed markedly from the dial settings on the Fluotec. The Fluotec is not recommended for use under such conditions; however, the Fluomatic can be used. The Vernitrol studies with halothane showed this new analyzer to be reliable.

Periodic checks of vaporizers in service are essential. All vaporizers must be calibrated before they are used.

---

(6) Anesthesiology 33:449-451, October, 1970.

Oxygen Fail-Safe Device for Anesthetic Apparatus is described by M. Rosen and E. K. Hillard[7] (Cardiff, Wales). Anoxia ensues if failure of the oxygen supply to an anesthetic apparatus is not noted immediately. Most available warning devices give only a visual or audible signal and rely on a second gas supply and/or batteries for their operation. A complete fail-safe system is operated by the oxygen supply alone. It stops all vapors from the anesthetic apparatus and opens the breathing circuit to the atmosphere. Warning of impending supply failure is given, with a further warning when failure occurs. It is not possible to administer an anesthetic unless the oxygen supply is restored after a failure. A device fulfilling these requirements has now been developed.

The device consists of two valves connected to the reduced pressure oxygen supply. The first valve begins to close when the oxygen pressure falls to 40 lb./sq. in., and a whistle sounds until the pressure falls to about 10 lb. Gas is cut off at an oxygen pressure of about 20 lb., and the one-way air inlet valve is released. The warning time is about $1\frac{1}{2}$ minutes with an oxygen flow of 5 L. per minute. In the air inlet, there is another whistle, with a different pitch, which sounds as air is drawn into the circuit. This signifies that the oxygen has failed or, when starting to anesthetize, that the oxygen supply has not been connected. The second valve, incorporated in a bag mount on the outlet of the anesthetic apparatus, prevents rebreathing after the safety valve has been activated. When a T-piece circuit is used, the patient rebreathes through the open path of the T-piece after the oxygen fails, and the whistle in the air inlet of the first valve does not sound. An automatic ventilator can be connected in place of the reservoir bag on the bag mount. The valves require no special servicing, and their action can be easily tested at any time.

▶ [Fail safe if no oxygen present! What we need is a fail safe when hypoxic mixtures are being delivered, for example, 5 or 10% oxygen.—Eds.]

Specifications and Recommendations for Nitrous Oxide-Oxygen Apparatus to Be Used in Obstetric Analgesia are presented by P. V. Cole, J. S. Crawford, A. G. Doughty, H. G. Epstein, I. D. Hill, W. N. Rollason and M. E. Tunstall.[8] In Great Britain, two types of machine have been devised to administer oxygen and nitrous oxide for obstetric analgesia, one having the gases in separate cylinders and the other having a single cylin-

(7)   Brit. J. Anaesth. 43:103-106, January, 1971.
(8)   Anaesthesia 25:317-327, July, 1970.

der containing premixed gas. A 50-50% mixture generally provides adequate pain relief during normal delivery. The need for portability for deliveries at home rules out the two-cylinder machine. With the one-cylinder type, the gases tend to separate when exposed to freezing temperatures. A need for machines delivering variable mixtures for use in hospitals persists; 70% nitrous oxide may be helpful in abnormal deliveries. Tests were carried out on both types of apparatus.

An apparatus with separate cylinders must operate on the demand principle, preferably with ability to adjust the oxygen output from 30 to 100%. Accuracy of oxygen delivery should be about ±5%. Maximal inspiratory resistance with equal gas flows should not exceed 25 mm. water at a flow rate of 20 L. per minute or 80 mm. water at a rate of 160 L. per minute. Maximal expiratory resistances at flow rates of 20 and 120 L. per minute should be 15 and 50 mm. water, respectively. If the oxygen supply fails, the apparatus should deliver room air only.

A portable apparatus should have a delivered oxygen concentration of 48-52%. A peak inspiratory flow rate of 300 L. per minute is desirable. Inspiratory resistance should not exceed 50 and 150 mm. water, respectively, at flow rates of 60 and 300 L. per minute, and expiratory resistance should not exceed the same figures at flow rates of 20 and 120 L. per minute. The device should operate on the demand principle. Precautions should be taken against freezing of gas in premixed cylinders, and appropriate warning labels should be shown.

▶ [Despite all these precautions, we must warn that premixing and variable and nonvariable control mechanisms are not fail safe.—Eds.]

Use of Entonox in the Ambulance Service during a pilot study in 1969 is described by Peter J. F. Baskett and Allan Withnell.[9] Entonox, a mixture of 50% nitrous oxide and 50% oxygen contained in a single cylinder, was used in nine ambulances in Gloucestershire, England, for self-administration by patients in pain. The cylinder was fitted with a noninterchangeable pin index valve in the yoke. The pin index valve was integral with the inhalation unit, consisting of a pressure gauge, reducing valve and demand valve connected to the expiratory valve and mask by wide-bore 60-in. flexible tubing. The demand valve insured that gas did not flow until negative pressure was produced; this was achieved by inhalation after an airtight seal was formed between the mask and the face of the patient. If

(9) Brit. M. J. 2:41-43, Apr. 4, 1970.

RESULTS OF FOLLOW-UP OF ENTONOX USE IN 50 PATIENTS

PATIENT REACTION	NO. OF PATIENTS
Pain much relieved	50
Anxiety relieved	30 (out of 30)
Felt sick	0
Felt drowsy	23
Fell asleep	0
Would like to have it again if similar circumstances reoccurred	50

consciousness was impaired during self-administration, the mask would fall away from the face and the demand valve would close.

Ambulance personnel received instruction on the therapeutic and side effects of nitrous oxide and the use of the Entonox inhalation unit before installation of the apparatus. They were told not to offer the gas to patients who had impaired consciousness, were overtly drunk or had maxillofacial or oral injuries.

In 3½ months, treatment was given to 26 female and 40 male patients, aged 9-89, with various injuries and illnesses. The table shows the effects of Entonox in 50 patients followed within 2-3 days of hospitalization. In no case did the admitting physician or surgeon complain that physical signs were masked. No patient complained of difficulty or fear in using the apparatus. As a result of the study, the Gloucestershire County Health Committee decided to extend the use of Entonox to the entire county ambulance fleet.

▶ [Nitrous oxide is a good analgesic and is rapidly eliminated and therefore may be preferable to the use of a narcotic analgesic by paramedical personnel. Since nitrous oxide is eliminated through the respiratory tract, its removal can be speeded by artificial respiration. Caution with such premixed gases is necessary in colder climates if the ambulance is not kept warm at all times. At lower temperatures, nitrous oxide will condense to a liquid in the cylinder, leaving an oxygen-rich gas phase. If this gas phase were used for one patient, a hypoxic mixture could be provided to succeeding patients. Once stratified by liquefaction, gas mixtures will not remix without vigorous agitation.—Eds.]

ANESTHETIC COMPLICATIONS

Malignant Hyperthermia, or hyperpyrexial syndrome, is a rare complication of anesthesia. Werner Kalow[1] (Univ. of Toronto) reviewed 65 reported cases of this syndrome. Rigidity

(1) Proc. Roy. Soc. Med. 63:178-180, February, 1970.

TABLE 1.—GENERAL ANESTHETICS WHICH HAVE BEEN ASSOCIATED WITH MALIGNANT HYPERTHERMIA

INHALATIONAL AGENT	No. DIED	No. SURVIVED	TOTAL No. CASES
Nitrous oxide	0	3	3
Halothane	24	10	34
Methoxyflurane	2	0	2
Ether	2	0	2
Cyclopropane	0	2	2
Various combinations	9	6	15
Unknown	1	6	7
Total	38	27	65

and hyperthermia are not always noted together, and rigidity is often present but not pronounced. A few patients had two independent hyperthermic episodes. Some surgeons have noted the heart to be stiff, like the skeletal muscles. Pronounced metabolic and respiratory acidosis is a constant feature of the syndrome. Alkali infusion is, with vigorous cooling, an important therapeutic measure. No particular premedicaments have been associated with occurrence of the syndrome. Anesthetics besides halothane have been implicated (Table 1). The syndrome can occur in the absence of any muscle relaxants. Relations to the use of succinylcholine are shown in Table 2. Typically a failure of succinylcholine to produce relaxation leads to a second dose, after which the rigidity becomes apparent.

The incidence of malignant hyperthermia appears to be 1/10,000 or at least greater than 1/100,000 and is similar in both sexes. The syndrome has not been noted in patients below age 3 (Table 3), but one third of all cases occur in the 1st decade of life. Of 65 cases analyzed, 43 were familial. Dominant inheritance appears to occur, with some skipping of generations,

TABLE 2.—CLASSIFICATION OF HYPERTHERMIA PATIENTS BY OCCURRENCE OF RIGIDITY, SURVIVAL AND USE OF SUCCINYLCHOLINE

	No. DIED	No. SURVIVED	TOTAL No. CASES
Rigidity:			
With succinylcholine	18	13	31
Without succinylcholine	7	3	10
Rigidity not observed:			
With succinylcholine	11	3	14
Without succinylcholine	2	8	10
Total	38	27	65

TABLE 3.—Cases of Hyperthermia Sorted by Age, Occurrence of Rigidity, Death and Survival

Age (Years)	Rigidity		Rigidity not Observed	
	No. Died	No. Survived	No. Died	No. Survived
1- 5	2	7	2	4
6-10	4	2	0	1
11-15	3	3	1	1
16-20	4	0	2	2
21-25	6	1	3	1
26-30	2	0	0	0
31-35	0	0	2	0
36-40	1	2	2	1
41-45	3	1	1	0
46-50	0	0	0	1
Total	25	16	13	11

but cases without a hereditary predisposition cannot be excluded.

The nature of the defect in malignant hyperthermia is not known. The lesion must be in muscle rather than in the central nervous system and must be distal to the neuromuscular end plate. In vitro studies showed an increased twitch response of normal human muscle with halothane, not reproducible in any laboratory animal. This may represent a species difference in excitation-contraction coupling. Halothane can affect human muscle in a way that requires close investigation.

Fulminating Hyperpyrexia during Anesthesia in a Member of a Myopathic Family. Fulminating hyperpyrexia, usually fatal, in the course of surgical anesthesia has been reported several times. Its cause is not clear, but sensitivity to succinylcholine has been postulated, and myopathy, infection and enzyme aberrations have been suggested as etiologic factors. A. J. W. Steers, John A. Tallack and Dorothy E. A. Thompson[2] (Romford, England) report a case with a possible myopathic association.

Male, 16, was admitted with signs suggestive of acute appendicitis. A strikingly muscular build was noted. His temperature was 100.2 F. Anesthesia was induced with thiopentone followed by suxamethonium. After the latter, there was unusually pronounced muscle twitching. Tubocurarine was given, but relaxation was poor, and a high oxygen concentration was required to prevent cyanosis. Persistent tachycardia developed. The axillary temperature was 107

(2)   Brit. M. J. 2:341-343, May 9, 1970.

F. after 15 minutes of anesthesia; a later rectal temperature was 108 F.

The appendectomy was rapidly concluded, and surface and intragastric cooling were instituted. Ventricular asystole was converted to fibrillation with epinephrine, and external electric defibrillation re-established normal rhythm. All limb muscles were rigid, and some opisthotonus was evident. Tendon reflexes were absent, fundal hemorrhages were noted, and the rectal temperature was 106 F. The temperature fell to subnormal overnight, but consciousness and spontaneous respirations did not return, and the patient died with persistent muscle rigidity. Autopsy showed only generalized venous congestion. The appendectomy site showed no abnormality.

The patient's father and 1 of 2 brothers were of a muscular build like the patient. In the father, weakness of the right leg with muscle wasting and localized areas of muscle hypertrophy were noted as well as asymmetrical hypertrophy of various muscles. The creatine phosphokinase (CPK) was 690 milli-I.U./ml. (normal, 5-50) and serum aldolase was 675 milli-I.U./ml. (normal, up to 6). Glucose tolerance was abnormal. Electromyography indicated primary muscle disease. Muscle biopsy showed changes of myopathy. The patient's brother had a CPK of 103 milli-I.U./ml. and a serum aldolase of 1.5.

Metabolic Error of Muscle Metabolism after Recovery from Malignant Hyperthermia. Malignant hyperthermia is characterized by a rapid rise of body temperature during general anesthesia. Although its etiology is unknown, indications are that it is not a single entity. W. Kalow, B. A. Britt, M. E. Terreau and C. Haist[3] (Univ. of Toronto) investigated the possible causes of malignant hyperthermia by studying biopsy specimens of quadriceps femoris muscle from 3 volunteer patients who survived an episode of hyperthermia and came from at-risk families.

Hyperthermia had been pronounced in 2 patients but absent in 1, as well as in his relatives. Contracture produced by caffeine in isolated muscle strips was measured. Normal human muscle was sampled at abdominal surgery, amputations and operations on the lower limb.

Caffeine caused isolated muscle to contract, with the maximal contracture occurring at 3-4 minutes; the effect lasted until the caffeine was washed out. The effect was potentiated by 1% halothane, which alone never caused contracture. Dose-effect curves showed a maximal effect at 2% halothane.

(3)   Lancet 2:895-898, Oct. 31, 1970.

Muscle from 1 patient without rigidity generally responded normally. Muscle from the 2 patients with rigidity showed increased susceptibility to caffeine and the effect was enhanced by halothane more than in normal muscle specimens. Halothane had little effect on calcium accumulation by isolated sarcoplasmic reticulum from normal muscle but it reduced the calcium content of reticulum from the 2 patients with malignant hyperthermia and rigidity.

Malignant hyperthermia with rigidity is apparently due to an inborn metabolic error in skeletal muscle, which renders it susceptible to disturbed intracellular calcium distribution. Calcium regulates the adenosine triphosphatase activity of actomyosin and the rigidity and hyperthermia may be linked. Malignant hyperthermia without rigidity is a different disease, although it is equally lethal and a precondition is inherited by autosomal dominance. Local anesthetics have been beneficial in patients with rigidity but may contribute to hyperthermia without rigidity.

Changes Underlying Halothane-Induced Malignant Hyperpyrexia in Landrace Pigs were studied by M. C. Berman, G. G. Harrison, A. B. Bull and J. E. Kench[4] (Univ. of Cape Town). Malignant hyperpyrexia is a rare but often fatal complication of inhalation anesthesia in man; halothane and other agents have been implicated. A similar syndrome has been described in a pure Landrace strain of pig (Harrison *et al.*, 1968). A rapid rise in body temperature to 42-45 C. occurs with muscle rigidity, severe acidosis and death, starting shortly after halothane administration. Cooling, alkalis and muscle relaxants do not prevent a fatal outcome. Halothane appears to act as a trigger in this syndrome. Uncoupling of oxidative phosphorylation has been suggested as a possible mechanism.

Studies were made of pure Landrace or Landrace-Large White cross strains of pigs. Susceptible pigs did not react adversely to thiopentone for up to $2\frac{1}{2}$ hours. Within 10 minutes of introducing halothane, however, organ temperatures rose except for that of skin, and a peak core temperature was reached at 30-45 minutes after halothane was stopped. Oxygen uptake increased, but a disproportionate rise in carbon dioxide output occurred, with a high respiratory quotient resulting. Oxygen consumption rose 20-40% per degree Celsius rise in core temperature. Water shifted to the intracellular space, and serum

(4) Nature, London 225:653-655, Feb. 14, 1970.

sodium and total protein levels increased. Calcium and magnesium shifted extracellularly. Inorganic phosphate was released into the plasma. Blood glucose increased, and uncompensated metabolic acidosis resulted from a rise in plasma lactate. Biochemical changes preceded the onset of pyrexia and were not secondary to heat injury to tissues.

It is not yet clear how halothane stimulates excess heat production in susceptible pigs, but this is not attributable to uncoupling of oxidative phosphorylation. Changes in water and electrolyte distribution and lactic acid production preceded the significant rise in temperature and not secondary to nonspecific heat damge. Known causes of defective tissue oxygenation cannot explain the degree of lactate production observed. A possible defect in mitochondrial electron transport is to be investigated.

Cerebrovascular Response during Progressive Hyperthermia in Dogs. Relatively little is known about cerebral blood flow during fever. E. M. Nemoto and H. M. Frankel[5] (State Univ. of New Jersey) determined cerebral blood flow at graded levels of hyperthermia in dogs anesthetized with pentobarbital. Flow was measured using $4\text{-}^{131}\text{I}$-iodoantipyrine and external brain scintillation detection. Temperature in a chamber was elevated to 40 C. and kept 2 or 3 degrees C. above the animal's rectal temperature for the rest of the study. The rectal temperature was elevated at a rate of about 2 degrees C. per hour.

Cerebral blood flow did not change significantly with progressive hyperthermia, although the mean arterial pressure decreased at rectal temperatures over 40.4 C. Heart and respiratory rates increased progressively with increased rectal temperature. Respiratory alkalosis occurred at higher temperatures. The $Paco_2$ reached a minimum of 19 mm. Hg. The arterial pH was 7.51 at 42 C. but dropped to 7.40 at 43 C., although the $Paco_2$ remained low. Cerebral blood flow and mean arterial pressure showed significant positive correlation in dogs with bilateral carotid artery ligation but not in nonligated animals. Cerebrovascular resistance was reduced significantly only in nonligated dogs at temperatures of 42 and 43 C. Cerebral blood flow increased significantly with increasing $Paco_2$ at normothermia. Apparent CO_2 sensitivity, or the ratio of mean cerebral blood flow to mean $Paco_2$, did not change significantly in

(5)   Am. J. Physiol. 218: 1060-1064, April, 1970.

controls but was significantly increased in nonligated dogs at rectal temperatures of 42 and 43 C.

During hyperthermia and its accompanying hypocapnia, stability of cerebral blood flow results in part from apparent change in the cerebral vascular sensitivity to CO_2.

Possible Predictive Tests for Malignant Hyperthermia during Anesthesia. Deaths from fulminant hyperpyrexia appear to have been reduced recently, probably because of greater awareness of this complication of anesthesia and of the need for rapid, vigorous treatment. J. Antonio Aldrete, Adrian Padfield, Clive C. Solomon and Marcus W. Rubright[6] report the successful management of a case of malignant hyperthermia in which a possibly predictive blood chemistry pattern was found.

Boy, 17, was admitted for closed reduction of an ankle fracture. The white blood cell count was 17,400/cu. mm. Propoxyphene hydrochloride was given for pain relief. Meperidine and atropine premedication were followed by methohexital sodium for induction and halothane with nitrous oxide-oxygen for maintenance. Succinylcholine was given to facilitate reduction of the fracture. The patient became "rigid," and the rectal temperature was 102.2 F. after the 21-minute operation. The temperature was 106.7 F. 45 minutes later, despite attempted cooling. Irregular heart sounds and an arterial pressure of 90/50 mm. Hg were noted. Sodium bicarbonate was given, but the temperature rose again, with an arterial pH of 7.16 and a P_{CO_2} of 46 mm. Hg. Generalized muscle rigidity was noted. The patient was unconscious, with a Babinski sign on the right and a larger right pupil. The neurologic deficit improved gradually. Muscle rigidity was not altered by curarization. Muscle hypertonicity persisted after recovery, and some muscle atrophy ensued.

The course of malignant hyperthermia in the patient was typical. Hyperkalemia was not noted, but determinations were not made at the time of the initial febrile episode. The patient subsequently had consistently elevated levels of creatine phosphokinase and inorganic pyrophosphate. The mother, brother and sister of the patient had elevated serum pyrophosphate levels, as well as slightly increased creatine phosphokinase levels. A maternal uncle and grandmother also had slightly elevated creatine phosphokinase levels. These determinations may help identify persons susceptible to malignant hyperthermia. The role of magnesium in the altered metabolism of malignant hyperthermia warrants further investigation.

▶ [Although it was recognized many years ago, the syndrome of malignant hyperthermia complicating anesthesia only began to receive widespread attention in the past 5 years. The Toronto group has acted as a

(6) J.A.M.A. 215:1465-1469, Mar. 1, 1971.

clearinghouse for the accumulation of data in the field. Kalow's article gives us important statistics summarizing the pertinent factors of this syndrome. It appears that there may be two or perhaps more forms of the syndrome whose primary common feature is temperature elevation but which vary in the occurrence of muscle rigidity, rhabdomyolysis and other features. An animal model is now available which may help us get to the root of this disorder. The animal form of the disease does appear to differ in that, once started, is irreversible.

A volume summarizing the proceedings of the Toronto conference on malignant hyperpyrexia is soon to appear. It will contain information of great importance to anesthesiologists.—Eds.]

Myopathy and Malignant Hyperpyrexia. M. A. Denborough, P. Ebeling, J. O. King and P. Zapf[7] (Melbourne) re-examined a family in which 3 deaths from malignant hyperpyrexia occurred and in which elevated creatine phophokinase levels were found in symptom-free relatives. The propositus, who survived a hyperpyrexial reaction, and 3 of the 16 relatives tested had high serum creatine phosphokinase levels; 2 of the 3 affected relatives had mild myopathy. Ten anesthetic deaths in all had occurred in this family; only the propositus survived.

This subject had a short neck and a rounded upper thoracic kyphosis with prominent trapezii. A sister had a short neck with prominent trapezii. A paternal aunt had had a life-long weak spine and lately, increasing difficulty in walking. Examination showed moderate weakness of the hip flexors and thinning of both quadriceps. There was excessive muscular contour of the legs below the knees, especially prominent laterally near the neck of the fibula. Electromyography showed minimal myopathic changes in the right quadriceps and tibialis anterior muscles. The father had similar but less severe findings.

Malignant hyperpyrexia on anesthetic exposure appears to occur in persons with an underlying disease of muscle. The disorder is inherited as a dominant characteristic. Anesthetics further damage the muscles of susceptible persons, leading to hyperpyrexia, convulsions and death. It is not clear whether involvement of the lower thigh muscles is characteristic of this type of myopathy. Serum creatine phosphokinase should be determined in all relatives of patients who have had malignant hyperpyrexia. Serum creatine phosphokinase should also be estimated in all persons having general anesthesia. When this cannot be done or when the creatine phosphokinase is elevated from another cause, body temperature should be monitored dur-

(7)   Lancet 1: 1138-1140, May 30, 1970.

ing anesthesia, so that hyperpyrexia can be corrected as early as possible.

▶ [According to the authors, every patient for general anesthesia should have a serum creatine phosphokinase estimation or have his temperature monitored. However, creatine phosphokinase elevation is not that definitive.—Eds.]

Recurrent Hepatitis in Patients Receiving Multiple Halothane Anesthetics for Radium Treatment of Carcinoma of the Cervix Uteri. Mary Hughes and L. W. Powell[8] (Royal Brisbane, Australia Hosp.), report 6 cases of severe acute hepatocellular jaundice seen during 1964-66, all in women who had received multiple halothane anesthetics for radium treatment of cervical carcinoma. Five patients had had recurrent episodes of fever, bilirubinuria or jaundice after separate halothane exposures. A prospective study was made of 50 patients given multiple nonhalothane anesthetics for radium therapy during 1965-69. No case of acute hepatocellular jaundice occurred after 1966, when use of halothane was discontinued.

There was a highly significant difference in incidence of late postoperative fever, starting more than 5 days after operation, between halothane and nonhalothane anesthetics. Eighteen patients in the prospective study had early postoperative fever, but none had fever more than 5 days after anesthetic administration. Liver function tests have remained normal in all these patients, except 1 with abnormal serum flocculation.

Strong circumstantial evidence implicates halothane as the cause of acute hepatocellular jaundice in the present 6 patients. In all patients, otherwise unexplained fever and/or bilirubinuria developed within a week after halothane anesthesia, and further exposure after a short interval resulted in acute hepatocellular jaundice. It is unlikely that recurrent exposure to halothane reactivated viral hepatitis in these patients. It is unlikely that radiotherapy contributed to the hepatic damage that occurred.

Development of fever later than the 5th day after halothane exposure is useful in detecting patients at risk of hypersensitivity reaction, and presumably liver disease, after multiple exposures to halothane. Halothane is best avoided in such patients and probably also in adults who require multiple anesthetics at very short intervals.

▶ [How often have you heard, "I've given multiple halothane anesthetics to patients many times and I've never observed hepatitis"? It is interesting

(8)   Gastroenterology 58: 790-797, June, 1970.

that all 6 patients acquired hepatitis and were quite sick but none died.—
Eds.]

Lymphocyte Stimulation Induced by Halothane in Patients with Hepatitis Following Exposure to Halothane. Fiorenzo Paronetto and Hans Popper[9] (City Univ. of New York) report additional evidence for sensitization to halothane in patients with liver damage after exposure to halothane. Interaction of lymphocytes and halothane was demonstrated in cell culture, using the uptake of ^{3}H-thymidine into DNA as a measure of lymphocyte stimulation. Study was made of 15 patients with hepatitis after exposure to halothane and 1 exposed to methoxyflurane. Three nonjaundiced patients exposed to halothane, 9 patients with liver disease and 6 healthy subjects were also studied. No patient had received blood before exposure to halothane. All but three of them survived. Phytohemagglutinin was used as a nonspecific lymphocyte stimulant. Australia antigen was detected by three agar-gel diffusion methods.

Healthy subjects and patients with liver diseases did not exhibit lymphocyte stimulation in the presence of halothane. Eight study patients exposed to halothane showed increased thymidine uptake on incubation of lymphocytes with halothane. Two others showed this effect when fetal calf serum was substituted for autologous plasma in the study, as did the patient exposed to methoxyflurane. Phytohemagglutinin reactivity also depended on fetal calf serum in these cases. Two nonreactive patients were hypersensitive to penicillin, and one was in hepatic coma and receiving steroids. Two patients showed stimulation when jaundiced but not when the bilirubin levels and transaminase activity were normal. Two of 3 patients with halothane hepatitis showed cross-reactive lymphocyte stimulation with methoxyflurane. The patient exposed to methoxyflurane did not show reactivity with halothane. The exposed patients without jaundice did not show reactivity to halothane. None of the study serums contained Australia antigen. Antimitochondrial antibodies were found in 10 study patients, as well as in control patients with primary biliary cirrhosis and chronic active hepatitis. Seven of the 10 positive study patients also had increased lymphocyte stimulation.

Stimulation of lymphocytes with halothane is helpful in distinguishing viral and halothane hepatitis. In some patients, halothane may be a sensitizing agent, with a pathogenetic role

(9) New England J. Med. 283-277-280, Aug. 6, 1970.

in hepatic damage. The failure to demonstrate Australia antigen in the serums of the patients with jaundice after exposure to halothane, also recently reported by others, militates against the hypothesis that the abnormality in these patients is viral hepatitis.

▶ [Paronetto and Popper claim that mere exposure of patients to halothane does not sensitize them, and that sensitization is not detectable before the appearance of jaundice. We seem to be on the track of identifying the problem.—Eds.]

Multiple Halothane Exposure and Hepatic Bromsulphthalein [BSP] Clearance. Clinical and statistical investigation of the role of halothane in postoperative liver dysfunction is hampered by inability to eliminate other potential causes of liver dysfunction. J. F. Biebuyck, S. J. Saunders, G. G. Harrison and A. B. Bull[1] (Univ. of Capetown) attempted to eliminate potential causes of liver dysfunction other than halothane by studying isolated perfused livers and liver homogenates from animals exposed to halothane on several occasions. Male albino rats were exposed to three or five 60-minute periods of 1% halothane or 4% diethyl ether vapor in oxygen on alternate days, and the livers were later isolated and perfused.

A significant increase in BSP retention was found 1 and 3 weeks after halothane exposures but not after ether exposures. A single halothane exposure did not alter BSP retention. The values returned to normal 6 weeks after halothane exposures, but re-exposure on three further occasions again led to rise in BSP retention after 1 and 3 weeks. Assays of BSP-glutathione conjugating enzyme in liver homogenates showed a significant decline in activity 2 and 3 weeks after halothane exposures. Levels after ether exposures did not differ significantly from control values.

The increase in BSP retention suggests a delayed hepatic effect of multiple halothane exposures. The precise mechanism of increased BSP retention is not clear. Possibilities include impairment of BSP conjugation, change in the character or serum albumin or a deficiency of the hepatic cytoplasmic organic anion acceptor protein Y.

▶ [Transient impairment of liver function is commonly observed after operations using general anesthesia with a variety of agents. Values usually return to normal promptly. This study, however, compares multiple halothane exposures with multiple ether exposures, both without surgical intervention, and shows that livers from halothane-treated but not ether-treated animals have a biochemical lesion that persists for at least 4

(1)   Brit. M. J. 1:668-671, Mar. 14, 1970.

weeks. It is of interest that this lesion did not appear after a single exposure to halothane.—Eds.]

Unexplained Postoperative Fever: Its Value as a Sign of Halothane Sensitization. The National Halothane Study suggested that "unexplained postoperative fever" alone, after previous halothane administration, might indicate sensitization, but the incidence and patterns of such fever have not been adequately delineated. Michael H. M. Dykes[2] (Harvard Med. School) examined the incidence and patterns of unexplained postoperative fever and evaluated its prognostic importance.

From the records of 200 consecutive nonobstetric patients given general anesthesia in May of 1969, only the records of those patients with a temperature above 98.6 F. orally within 1 week after operation were reviewed to determine whether or not there was a bona fide cause for the elevation. The hospital records of 61 additional patients—four groups of 20 consecutive patients with unexplained fever after abdominal hysterectomy, cholecystectomy, radical mastectomy and leg surgery—were obtained and evaluated similarly. Pulmonary physiotherapy was given before and after abdominal operations.

Of 162 patients with available postoperative temperature records, 133 had a temperature above 98.6 F. orally. This appeared to be a continuation of pre-existing fever in 29 cases and a bona fide postoperative complication in 31. There remained 73 patients with an unexplained postoperative temperature elevation. Such fever developed in all 57 who had temperatures recorded for at least 3 days postoperatively and in 16 who had temperatures recorded for less than 3 postoperative days. Pneumonitis, pneumonia, atelectasis, urinary tract infection, wound infection or hematoma accounted for 27 of the 31 cases with bona fide postoperative complications. In the selected groups with unexplained fever, the mean temperatures fell steadily from 99.5-100.4 F. on the 1st postoperative day to 98.6-99.1 F. on day 7. The peak temperature exceeded 99.9 F. in 48 cases and above 100.9 F. in 20. Patients given halothane showed a pattern of temperature elevation similar to that of other patients. The temperature elevation was bimodal in about a quarter of the 80 patients and persistent in about the same proportion.

An elevation in body temperature appears to be the normal response to all but the least traumatic surgical procedures and to be even after atraumatic procedures. A recognizable pattern of unexplained postoperative fever may ultimately be associated statistically with halothane sensitization, but it might prove of little practical help if the association is not a strong one. Unexplained fever alone after a prior administration of halothane cannot be considered a contraindication to the subsequent use of the agent. The epidemiologic consequences of withholding halothane from nearly all patients returning for a second operation might well be the opposite of those intended, because of the possible greater over-all safety of giving two halothane anesthetics as opposed to one such anesthetic, followed or preceded by a nonhalothane anesthetic.

▶ ["Control" data such as these are invaluable.—Eds.]

Renal Dysfunction Associated with Methoxyflurane Anesthesia: A Randomized, Prospective Clinical Evaluation was carried out by Richard I. Mazze, Gary L. Shue and Stephen H. Jackson[3] (Stanford Univ.) in male patients scheduled for elective surgical procedures.

METHOD.—Twelve patients received methoxyflurane and 10, halothane. Criteria for inclusion in the study were a preoperative blood urea nitrogen under 35 mg./100 ml., serum creatinine under 1.6 mg./100 ml., endogenous creatinine clearance of 50 ml. per minute or higher and urine concentrating ability of over 600 mOsm./kg. water after overnight dehydration. Medications were stopped before operation. Atropine alone was given for premedication. Anesthesia was induced and maintained with methoxyflurane and oxygen, 6 L. per minute in a semiclosed circle system. The control anesthetic was halothane in oxygen, 6 L. per minute. Succinylcholine was used for intubation and curare for muscle relaxation during operation. A ventilator was used to maintain a Pco_2 of 35-40 mm. Hg. Lactated Ringer's solution was given intraoperatively and, with KCl added, after operation.

The two groups were similar preoperatively. Postoperatively, halothane patients had mild but significant hyponatremia and serum hypo-osmolality, with slight weight loss. Two patients had an inappropriate response to antidiuretic hormone on the 2d postoperative day. Methoxyflurane patients had significant increases in serum sodium, urea nitrogen, uric acid and osmolality. Uric acid clearance was significantly reduced. Marked weight loss and delayed return of renal concentrating ability to preoperative levels were also noted. Both groups had proteinuria and, less often, glycosuria on the day of operation but rarely thereafter. Potassium excretion was greater in the methoxyflurane group.

(3) J.A.M.A. 216:278-288, Apr. 12, 1971.

Although current opinion among anesthesiologists seems to be that renal dysfunction due to methoxyflurane is rare, it must be considered a nephrotoxic agent. The changes resulting from methoxyflurane were clinically significant. Severe thirst was a problem in many patients, and postoperative fluid homeostasis was sometimes severely compromised. Extrarenal fluid loss may contribute to symptoms but does not appear necessary for development of the renal dysfunction. The mechanism by which methoxyflurane produces renal dysfunction is not clear. The agent is known to undergo extensive breakdown in the liver. Until further information is available, methoxyflurane should be withheld from patients with known renal disease and those having operations associated with a high incidence of postoperative renal complications.

▶ [Are these 12 closely observed patients unusual or are they universal; if they represent our usual patients, why don't we observe more renal difficulties?—Eds.]

Renal Oxalosis and Azotemia after Methoxyflurane Anesthesia. Calcium oxalate crystals have been noted in the kidneys of a few patients dying in renal failure after operation under methoxyflurane anesthesia, but oxalate deposition has not been attributed to administration of this anesthetic. Joseph A. Frascino, Parker Vanamee and P. Peter Rosen[4] (New York) report observations in 11 patients with renal failure after methoxyflurane anesthesia, indicating a distinct relationship between methoxyflurane and renal oxalosis. The patients had had major operation, usually radical cancer operation, with exposure to methoxyflurane for 2.75-7.5 hours. All had normal serum creatinine levels preoperatively. Four patients had creatinine levels of 8.7-12.6 mg./100 ml. postoperatively. Four had moderate renal failure, with creatinine levels of 2.0-4.8 mg./100 ml. Two had mild renal failure, with creatinine levels of 1.2-1.9 mg./100 ml. One had an uneventful course after exploration with methoxyflurane anesthesia.

All patients had elevated urinary oxalate excretion, with a range of 96-480 mg./24 hours (normal, 5-45 mg.). The mean level 5-10 days postoperatively was 320 mg./24 hours. All biopsy specimens showed sheaves of birefringent intratubular crystals; histochemical tests showed them to be calcium oxalate. The crystals were deposited primarily in proximal tubules, where they occasionally elicited giant cell reactions. Prominent

(4) New England J. Med. 283:676-679, Sept. 24, 1970.

associated findings included tubular dilatation and epithelial cell degeneration and necrosis. Crystal deposition and tubular damage closely paralleled the degree of azotemia present. Crystals were present in about 10% of tubules in mild cases and in 35% in severe cases of renal failure. Severity of the lesions was not related to the duration of exposure to methoxyflurane. Autopsy findings included marked interstitial inflammation and fibrosis and tubular atrophy.

Intrarenal oxalate precipitation is a characteristic complication of postoperative renal failure in patients anesthetized with methoxyflurane. The oxalosis may contribute to the severity and duration of the renal failure, especially in patients with acute tubular necrosis, who can least tolerate an added renal insult if recovery of renal function is to occur.

▶ [Seven of these 11 patients had radical cystectomy and urinary diversion. These are long operations accompanied by significant blood loss, fluid translocation and electrolyte disturbances. How much of a causal role was played by methoxyflurane in producing renal oxalosis is not clear, but it is quite certain that blood volume and fluid and electrolyte therapy must be meticulously monitored in such cases.—Eds.]

Hepatic Coma Associated with Methoxyflurane Anesthesia: Report of a Case is presented by Seymour Katz[5] (Albert Einstein College of Medicine). Evidence of hepatic dysfunction after exposure to methoxyflurane has been largely limited to reports of mild abnormalities of liver function tests. Only 6 cases of severe liver damage have been reported; 4 of the patients died. The patient in the present case recovered after exchange transfusion.

Woman, 22, an operating room nurse, was admitted because she had been confused and sleepy for 3 days. Twenty-four days earlier, at another hospital, she had undergone dilatation and curettage for incomplete abortion with methoxyflurane anesthesia without premedication. Two units of blood had been given for a hypotensive episode. Two weeks later, chills, dark urine and vomiting developed, followed by icterus and delirium alternating with somnolence.

The patient was obese and somnolent and screamed episodically. Icterus was apparent. The urine contained bilirubin and urobilinogen. An EEG was compatible with toxic-metabolic encephalopathy. The patient progressed to a decorticate state despite administration of fluids, neomycin and corticoids. The white blood cell count rose although the serum bilirubin fell.

On the 5th and 6th days, whole blood exchanges were performed, 12 units of fresh whole blood being given each day through a surgical arteriovenous fistula of Silastic catheters connecting the right radial artery and brachial vein. γ-Globulin was then administered.

(5) Am. J. Digest. Dis. 15:733-739, August, 1970.

The mental state improved dramatically after the first exchange. There was a subsequent brief period of oliguria and bradycardia. An EEG, taken before discharge with the patient on a normal-protein diet, was normal.

Identification of the true hepatotoxin in a particular case is difficult. Although this patient was undoubtedly exposed to hepatitis virus as well as to halogenated hydrocarbon anesthetics in her work as an operating room nurse, methoxyflurane toxicity is likely. Mechanisms postulated for liver injury in these cases include a direct hepatotoxic effect, a drug-potentiated hemodynamic change and hypersensitivity. Experience with exchange transfusions in cases of drug-related liver failure has been gratifying, but it has been poor in cases of viral hepatitis.

► [Methoxyflurane toxicity may seem likely to the author but without better evidence it doesn't to the editors.—Eds.]

Plasma Levels of Antidiuretic Hormone in Man during Methoxyflurane Anesthesia and Surgery were studied by T. Oyama and K. Sato[6] (Hirosaki Univ.) in 10 patients, aged 27-69. All had elective operations; none had hepatic, renal or endocrinologic disease. All patients but 2 had laparotomy.

Pentobarbitone and pethidine with atropine were given for premedication, and anesthesia was induced with nitrous oxide-oxygen in a semiclosed system. Methoxyflurane was given via a Pentec vaporizer. After a blood sample was taken, tracheal intubation was facilitated with suxamethonium, and 3d stage, plane 2-3 anesthesia was maintained. Respiration was assisted throughout the procedure. Anesthesia alone lasted preoperatively for at least $1\frac{1}{2}$ hours in each case. Patients were fasted and water-deprived for 10 hours before anesthesia induction. They received 5% fructose, 1.4-2 ml. per minute, starting 30 minutes before induction to the end of operation. Bioassays were done in male rats using USP posterior pituitary reference standard as a standard.

The mean preoperative plasma antidiuretic hormone (ADH) level was 2.5 ± 0.2 μU./ml. The level was elevated to 5.1 μU. after 30 minutes of methoxyflurane anesthesia alone. After 1 hour of anesthesia it was 3.4 μU., and $1\frac{1}{2}$ hours later it was 3.9 μU. The level was 20.5 μU. 10 minutes after the start of operation (Fig. 14). Urine volume was 3.5 ml. per minute shortly after fructose infusion and dropped to 1.2 ml. shortly after induction. The value 1-$1\frac{1}{2}$ hours after induction was 0.5 ml. per

(6) Anaesthesia 25:500-507, October, 1970.

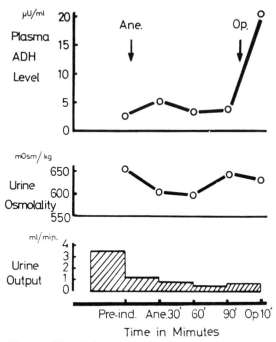

Fig. 14.—Plasma antidiuretic hormone levels and changes in urine osmolality and urine output in 10 patients. *Ane.*, anesthesia; *Op.*, operation. (Courtesy of Oyama, T., and Sato, K.: Anaesthesia 25:500-507, October, 1970.)

minute. The volume was 0.5 ml. 10 minutes after the start of operation. Urine and serum osmolalities did not change significantly.

Antidiuretic hormone plays a part in reducing urine output at anesthesia and operation. The elevation in plasma ADH was more marked at laparotomy than at operation on an extremity or orthopedic surgical procedures. The elevated ADH secretion at anesthesia and operation contribute to the decreased urine formation observed.

▶ [Might an increase in renal tubular reabsorption of water tend to concentrate fluoride ions in the tubular cells?—Eds.]

Emergency Treatment of Pneumothorax: A Simple Catheter Technic for Use in the Radiology Department is described by E. Nicholas Sargent and A. Franklin Turner[7] (Univ. of Southern California). All symptomatic pneumothoraxes, even small ones, are best managed by removing air from the pleural space.

(7)   Am. J. Roentgenol. 109:531-535, July, 1970.

The newly designed pneumothorax catheter used consists of a thin-walled Teflon no. 9 F. radiopaque catheter with a 3-mm. outside diameter and a 2.08-mm. inside diameter. The tubing is 14 in. long and has a Luer-Lok connector at its proximal end. The distal 3 inches has multiple perforations. An 8-in. no. 18 cannula, with an obturator, is inserted through the most proximal side opening, about 3 in. from the tip of the tube.

The catheter is optimally inserted at the 2d anterior interspace in the midclavicular line. It can also be placed in the needle track of a pulmonary biopsy. The procedure is done under aseptic conditions, using 2% lidocaine for block anesthesia. A stab wound is made for catheter insertion. When the catheter tip is within the pleural cavity, the catheter is "milked" forward as the cannula is slowly withdrawn. After the air is withdrawn, the catheter is connected to a Heimlich drainage valve, and an antibiotic is given for 2 days.

A roentgenogram is taken just after the procedure and another an hour later. If there is a persistent air leak, the distal tip of the drainage valve should be attached to a watersealed drainage system. This one-way system depends on changes in intrapleural pressure to evacuate the pleural space. Negative pressure may be applied to the system if the rate of air leakage is extremely rapid. An Emerson Postoperative Pump is conveniently used, with 25-30 cm. suction water pressure.

The catheter is not used if much fluid or blood is present, except for temporary emergency relief. A recheck x-ray is obtained in 24 hours. If the lung is not fully expanded then, the tube is left in place for 24 hours longer. The catheter is withdrawn as the patient holds his breath in forced expiration.

This procedure is recommended as a reliable expedient for the immediate treatment of any pneumothorax that may present as an emergency in the radiology department.

▶ [Why just the radiology department? Seems as if anesthesiologists might often find use for this technic.—Eds.]

Sensory Polyradiculoneuropathy Following Spinal Anesthesia: A Clinicopathologic Study. Hiroshi Tsukagoshi, Haruki Mori, Akira Enomoto, Kiku Nakao and Noriko Fukushima[8] (Univ. of Tokyo) describe a man with sensory polyradiculoneuropathy involving almost all areas of the body.

Man, 30, underwent appendectomy elsewhere with spinal anesthesia with 0.3% dibucaine in 5% saline. Headache and dizziness occurred at operation and persisted afterward. Two or 3 days later,

(8) Neurology 20:266-274, March, 1970.

weakness and paresthesias appeared in the distal part of the lower limbs, with hypalgesia and thermohypesthesia of the body and extremities. He was discharged 10 days after operation with mucous diarrhea with tenesmus and occasional incontinence.

About a month later, he was admitted to this institution. Tonic pupils, dysarthria and dysphagia, impaired sensation in most areas of the body, hypohidrosis and an ataxic gait were noted. Deep tendon reflexes were abolished in the upper and lower limbs. Cerebrospinal fluid was under normal pressure and contained 60 mg. protein per ml. An EEG and electromyogram were normal.

At a subsequent admission about 2 years later, bradylalic speech and reduced muscle tone were noted. Hypohidrosis, impotence, diarrhea and bladder disturbance persisted. The patient was found dead about 5½ years after operation.

Autopsy showed cardiac dilatation and moderate pulmonary edema. Nerve cells in the cerebral cortex and putamen were ischemic and shrunken. Leptomeningeal thickening was noted in various areas. In the cervical cord, the bilateral posterior funiculi showed demyelination and atrophy. Lissauer's tract could not be identified. The dorsal roots showed prominent demyelination and fibrosis. Similar changes were found at lower cord levels. In the cauda equina, about half of the nerve fiber bundles were severely disintegrated and scarred. All dorsal root ganglions examined showed severe degeneration of nerve cells and fibers. The sciatic nerve showed disintegration of myelin sheaths and swollen axis cylinders. Nerve cells in the ganglia of the sympathetic trunk were disintegrated; nerve fibers showed marked degeneration. The brachial and quadriceps muscles were normal.

Neurologic complications of spinal anesthesia appear to be infrequent except for aggravation of coincidental disorders. A lesion of the dorsal root ganglion and sympathetic ganglion has rarely been reported. The present case is attributed to a toxic effect of dibucaine.

▶ [Can we really attribute this to dibucaine?—Eds.]

Electrocautery Simulating a Laboratory Effect of Myocardial Infarction. J. W. Mostert, R. J. Trudnowski, G. H. Hobika, R. Rico and R. Moore[9] (Roswell Park Mem'l Inst.), having recently found that serum creatine phosphokinase (CPK) is elevated within 7 hours postoperatively after electrocautery of bleeding tissues, obtained results beyond 7 hours. Venous blood was taken for CPK determination before and 7, 24 and 48 hours after operation in patients having major cancer surgical procedures. Thirteen patients had electrocoagulation of bleeding tissues, 9 at thoracotomy and 4 at abdominoperineal resection of the rectum, and 15 patients did not have electrocautery. Drugs that might affect the serum CPK such as succinylcholine were

(9) J. Med. 1:188-191, 1970.

not used. Anesthesia was with droperidol, fentanyl, diazepam, nitrous oxide or intermittent tubocurarine and meperidine.

All patients who had electrocautery had a marked rise in CPK within 6 hours after operation. Peak levels occurred at 24 hours and were quantitatively indistinguishable from those expected after myocardial infarction. Control patients showed only the expected mild rise in serum CPK activity after operation.

Electrocoagulation causes marked elevation of serum CPK activity, indistinguishable temporally and in magnitude from that associated with myocardial infarction. The rise is apparently related to the amount of energy of the electric discharge in muscle tissue. Leakage of CPK in itself does not necessarily indicate necrosis; severe exercise causes elevation of serum CPK.

▶ [Very interesting and worth keeping in the back of one's mind.—Eds.]

Operating Room Temperature and Anesthetized, Paralyzed Patient. Roger H. Morris[1] (Harvard Med. School) sought a correlation between room temperature and body temperature after anesthesia and examined the effect of time on the relation between ambient and body temperatures. Esophageal and room temperatures were measured during 25 intra-abdominal and 20 extra-abdominal operations in patients aged 20-85 years. The skin was prepared with hexachlorophene, isopropyl alcohol and distilled water, followed by ether. Draping was with four thicknesses of cotton. Patients were anesthetized with endotracheal nitrous oxide-oxygen, supplemented by 1-3% ether, 0.5-0.75% halothane, 0.3-0.5% methoxyflurane, or a narcotic. They were paralyzed with tubocurarine or gallamine, and mechanically ventilated. Temperatures were measured at 15-minute intervals during operation.

The mean oral temperature preoperatively was 36.9 C. Room and esophageal temperatures were significantly correlated 1, 2 and 3 hours after anesthetic induction. All patients became hypothermic in rooms at 17-21 C., compared with 30% at 21-24 C., whereas at 24-26 C. all patients remained normothermic. At 18-21 C., the mean body temperature fell significantly to 35.6 C. in the 1st hour of anesthesia and fell further to 35.3 C. at 2 hours. A further drop of 0.1 C. occurred in the 3d hour. At 21-24 C., the mean body temperature fell significantly to 36.2 C. in the 1st hour and then remained stable.

(1)   Arch. Surg. 102:95-97, February, 1971.

Findings were similar in patients undergoing intra- and extra-abdominal operations, and no significant differences were found with different anesthetic agents.

The greatest fall in body temperature occurs in the 1st hour of anesthesia and operation. Patients in rooms at below 21 C. will almost always become hypothermic unless the procedure is brief. Falls in temperature of as little as 0.3 C. may be followed by postoperative shivering and increased cardiorespiratory demands. Operating room temperatures should be kept at 21-24 C. (70-75 F.). In rooms colder than 21 C., patients should be warmed with heating blankets and/or fluid warmers. Body temperature should be monitored during all major operations.

▶ [How often have you heard the patient complain of the cold temperature of the operating room as he moves from litter to operating table?—Eds.]

Septicemia from Intravenous Infusions. Hospital-acquired infections associated with therapeutic equipment occur almost daily in "modern" general hospitals. Ventilatory equipment, urinary tract drainage tubes and indwelling intravenous catheters have been implicated in such infections. Richard J. Duma, John F. Warner and Harry P. Dalton[2] (Med. College of Virginia) documented another source that may be common, intravenous fluids and volume-control sets. Study of a fatal case of escherichia septicemia showed the same organism in an infusion set, and 2 other patients with similar infections were recalled. All these patients had been "toxic," with multiple positive blood cultures. All improved after intravenous infusions were removed. All intravenous infusion sets in use were then inspected and cultured in 27 wards caring for 553 patients. The commonest devices used are the Abbott SOLUSET-100 and Additive SOLUSET. Forty unused sets and 40 unused liter bottles of fluids were also tested for sterility.

Of 68 sets used in 63 patients, 35% were contaminated; they had been used in 24 patients on 15 wards. Of the contaminating organisms, 60% were gram-negative bacilli. Most contaminated sets were considered to be in unsatisfactory working condition. The commonest defects were loose or absent air filters and dirty medication injection sites. Most uncontaminated sets were also in unsatisfactory condition. Contaminated sets had been used continuously for an average of 4.4 days, compared with 2 days for uncontaminated sets. Positive cultures were obtained in 10% of unused bottles of fluid and in 12% of unpackaged SOL-

(2)   New England J. Med. 284:257-260, Feb. 4, 1971.

USETs. A patient with serratia septicemia was found; the infection was definitely related to a contaminated infusion. A probable relation was found in another patient, with candida fungemia.

Contamination occurs after packaged materials are opened and used. Contamination occurs at the level of the bottle screw cap. Many "breaks" in aspetic technic for changing volume-control sets and fluid bottles were identified. The design of the sets also appeared to abet contamination. Location of medication injection sites and air filters on the cylinders of sets is not ideal. It is unclear why contaminants consist predominantly of gram-negative bacilli.

▶ [Since publication of this article, much has appeared in the medical and lay press regarding the problems with Abbott Laboratories' intravenous infusion fluids and sets. The screw cap system was the main fault. Abbott Laboratories has withdrawn this type of set from the market. Regardless of the particular fault, an editorial comment bears repeating: ". . . the principal impact of the Duma report is to remind all concerned with intravenous therapy that asepsis must be maintained with near religious fervor, that there are no foolproof systems that permit the disregard of meticulous technic."—Eds.]

Statistical Analysis of Relationship of Physical Status to Postoperative Mortality in 68,388 Cases. Charles J. Vacanti (Naval Hosp., Portsmouth, Va.), Robert J. VanHouten and Robert C. Hill[3] (Nat'l Naval Med. Center, Bethesda, Md.) examined 32 items of data relevant to anesthetic administration in 63,388 procedures performed in eleven Naval hospitals during 1964-66. There were 266 deaths, for a mortality rate of 0.39%. The mortality rate was 0.08 in 50,703 procedures on healthy patients (ASA class I); 0.27% in 12,601 on patients with mild to moderate illness (class II); 1.8% in 3,636 on patients with severe systemic disease (class III); 7.8% in 850 done on patients with incapacitating systemic disease (class IV); and 9.4% in 608 done on moribund patients (class V). Respective mortality rates for elective procedures in these groups ranged from 0.07 up to 8.1%, and for emergency procedures, from 0.16 to 9.5%.

These figures support the generally accepted belief that postoperative mortality increases as physical status declines and that mortality is significantly increased in emergency procedures. Mortality was higher after emergency than after elective operation in all five classes of patients considered in the present analysis. Increased efforts are needed to give every atten-

(3) Anesth. & Analg. 49:564-566, July-Aug., 1970.

tion possible to emergency surgical patients before anesthesia.
▶ [Interesting how similar these data are to those in our 1961 study.—
Eds.]

**Special Committee Investigating Deaths under Anesthesia:
Report on 745 Classified Cases,** 1960-68.[4] Review was made of
deaths associated with anesthesia and operation that occurred
in New South Wales in Australia in 1960-68. Information was
obtained on 1,462 of 1,603 such deaths that occurred in this
period, and of these, 745 were associated closely enough to warrant detailed review. Deaths occurring during or within 24
hours after anesthetic administration were considered. "True"
anesthetic deaths, deaths in which the anesthetic appeared to
have played a role, totaled 286. The number of such deaths declined slightly each year during the review period. Anesthetic
mortality ranked ahead of influenza, childbirth complications
and nonmeningococcic meningitis as a cause of death.

The incidence increased sharply in the later decades of life
(Table 1). Table 2 illustrates the preponderance of emergency
procedures over the elective situations, but nearly 40% of the
deaths occurred in elective situations. The most common operations are shown in Table 3. Just over one third of the true anesthetic deaths occurred outside metropolitan areas. Proportionately more younger patients were involved in country than in
metropolitan institutions. Specialists appeared responsible for
about one quarter of the deaths and non-specialists for about
three fifths of the total. Rural practitioners administered anesthetics in more emergencies than did specialists in metropolitan

TABLE 1.—AGE GROUPS, PERCENTAGE INCIDENCE OF ANESTHETIC MORTALITY
AND INCIDENCE PER 100,000 POPULATION

AGE GROUP (YEARS)	NO. CASES	% OF TOTAL	AVERAGE INCIDENCE (DEATHS PER 100,000 POPULATION PER YEAR)
0- 4	19	7	0.5
5- 9	14	4	0.45
10-19	15	4.5	0.23
20-29	25	9.5	0.45
30-39	20	7	0.4
40-49	23	8	0.5
50-59	32	11	0.87
60-69	51	18	2.0
70-79	59	21	3.6
80-over	28	10	6

(4) M. J. Australia 1:573-594, March 21, 1970.

TABLE 2.—TRUE ANESTHETIC DEATHS (URGENCY OF PROCEDURE)

PROCEDURE	No. CASES	%
Elective	111	39
Emergency	155	54
Indeterminate	20	7
Total	286	100

TABLE 3.—THE 10 COMMONEST PROCEDURES ("TRUE" ANESTHETIC DEATHS)

ORDER	OPERATION	No. CASES	%
1	Intestinal obstruction	37	12.5
2	Laparotomy for peritonitis	24	8.4
3	Cesarean section	11	3.9
4	Appendectomy	11	3.9
5	Laparotomy for hemorrhage	10	3.5
6	Hysterectomy	8	2.5
7	Gastrectomy	8	2.5
8	Forceps delivery	7	2.4
9	Tonsils and adenoids	7	2.4
10	Cholecystectomy	7	2.4
	Cystoscopy	7	2.4

areas. Muscle relaxants contributed to half of the anesthetic deaths in which they were used. Forty deaths were related to the use of ether; 25 patients given open ether died of overdosage. Only 10% of deaths occurred during induction; about one quarter occurred in the postanesthetic period and the rest during anesthesia. A regional technic was used in 12 cases. Nonspecialists were twice as likely as specialists to use dangerously hypoxic gas mixtures. The commonest management errors were listed as incorrect choice of anesthetic technic, inadequate preparation, resuscitation, ventilation, inadequate management of a crisis situation and overdosage.

Errors responsible for anesthetic deaths are due, for the most part, to neglect of established principles of preanesthetic preparation, choice of anesthetic and dosage, intraoperative observation and postoperative care. Anesthetics themselves are not lethal except when used improperly. A committee that studies case data and corresponds confidentially with anesthetists exerts a restraining influence on anesthetic mortality.

▶ [This long, complex article is not easy to understand and even more difficult to abstract. The article contains a wealth of information obtained by a very careful and complete study of each death. The study committee consisted of anesthetists, surgeons, general practitioners and obstetricians and gynecologists. All records provided to the committee were confidential and could not be released.—Eds.]

MUSCLE RELAXANTS AND COMPLICATIONS

Strabismus as a Possible Sign of Latent Muscular Disease Predisposing to Suxamethonium-Induced Muscular Injury. Suxamethonium has been noted occasionally to cause signs of transient muscle injury-myoglobinuria and increased serum creatine phosphokinase (CPK) activity—during halothane anesthesia in ophthalmic patients operated on for strabismus. However, since others noted a lower incidence of increase in CPK values, a high incidence of latent muscle disease in the ophthalmic series was considered.

T. Tammisto, P. Brander, M. M. Airaksinen, V. Tommila and J. Listola[5] (Univ. of Helsinki) studied CPK activity in 23 boys and 9 girls with a mean age of 7.3 years, 9 of whom were anesthetized for dental extractions and 23 for minor plastic procedures. Premedication was with atropine, promethazine and pethidine. Anesthesia was induced with nitrous oxide and halothane. Suxamethonium, 1 mg./kg., was given for tracheal intubation and doses of 0.5 mg./kg. were repeated at intervals of 5-10 minutes to a total of 4 doses (2.5 mg./kg.). Saline or sucrose solution, about 30 ml./kg., was given by infusion. Serum CPK was measured just before anesthesia and 24-28 hours later.

The increase in CPK activity was similar after both types of operation. Males tended to have higher postoperative levels than did females. The highest increase, 126 I.U./L., occurred in association with administration of 300 ml. of whole blood. Three patients had positive Hemastix reactions in postoperative urine, but none had red cells in the urine. In 11 patients, increase in CPK exceeded 10 I.U./L., the median increase being 6.7 I.U./L.

Increases in CPK were about 4 times greater in the previous series of 34 ophthalmic patients operated on for strabismus who were given 4 doses of suxamethonium during halothane-nitrous oxide anesthesia. The increase exceeded 10 I.U./L. in 80% of the strabismus patients, compared with 34% in the present series; the incidence of probable myoglobinuria was 37 and 9%, respectively. The differences were apparent even in patients having thiopentone induction. All 6 patients with complicated strabismus had a clearly abnormal rise in CPK activi-

---

(5)   Ann. Clin. Res. 2:126-130, June, 1970.

ty, and 4 of them had a positive Hemastix test. It is suggested that strabismus may sometimes be a sign of a latent general disturbance of the muscular system, manifested only through muscular overstrain, such as suxamethonium-induced fasciculations during halothane anesthesia.

▶ [Interesting! Is a person with strabismus more likely to acquire myoglobinuria after severe exercise, e.g., running?—Eds.]

New Technics of Measurement of Relaxants and Their Antagonists. Measurements in patients are often made on the small muscles of the hand, which may not necessarily reflect the state of neuromuscular blockade in other muscle groups. Leon Kaufman[6] (Univ. College Hosp., London) describes three technics of assessment.

The effects of depolarizing relaxants were studied during strabismus surgery by attaching the resected muscle by a fine wire to a strain gauge. Intravenous suxamethonium, 25-50 mg., increased tension in the rectus muscle within 25 seconds, the peak tension produced being an increase of 20 Gm. The rise was maintained for 7 minutes. The rise preceded onset of apnea and also outlasted it. Decamethonium produced apnea for 20 minutes and a rise of muscle tension for 24 minutes. Prior administration of tubocurarine failed to prevent the rise in muscle tension.

The effects of neostigmine on the bowel were investigated by measurement of pressure within the ileum with a balloon after ileorectal anastomosis or in established ileostomies. Pressure rose within 1 minute of intravenous injection of 1.2-5 mg. neostigmine. Prior administration of atropine, 0.5 mg., delayed onset of this increase for 10-15 minutes. Halothane anesthesia prevented the pressure response to neostigmine.

The effects of muscle relaxants on intramuscular pressures were studied by means of a 23-gauge needle inserted in the muscle belly. The system is saline-filled and its pressure kept constant by a slow saline drip. The same needle is used to stimulate and to record pressures. The tetanus-twitch ratio was 4:1 (normal) and the refractory period, 2 msec. A dose of 20 mg. gallamine produced marked decreases in pressure, restorable by a burst of tetanus or by neostigmine. Tubocurarine had similar effects. Pancuronium produced an intense neuromuscular blockade. Time-to-peak was reduced by nondepolarizing drugs, which also produced poorly sustained tetanus and post-

(6) Proc. Roy. Soc. Med. 63:696-697, July, 1970.

tetanic facilitation. With decamethonium, tetanus was well sustained. Most of these measurements were made from the extensor forearm muscles, but the intercostal muscles were also examined.

These technics permit a wider variety of muscles to be examined, including those of respiration. The results are constant and immediately available. Studies on the effects of relaxants on time-to-peak are in progress.

▶ [The technics described for measuring the effects of relaxants on eye muscle and on ileal pressure have rather limited application. However, the third technic, in which a small needle is inserted directly into the muscle of interest, appears generally useful. The technic is more complex than the use of a Block-aid stimulator on the ulnar nerve.—Eds.]

Residual Postoperative Paralysis. Many patients have ptosis and nystagmus for several hours after anesthesia in which a nondepolarizing muscle relaxant is used. The extent of ocular diversion is a very sensitive measure of the effects of small amounts of relaxant. J. G. Hannington-Kiff[7] (Royal Infirm., Bristol), with the use of the Maddox wing, which measures the relative position of the eyes in prism diopters, assessed medial rectus tone in 91 patients anesthetized for gynecologic operations. Minor procedures were done in 52 cases, and major ones in 39, the latter lasting about an hour. Premedication was with pethidine and atropine. General anesthesia was induced with thiopentone and, in minor cases, maintained with 1.5-2.0% halothane and nitrous oxide. In major cases; the trachea was intubated after intravenous injection of suxamethonium 0.8 mg./kg., and anesthesia maintained with 0.5% halothane and nitrous oxide. Intravenous gallamine, 1.9 mg./kg., was given, and patients were ventilated at 8-10 L. per minute. Neostigmine and atropine were given at the end of operation.

Greater ocular divergence was found in major than in minor cases in the first 4 postoperative hours, the difference being highly significant. A significant difference persisted at 5-12 hours. Five major cases had appreciable exophoria for the next 2 days. Initially, recovery occurred shortly after anesthesia in both groups, but, in major cases, divergence reappeared within 30 minutes of neostigmine injection. The test was highly sensitive. Patients given tubocurarine, 0.4 mg./kg., had similar findings. Residual divergence appeared to be related to restlessness. Suxamethonium, 0.8 mg./kg., did not lead to residual postoperative paralysis in patients having minor surgical procedures.

(7)   Proc. Roy. Soc. Med. 63:73-76, January, 1970.

Recurarization can occur following neostigmine when its effect wanes in postoperative patients. The Maddox wing may provide a useful means of measuring the rate of decay of drugs used to reverse muscle relaxants. Use of a potent analgesic may be hazardous when patients are kept in the recovery area for only 30 minutes after operation.

► [This is worthwhile clinical observation, which won the author the Registrar's Prize in England.—Eds.]

A New Theory of Termination of Action of Muscle Relaxants is proposed by Stanley A. Feldman and M. F. Tyrrell[8] (Westminster Hosp., London). It has been suggested that the neuromuscular block induced by relaxant drugs results from competition between acetylcholine and curare-like drugs for receptor sites, the point of equilibrium depending on rate of reaction between drug and receptor. The equilibrium dose ratio should then be a constant and the rates of association and dissociation of the same order if entropy in the system is constant. It has been assumed that degree of paralysis depends on the blood and hence the extracellular fluid level of the drug and that reducing this level would reverse the paralysis. The present work suggests that this assumption is not valid in anesthetized human patients.

Anesthesia was induced by thiopentone and maintained with 1% halothane, oxygen and nitrous oxide. The force of adductor pollicis longus contraction was recorded after ulnar nerve stimulation as small doses of the drug were given under tourniquet control.

Results were similar with 3 mg. curare and 8 mg. gallamine; duration of paralysis was over 90 minutes and 23 minutes, respectively. Paralysis induced by 0.5 mg. decamethonium was of short duration. Individual patients had constant 25-75% recovery times with gallamine and curare, although these varied between patients, suggesting that these drugs are strongly bound to the receptor sites. Even when the blood and extracellular fluid curare level is reduced to zero, about 16 minutes are required to reduce the drug receptor occupancy by 10-20%; 10 minutes are required with gallamine. Decamethonium is apparently not bound to the receptor site in this way.

The difference between a depolarizing and a nondepolarizing drug appears to be due principally to the strength of the drug-receptor combination. Drugs bound at the end-plate have an

(8)   Proc. Roy. Soc. Med. 63:692-695, July, 1970.

action that is not ended by reducing the blood level and are curare-like in activity. Drugs that do not form a strong bond with receptor sites will not obstruct access of acetylcholine to the end-plate and act as depolarizing muscle relaxants. A drug like decamethonium could have both modes of action at the myoneural junction. Probably the random release of packets of acetylcholine in normal anesthetized persons causes a slow disruption of the curare-receptor bonding.

These results do not support the concept of dynamic competition between curare and acetylcholine for occupancy of the receptor site. The new theory is summarized as follows: (1) A drug may form a loose receptor complex, resulting in rapid association and dissociation in accord with the extracellular fluid concentration; examples are acetylcholine, decamethonium and suxamethonium. (2) Drugs such as curare may bind with the receptor substance to form a stable complex, preventing access of acetylcholine to the receptor site. (3) Drugs may have a limited ability to form a stable receptor complex. (4) Displacement of drug from the receptor complex by acetylcholine depends on the total quanta of acetylcholine to which the complex has been exposed, not on the acetylcholine concentration present at a given moment.

Heart-Rate Changes after Atropine and Neostigmine Given for Reversion of Muscle Paralysis. M. Kjellberg and T. Tammisto[9] (Univ. of Helsinki) attempted to find the mode of neostigmine-atropine administration with the least effect on pulse rate and cardiac irritability. Study was made of 120 patients with normal cardiovascular function, except for slight hypertension in patients over age 50 years. Premedication consisted of meperidine, 1-1.5 mg./kg., promethazine, 1 mg./kg. up to 50 mg., and atropine, 0.01 mg./kg. Anesthesia was induced with thiopental, and tracheal intubation performed with 50-100 mg. of succinylcholine. d-Tubocurarine was given for subsequent muscle relaxation. Anesthesia was maintained with nitrous oxide and oxygen; meperidine was given when required. Respiration was controlled manually or with a Manley or Bennett ventilator. Patients were given neostigmine, 0.03 mg./kg., and atropine, 0.015 mg./kg., intravenously after all surgical stimuli had ceased and were ventilated with oxygen as the ECG was monitored.

Atropine increased the pulse except when injected slowly im-

(9) Acta anaesth. scandinav. 14:203-210, 1970.

mediately after neostigmine. The increase was more pronounced when atropine was given before neostigmine, and less when it was mixed with neostigmine. The pulse then fell below baseline, least markedly when atropine was given just after neostigmine. The most marked drop in pulse rate occurred when atropine was given 10 minutes before neostigmine. Rapid pulse rates tended to decrease more than slow ones. Arrhythmias occurred in all groups. Two cases of cardiac standstill lasting 2-4 seconds occurred when neostigmine was given 2 minutes before atropine, as did three episodes of 1:2 A-V block and one of wandering pacemaker. These arrhythmias were transient and occurred $1\frac{1}{2}$-$2\frac{1}{2}$ minutes after the start of neostigmine injection.

Both atropine and neostigmine may cause seriously disturbed cardiac action when the CO_2 tension is increased or when cardiovascular disease is present. Otherwise the mode of antidote administration does not seem to be crucial when neostigmine is preceded by atropine, when both drugs are given together or when neostigmine is followed immediately by atropine. It is not clear whether the actions of these drugs on other autonomic functions are similar to that on cardiac function.

▶ [A nice study that says atropine is important, it probably should be given simultaneously with neostigmine, but one must continue proper ventilation.—Eds.]

Reversal of Curarization with Atropine-Neostigmine Mixture in Patients with Congenital Cardiac Disease. Because of reports of cardiac arrest and arrhythmia after neostigmine injection, anesthetists have been reluctant to reverse the effects of tubocurarine in patients with cardiovascular disease. Information regarding reversal of curarization in infants and children with heart disease is lacking. M. R. Salem, L. B. Ylagan, J. J. Angel, V. S. Vedam and V. J. Collins[1] (Cook County Hosp.) studied the ECG changes produced during reversal in pediatric patients with congenital heart disease, using a mixture of atropine, 0.02 mg./kg., and neostigmine, 0.05 mg./kg. Study was made of 41 patients, aged 5-days to 13 years (including 18 in the 1st year of life) having operations for various congenital cardiac abnormalities. Open heart procedures were done with bypass in 12 patients. Patients below age 1 year received only hyoscine for premedication; others received morphine as well. Anesthesia was induced with thiopental or halothane-nitrous oxide, and

(1)   Brit. J. Anaesth. 42:991-998, November, 1970.

maintenance was with 0.4-0.5% halothane in oxygen. Intermittent doses of tubocurarine were given as needed. The trachea of all patients were intubated. Reversal was carried out after halothane was discontinued as lead II of the ECG was monitored.

Injection of atropine and neostigmine increased the heart rate slightly, with a peak of 148 a minute after the injection. The initial heart rate was significantly correlated negatively with the maximal increase in rate. The rise in rate was less in cyanotic than in acyanotic patients after injection of the reversal mixture. Twelve patients showed ECG changes during reversal. Three had a change from normal sinus rhythm to an abnormal rhythm; 6 changes from an abnormal to normal sinus rhythm just after reversal; and 3 had continued abnormal rhythm or a change to a different abnormal rhythm during the period of reversal.

Routine reversal of curarization with atropine and neostigmine does not appear to have any particular hazards for pediatric cardiac patients. Reversal should not be withheld for fear of dangerous cardiac arrhythmias. However, many factors influence the termination of curarization, especially in patients with heart disease, and these must be carefully considered before patients are permitted to breathe spontaneously.

▶ [There were 14 cyanotic patients in this study, and 3 of these had temporary, abnormal rhythms after reversal. If one has to use curare in these patients, the method outlined appears to be a good one. One must question the necessity of using curare in the first place if a potent volatile agent is the primary agent.—Eds.]

Sympathomimetic Effect of Gallamine on the Heart. Gallamine is a widely used neuromuscular blocking drug which, like *d*-tubocurarine, is a quaternary ammonium compound belonging to the group of nondepolarizing competitive antagonists of acetylcholine. Burnell R. Brown, Jr., and J. Richard Crout[2] (Univ. of Texas Southwestern Med. School) found that gallamine has a sympathomimetic effect on guinea pig atrium in vitro and on cat ventricle in vitro and in vivo, mediated by the release of norepinephrine from adrenergic nerve endings. In vitro studies were conducted on electrically driven guinea pig left atria, paced at a rate of 60 beats per minute at just above threshold. Cat atria and right ventricular papillary muscles were also examined. The effects of gallamine were studied in cats, with opened chests, anesthetized with pentobarbital.

---

(2) J. Pharmacol. & Exper. Therap. 172:266-273, April, 1970.

Stretched guinea pig ileal segments were also exposed to gallamine. The uptake of norepinephrine-^{3}H by guinea pig atrium was determined.

Gallamine increased the cardiac rate and contractile force of guinea pig and cat atria in vitro. The heart rate and right ventricular contractile force were increased in vivo in the cat. Positive inotropic responses to the drug were inhibited in vitro by 2×10^{-6}M propranolol and in vivo by pretreatment with propranolol in a 0.5 mg./kg. dose. Guinea pig atria pretreated with reserpine failed to respond to gallamine or responded only poorly. The positive inotropic response of guinea pig atria in vitro was not inhibited by 1×10^{-7}M atropine, 1×10^{-4}M d-tubocurarine, 1×10^{-5}M hexamethonium or 2.9×10^{-5}M cocaine.

Tachyphylaxis to gallamine developed rapidly in vitro and could be reversed by exposure to 1×10^{-7}M norepinephrine for 10 minutes. Cross-tachyphylaxis did not occur between gallamine and tyramine. Gallamine, 5×10^{-4}M, did not inhibit the initial uptake of labeled norepinephrine by guinea pig atria in vitro.

Gallamine releases norepinephrine from adrenergic nerve endings in the heart by an unidentified mechanism that is not identical to that of tyramine, nicotine or bretylium. The sympathomimetic effect of gallamine on the heart explains the cardiac arrhythmias and increased cardiac output that may accompany use of the drug during clinical anesthesia.

▶ [Would gallamine administration to patients receiving monoamine oxidase inhibitors be hazardous?—Eds.]

Effects of Modern Intravenous Local Analgesics on Respiration during Partial Neuromuscular Block in Man. Local analgesia given intravenously after operation causes respiratory depression in some patients. These agents may increase the action of neuromuscular blocking drugs. Direct respiratory center depression is also possible. L. Telivuo (Helsinki Univ.) and R. L. Katz[3] (Columbia-Presbyterian Med. Center) attempted to determine the relative importance of these two effects by recording the degree of neuromuscular block and tidal volume in patients with partial block given local analgesics intravenously.

Study was made of 44 anesthetized patients preoperatively. Only atropine was given for premedication. Anesthesia was induced with thiopentone and maintained with halothane,

---

(3)   Anaesthesia 25:30-35, January, 1970.

0.5-0.7 vol.%, and nitrous oxide-oxygen in a nonrebreathing system. Thumb adduction was measured on ulnar nerve stimulation. Tidal volume was measured with a pneumotachograph and electromanometer and with a Wright respirometer. Partial neuromuscular block was induced by injecting 2 mg. nortoxiferine (Alloferin) intravenously; another 2-3 mg. was injected if needed. Local analgesic was then injected into the basilic vein. Mepivacaine, bupivacaine, lignocaine and prilocaine were tested; bupivacaine was given in a dose of 0.75 mg./kg. and the other agents, in a dose of 3 mg./kg.

A total of 3-5 mg. nortoxiferine was given, reducing twitch amplitude to 14-96% of the original value. The analgesics reduced the amplitude only slightly more; the mean drop from pre-nortoxiferine levels was 5-8%. The mean drop in tidal volume was 23.7-40.2%. The fall was greatest in patients given lignocaine and least in those given bupivacaine. The longest depressant effect was after bupivacaine and lignocaine and the shortest after mepivacaine and prilocaine. Changes in end-tidal CO_2 levels corresponded to changes in tidal volume. All the parameters returned to normal in 2-9 minutes. No side effects were noted.

The local analgesics tested produced only a small further decrease in twitch height, but a marked drop often occurred in the respiratory tidal voulme. The major cause of respiratory depression was the central nervous system depressant action of the analgesics. If patients are given local analgesics as antiarrhythmic agents in the immediate postoperative period, respiration should be carefully monitored.

▶ [It should go without saying that one must monitor carefully all vital functions when treating arrhythmias, but there is a tendency to treat the oscilloscope and ignore the patient in the process. The acidosis resulting from depressed respiration would nullify any benefit from the antiarrhythmic drug injected.—Eds.]

Systemic Reaction to Succinylcholine: Case Report. Carl Redderson, Haven M. Perkins, W. H. Adler and J. S. Gravenstein[4] describe a patient in whom sustained hypotension, erythema and muscle tenderness that followed succinylcholine injection were attributed to a rare hypersensitivity reaction to this drug.

Man, 50, admitted for repair of a recurrent hernia, had had two previous operations with succinylcholine within a week of each other 3 years previously and had had urticara and erythemia after spinal anesthesia, attributed to morphine. Examination showed no

    (4)   Anesth. & Analg. 50:49-52, Jan.-Feb., 1971.

abnormalities. Pentobarbital and atropine were given an hour before induction of anesthesia with thiopental. A dose of 80 mg. succinylcholine was given intravenously with more thiopental during 100% oxygen inhalation, and the trachea was intubated, followed by anesthesia with nitrous oxide-oxygen. The patient became flushed immediately after intubation and cutis anserina developed. Blood pressure fell to 40 mm. Hg systolic, where it remained for 20 minutes despite ephedrine, phenylephrine and norepinephrine. The pressure recovered after hydrocortisone was given intravenously. The operation was canceled. Bronchospasm did not develop during the episode. An ECG showed only sinus tachycardia. Spontaneous respirations had reoccurred about 3 minutes after succinylcholine injection. Muscle tenderness was reported in the operating room, subsiding over 5 hours along with the cutaneous flushing. The urine contained 2+ glucose and moderate hemoglobin as well as coarse granular casts and 15 red blood cells per high-power field. Serum histamine was normal.

Skin tests and chemical studies of blood and urine provided no explanation of this episode. Isolation of leukocytes and their challenge in culture with succinylcholine a week after the episode showed significantly greater incorporation of labeled thymidine than control leukocytes or than the patient's leukocytes taken a month after the episode. The reaction was attributed to hypersensitivity to succinylcholine. This drug has a low degree of immunogenicity; the patient's response was idiosyncratic.

▶ [It is unfortunate that a comparison of the effect of thiopental on thymidine incorporation by leukocytes was not also performed since the patient's response was temporarily related to administration of that drug as well.—Eds.]

Effect of Gallamine on Cholinergic Receptors. Flora J. Rathbun and John T. Hamilton[5] (Univ. of Western Ontario) sought a true antiacetylcholine action of gallamine on the heart. Studies were done on male rats with doses of propranolol sufficient to block cardiac sympathetic receptors. The antiacetylcholine activity of gallamine was estimated in spontaneously beating, sympathetically blocked hearts. Gallamine was given in doses of 8, 16 and 64 mg./kg. intravenously in saline. Half the rats were pretreated with 1.5 mg. propranolol. Dose-response curves were obtained in rats given 0.125, 0.250 or 1 mg. atropine per kg. without propranolol. Curves were recorded after pretreatment with 4 mg. hexamethonium per kg. and 16 mg. gallamine per kg. or 0.250 mg. atropine per kg. Cats were given 1, 4 or 16 mg. gallamine per kg., with or without 2 mg. atropine per kg. and 1 mg. propranolol per kg. Some cats also were pre-

---

(5) Canad. Anaesth. Soc. J. 17:574-590, November, 1970.

treated with 4 mg. hexamethonium per kg., followed by 2 mg./ kg. every 30 minutes. Propranolol was given in a dose sufficient to reduce the tachycardia induced by 4 μg. isoproterenol to 10% or less. In vitro studies were done on guinea pig ileum and on ileal longitudinal muscle strips, using carbachol as a stimulant, in the presence of 1×10^{-4}M hexamethonium.

Gallamine shifted the acetylcholine dose-response curve to the right in rats. Results were analogous in spinal cat preparations pretreated with gallamine and in spinal cats given atropine. Hexamethonium shifted the control and gallamine curves to the right in pithed rats. This effect was not noted in the spinal cat with control or atropine curves, but hexamethonium shifted the gallamine curve significantly to the left. Gallamine had a very low affinity for gut receptors, compared with atropine. Atropine had a greater affinity for gut than for cardiac receptors.

The antiacetylcholine activity of gallamine on the heart fulfills many of the requirements for competitive antagonism. If atropine acts on the acetylcholine receptor competitively, gallamine likely does also. Anticholinergic actions of gallamine on the heart were noted in both species with doses necessary for muscle relaxation, and a true atropine-like action may complement any sympathomimetic action of gallamine in producing the tachycardia seen clinically.

Succinylcholine-Induced Hyperkalemia in Neuromuscular Disease. Transient hyperkalemia follows succinylcholine administration to anesthetized patients, and the rise may be marked, leading to serious cardiac arrhythmias, in patients with burns or extensive soft tissue injury. Lee H. Cooperman[6] (Univ. of Pennsylvania) studied 37 patients having general anesthesia for various operations. Most had hemiplegia after a stroke or paraplegia secondary to spinal cord injury or tumor. Nine had multiple sclerosis, Parkinson's disease or muscular dystrophy.

Anesthetics included secobarbital and atropine for premedication, thiopental for induction and nitrous oxide with either halothane or methoxyflurane, given in a semiclosed system. Succinylcholine was given intravenously 10-15 minutes after induction in a dose of 1 mg./kg. Four patients had a second general anesthetic for a later operation; at that time, 6 mg. tubo-

---

(6) J.A.M.A. 213:1867-1871, Sept. 14, 1970.

curarine was given intravenously 5 minutes before succinylcholine.

Increases in plasma potassium after succinylcholine was given ranged up to 6 mEq./L.; the peak levels occurred 3 minutes after injection and dropped after 7 minutes. Of the 15 patients with a rise of 1 mEq./L. or more, 13 had muscle paralysis preoperatively, and 9 had had neuromuscular disease for less than a year. Patients with low potassium levels had been ill longer and often had less muscle involvement.

The patient with the largest rise in potassium had ventricular fibrillation. More often when plasma potassium levels were increased, the height of the T wave was increased. Sometimes the QRS was widened. Blood pressure and heart rate did not change significantly during hyperkalemia except in the patient with ventricular fibrillation. The 4 patients who had a second general anesthetic all had tubocurarine therapy before succinylcholine; all had a smaller rise in potassium after succinylcholine.

Neuromuscular disease is another condition in which succinylcholine may cause hyperkalemia. Susceptibility seems to occur within the first 6 months after the acute onset of hemiplegia or paraplegia and to extend longer in patients with progressive disease. Skeletal muscle apears to be the source of potassium. Tubocurarine will moderate the rise in potassium caused by succinylcholine.

▶ [This article confirms and extends the previous work of Tobey in service-connected spinal injuries.—Eds.]

Neuromuscular Blocking Action of Pancuronium in Man during Anesthesia. J. Norman, R. L. Katz and R. F. Seed[7] (Royal Postgrad. Med. School, London) studied the degree and rate of onset of neuromuscular blockade induced by pancuronium, the duration of blockade and the effects of repeated doses. Most patients were premedicated with atropine or hyoscine, pethidine or papaveretrum and, occasionally, droperidol. Anesthesia was induced with thiopentone and maintained with nitrous oxide and halothane. Suxamethonium was used for tracheal intubation. Pancuronium was not given until the twitch response had returned to its maximum after suxamethonium. Ventilation was usually controlled, with a $Paco_2$ of about 30 mm. Hg. Pancuronium was given intravenously. The ulnar

(7)   Brit. J. Anaesth. 42:702-710, August, 1970.

nerve was stimulated at supramaximal intensity and at twitch rates of one pulse every 3-4 seconds; tetanic stimulation was also applied and thumb adduction force recorded.

The mean time from injection of pancuronium, 0.02 mg./kg., to the first effect in 14 patients was 1.3 minutes, with a peak effect occurring 4.5 minutes later. The block averaged 68%. The mean 50 and 90% recovery times from the time of first effect were 12.2 and 23.0 minutes, respectively. A dose of 0.05 mg./kg. was effective in 0.7 minute, with a mean time to peak effect of 2.7 minutes. The average block was 99%. The average 50% recovery times was 36.8 minutes. Complete block was produced by a dose of 0.1 mg./kg. when no suxamethonium was administered. In 3 patients, the twitch response was visible from 46 to 80 minutes after the onset of drug action. Repeated doses of pancuronium produced a greater duration of action and a somewhat greater intensity of block. Respiratory acidemia occurred during recovery from the drug; respiratory alkalemia increased the rate of recovery. The effects of pancuronium, 0.02 mg./kg., were about the same as those of tubocurarine, 0.1 mg./kg., noted in a previous study.

New Steroid Muscle Relaxant: Dacuronium—NB 68. S. A. Feldman and M. F. Tyrrell[8] (London) report preliminary experience with a new steroid muscle relaxant, dacuronium bromide, similar in structure to pancuronium bromide. The drug is a nondepolarizing agent, its action being completely reversed by neostigmine. It does not release histamine significantly in animals and has weak anticholinesterase activity. Studies with subparalytic doses in conscious subjects indicated that the drug is slightly weaker than gallamine. A preliminary study in surgical patients confirmed that the drug is a nondepolarizing relaxant. A clinical trial was conducted in 30 patients, 28 having abdominal operations and 2, endoscopy. Anesthesia was induced with thiopental. Tracheal intubation was facilitated with suxamethonium in all but 5 patients. Patients were moderately hyperventilated with 0.5% halothane, nitrous oxide and oxygen. When spontaneous ventilation returned, 2-2.2 mg. dacuronium per kg. was given intravenously. Atropine, 1.2 mg., was given with 2.5 mg. neostigmine near the end of the procedure.

Dacuronium was marginally weaker than gallamine, in a ratio of 1.2:1. The 25-75% recovery time for the two drugs did not differ greatly. The drugs showed no difference in respira-

---

(8)   Anaesthesia 25:349-355, July, 1970.

tory muscle "sparing" effect. Adequate muscle relaxation was always obtained. Drug effects were completely reversed by 2.5 mg. neostigmine. No patient reported muscle weakness or postoperative diplopia. Relaxation lasted 10-40 minutes. Second doses showed a cumulative effect. The largest total dose given was 220 mg. in 3 hours. Tachycardia developed in 24 patients, without consistent blood pressure change. The average pulse rate rise was 18.5 beats per minute.

Dacuronium is a nondepolarizing muscle relaxant with clinical effects similar to those of gallamine. It does not release histamine or cause marked changes in blood pressure. Like gallamine, it has vagolytic properties.

▶ [Seems to offer little if any improvement over gallamine.—Eds.]

ENDOTRACHEAL TECHNICS AND COMPLICATIONS

Nasal Endotracheal Intubation by External Visual Technic is described by Jay Jacoby[9] (Philadelphia). The term "blind" seems appropriate for attempted passage of an endotracheal tube through the nose. Patients may be made hyperpneic in a light plane of anesthesia to "suck the tube in," or the neck may be flexed during light anesthesia to make the patient take a deep breath on release of the obstruction. Most anesthesiologists cannot reliably intubate patients by these methods. Nasal hemorrhages may occur. The nasal route may be indicated to avoid interference by the tube in the operative field. The tube is anchored more securely and is better tolerated when the patient wakens from anesthesia. There are specific advantages to blind insertion of the nasotracheal tube, and these pertain particularly to the avoidance of laryngoscopy. Each of these may constitute an indication to use the technic. Indications include inability to open the mouth, dental difficulties, avoidance of head or neck movement, contraindication of muscle relaxants and a need for airway protection until the patient is fully awake.

A new technic of nasotracheal intubation has been used for 15 years and taught to residents, who can easily achieve 80% success. Wherever the tube impinges internally, a slight movement is noted at the overlying skin, and rotation of the external

(9)   Anesth. & Analg. 49:731-739, Sept.-Oct., 1970.

portion permits guidance of the tube into the larynx. A full-length tube with a rounded tip, with or without a cuff, is used. Anesthesia is induced with repeated small doses of intravenous barbiturate. Tubocurarine is not required. The nose is sprayed with 4-10% cocaine solution. Denitrogenation is carried out, followed by tracheal intubation. The oral route is used if undue pressure is required to pass a nasal tube. The patient breathes spontaneously throughout the procedure. If there is difficulty, he breathes oxygen through the tube. The breath sounds are not used in guiding the tube. The tube is advanced swiftly at the vocal cord level. Conscious patients can be intubated in this way with the repeated use of local anesthesia. Trauma is rare if gentleness is exercised. Laryngeal spasm is very infrequent. Hoarseness and sore throat are slightly more frequent postoperatively than after orotracheal intubation.

Nasotracheal intubation has been found to be especially useful where laryngoscopy would be traumatic or very difficult, and where an orotracheal tube would not be well tolerated on emergence from anesthesia or coma. The technic is useful in patients whose jaws are wired, or who have had such operations as radical neck resection that require bulky dressings about the neck. Transillumination may be used as an aid in localizing the tip of the tube.

▶ [We suspect many will be surprised to learn that this is a "new" technic. —Eds.]

Blood Gases during Intubation Following Two Types of Oxygenation. During the period of paralysis when an endotracheal tube is being inserted, there is a time when no respiratory exchange occurs. Oxygenation before apnea is produced protects against arterial oxygen desaturation. William L. Cole and V. K. Stoelting[1] (Indiana Univ.) assessed the protection against desaturation gained from two common methods of preoxygenation. Study was made of 37 adults requiring endotracheal anesthesia, aged 16-83 years. Arterial blood was sampled after premedication with morphine and either atropine or scopolamine. Some then breathed 100% oxygen by mask, delivered through a semiclosed-circle absorption system, at flows of 8-10 L. per minute. After $4\frac{1}{2}$ minutes of oxygenation they received thiamylal, 3 mg./kg., intravenously, followed by succinylcholine, 1.5 mg./kg. The other patients received thiamylal and succinylcholine before being hyperventilated with 100% oxygen by

(1)   Anesth. & Analg. 50:68-72, Jan.-Feb., 1971.

mask at a rate of 8 L. per minute for 1 minute. These patients were ventilated 18 times during the oxygenation period. There were 20 patients in the 1-minute-test group and 17 in the 5-minute-test group. No supplemental oxygen was given during tracheal intubation.

The Pao_2 was well above that of room air after 3 minutes of apnea, regardless of the type of oxygenation. The $Paco_2$ was not excessively high nor was arterial pH excessively low in either group. No patient exhibited a base deficit at any time. One patient in the 1-minute group showed a bigeminal rhythm, with a return to normal sinus rhythm shortly after the start of artificial ventilation with 100% oxygen. Poor mask fit and obesity were factors in this case. Hyperventilated patients had a lower $Paco_2$ at the end of oxygenation. The rise in $Paco_2$ was higher in both groups in the first minute of apnea than in succeeding minutes; after the first minute, the rise continued at a rate of about 4 mm. Hg per minute.

With both methods, Pao_2 after 3 minutes of apnea was higher than room-air control levels. The $Paco_2$ was not excessively high during the period without ventilation, and the arterial pH was not excessively low.

▶ [They should have compared a third group breathing 70% N_2O and 30% oxygen. The need for preoxygenation is directly dependent on the facility with which the trachea can be intubated.—Eds.]

Tracheal Rupture, Complication of Cuffed Endotracheal Tube is reported by Svante S. Törnvall, Kenneth H. Jackson and Enrique Oyanedel T.[2] (Univ. of Chile). Tracheal rupture may occur during intubation, especially if a stylet is used. Use of no-return valves that become sticky in the inspiratory position may also cause tracheal or bronchial rupture.

Woman, 49, with biliary colic, was admitted for cholecystectomy. After atropine and meperidine, anesthesia was induced with thiopental and curare, and the trachea was intubated with a cuffed no. 36 Foregger tube without a stylet. Anesthesia was maintained with ether and oxygen. Oxygen was temporarily connected to the deflated cuff of the endotracheal tube after operation. Emphysema of the face and neck appeared at 21 hours and was more marked 2 hours later, when dyspnea, hypertension and cyanosis were evident. Extreme respiratory distress ensued. Fluoroscopy showed 70% right pneumothorax, and two endopleural tubes were inserted, with improvement in the dyspnea and blood pressure. Bronchoscopy showed laceration of the right side of the trachea extending 3 cm. above the carina to 1 cm. below into the right bronchus. The lung was found to be collapsed and pneumomediastinum was present at exploration

(2) Chest 59:237-239, February, 1971.

with high tracheal intubation. A tracheal rupture about 7 cm. long was found, and a flap of pericardial fat was used to cover the suture line. Bronchography 3 months later showed a good tracheal lumen but an irregular right contour. The patient was well a year later, with no respiratory complaints. Bronchography most recently showed megatrachea.

This is an unusual complication of intubation with a cuffed endotracheal tube. The delayed onset of symptoms is attributed to the effects of anesthesia and sedation. Initial air leakage was probably into the pleural space. Hemoptysis is not a reliable sign of tracheal rupture. The diagnosis is confirmed by endoscopy. Tracheostomy may suffice if the rent is small, but drainage and suction are indicated in the presence of penumothorax, and early operation to prevent infection is indicated if the rent is large.

▶ [Daily someone is heard to say, "Now I've heard them all." Oh, really? —Eds.]

Ethylene Oxide Toxicity: Study of Tissue Reactions to Retained Ethylene Oxide. Ethylene oxide is a common sterilizing agent in hospitals. It is very soluble and readily penetrates most porous materials, actually dissolving in some solids, such as rubber and plastics. Shirley R. Andersen[3] (New York Univ.) studied the duration of retention of ethylene oxide in medical materials, and the levels that are toxic to tissues. Specimens used included plasticized polyvinyl chloride tubing with external and internal diameters of 5 and 3 mm, respectively; rubber tubing 6 mm. wide and 1 mm. thick; polyethylene balls 0.5 cm. in diameter; and flat Teflon disks 1 mm. thick and 1 cm. in diameter. Specimens were exposed to pure ethylene oxide at 68-82 F. and atmospheric pressure. Specimens were implanted in mice, and test sites were observed for up to 120 hours. "Blind" studies were done in 11 mice implanted with specimens containing 0.2-2.8 mg. ethylene oxide per gram of polyvinyl chloride or natural rubber.

Large amounts of ethylene oxide were absorbed by polyvinyl chloride tubing, but the gas desorbed quickly. Retained ethylene oxide present at various times after exposure is shown in Figure 15. Natural rubber absorbed less ethylene oxide and eluted the gas more rapidly. Polyethylene and Teflon absorbed very little ethylene oxide. None remained in Teflon specimens in place from $1\frac{1}{2}$ to $3\frac{1}{3}$ hours. Mild reactions to implanted ethylene oxide consisting of slight edema occurred with 2-7.2

(3)   J. Lab. & Clin. Med. 77:346-356, February, 1971.

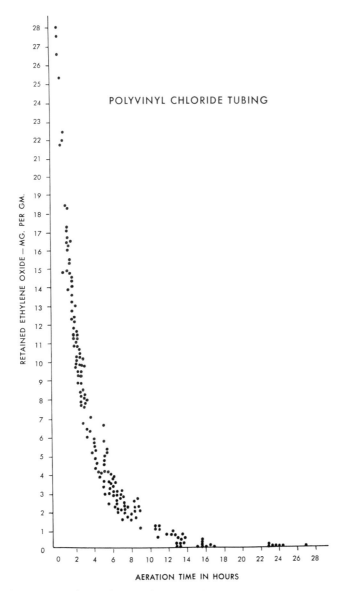

Fig. 15.—Desorption of ethylene oxide retained in polyvinyl chloride tubing. (Courtesy of Andersen, S. R.: J. Lab. & Clin. Med. 77:346-356, February, 1971.)

ethylene oxide per gram of material, whereas moderate reactions occurred with 5.2-8.6 mg. and severe reactions, including edema, necrosis and ulceration, with 5.6-12.2 mg. No reaction occurred with specimens containing less than 2 mg. ethylene oxide per gram. In the "blind" studies, a reaction was seen only with a rubber implant containing 2.8 mg. ethylene oxide per gram. There were notable differences in degree of reaction in individual mice.

Ethylene oxide dissolved in polyvinyl chloride, natural rubber, polyethylene and Teflon diffuses from these materials at a reproducible rate. A number of factors may affect the desorption of ethylene oxide. In the system used in the present study, 24 hours of aeration would provide a generous margin of safety. Little aeration seems to be necessary for polyethylene and Teflon sterilized by this system.

Safe Use of Ethylene Oxide Sterilization in Hospitals. According to L. Rendell-Baker and Robert B. Roberts[4] (Mount Sinai School of Medicine), ethylene oxide sterilization is an effective, reliable method particularly applicable to plastics and rubber, which may be destroyed by heat, and to bulky equipment. The major hazard is inadequate poststerilization aeration, with failure to remove residual ethylene oxide and its byproducts, ethylene glycol and ethylene chlorhydrin, which are highly irritating to tissues. Typical conditions for effective ethylene oxide sterilization are 3 or 4 hours' exposure at 120-135 F. and over 50% relative humidity. Maximum tolerable levels of the residuals are not known, and every effort must be made to remove them completely.

Polyvinyl chloride plastics and rubber materials sterilized with ethylene oxide, if stored at room temperature, should not be used for at least a week. Two days suffice for plastics such as polyethylene and polypropylene. The time for elimination is reduced to 12 hours if plastic and rubber items are aerated at 122-140 F. after ethylene oxide sterilization. Polyethylene wrap is satisfactory for packaging and protects the sterility of products if it remains intact. Nylon film and polyvinyl chloride wrap should not be used. Any polyvinyl chloride sterilized by gamma-irradiation should never be treated with ethylene oxide. Visible water droplets should be wiped off equipment before sterilization to avoid formation of persistent ethylene glycol. Biologic indicators, such as paper strips impregnated with Bacillus ste-

(4)   Anesth. & Analg. 49:919-921, Nov.-Dec., 1970.

arothermophilis or B. subtilis, should be used with ethylene oxide sterilization, at least for spot testing.

Use of disposable items presterilized by the manufacturers should be encouraged in all areas of the hospital, especially in intensive care areas. Sterility of the equipment used on and in patients is vital and must be beyond suspicion.

Vocal Cord Paralysis after Tracheal Intubation is reported by H. Steele Holley and James E. Gildea[5] (Northwestern Univ.) in 4 patients. Tracheal intubation at anesthesia is relatively safe, but laryngeal complications may follow intubation, although they are usually transient and minor. A few cases of vocal cord paralysis after endotracheal anesthesia have been reported previously.

Man, 45, underwent craniotomy for a frontal lobe mass. He had had poliomyelitis at age 1, with no apparent sequelae. Anesthesia was inducted with thiopental and maintained with halothane and 50% nitrous oxide and oxygen. Succinylcholine chloride was given after curare, with two additional doses of 40 mg. because of inadequate relaxation. The trachea was intubated with a no 36 polyethylene tube, and reintubated with a no. 38 cuffed tube after the cuff on the first tube leaked. The procedure lasted 6 hours. Marked inspiratory stridor and inability to say "E" were noted an hour postoperatively. A nasotracheal tube was inserted, and 40% oxygen was given with a heated aerosol. The patient vomited and dislodged the tube about 6 hours later. The lungs were ventilated using a bag and mask, and an oral endotracheal tube was inserted. A tracheostomy was done the next day. Mirror examination showed a 2- to 3-mm. glottic chink and no movement of the slightly edematous cords on phonation. The patient died of his disease 27 days after tracheostomy. At autopsy, portions of the vagus nerves showed myelin degeneration, of undetermined cause.

The usual cause of vocal cord paralysis after neck surgery is direct injury to one or both recurrent laryngeal nerves by severing or stretching them. The commonest cord position after bilateral injury is in the midline. Bilateral cord paralysis does not appear to be related to the duration of intubation. The endotracheal tubes used in the 4 cases all were polyethylene, with a latex rubber cuff. All tubes had been sterilized with a mixture of 12% ethylene oxide and 88% dichlorodifluoromethane. The vocal cords showed minimal inflammation and no edema or ulceration in all 4 cases. In only 1 case was the head turned to the side during operation. All intubations were done with the neck extended using a curved Macintosh blade.

Cord paralysis is a rare but potentially dangerous complica-

(5) J.A.M.A. 215:281-284, Jan. 11. 1971.

tion of intubation. The usual methods of treating upper airway obstruction are ineffective, but assisted ventilation provides immediate relief. Often tracheal intubation followed by elective tracheostomy is necessary.

▶ [Sounds like the ethylene oxide was responsible.—Eds.]

MONITORING

Reliability of Central Venous Pressure as an Indicator of Left Atrial Pressure: Study in Patients with Mitral Valve Disease. Central venous pressure measurement has been used extensively to guide the treatment of critically ill patients. Its clinical usefulness depends on the relation between the left and right atrial pressure. Hubert Bell, David Stubbs and David Pugh[6] (Univ. of Kansas) studied the relation of central venous pressure to left atrial pressure in 200 consecutive patients with mitral valve disease who underwent cardiac catheterization. The series included patients with relatively pure mitral stenosis or mitral insufficiency and patients with "mixed" mitral valve disease, but those with associated aortic or tricuspid valve disease were excluded. A left atrial catheter was introduced transseptally. A significant rise in atrial pressure was induced by transvenous pacing, isoproterenol infusion, phenylephrine or volume expansion in 25 patients. The catheter was withdrawn into the right atrium as pressures were monitored; pulmonary artery pressure was also continuously recorded. The rise in left atrial pressure was sustained for at least 15 minutes. Volume expansion was achieved using 5% dextrose in water. Pacing was done at a rate of 100-150 per minute from the right atrium or right ventricle. Isoproterenol was infused at a rate of 5-10 μg. per minute and phenylephrine in a total dose of 2-3 mg. over 5-10 minutes.

The correlation coefficient of left and right atrial pressure was 0.48. Right atrial pressure equaled 0.228 of left atrial pressure. Four patients with a markedly elevated left atrial pressure had a low right atrial pressure, as did 18 with a left atrial pressure of 20 mm. Hg or greater. Three patients with a left atrial pressure of 12 mm. Hg or less had a right atrial pressure of 8 mm. Hg or higher. Mean pulmonary artery pressure was ele-

(6) Chest 59:169-173, February, 1971.

vated in all but 1 of 91 patients with a left atrial pressure of 20 mm. Hg or higher. The correlation coefficient of left atrial and mean pulmonary artery pressure was 0.70. The mean pulmonary artery pressure equaled 1.23 of left atrial pressure. No consistent pattern of right atrial or pulmonary artery pressure change was noted in response to a left atrial pressure rise. Sixteen patients had a rise in right atrial pressure with a rise in left atrial pressure, but 4 of these had a left atrial pressure rise of 10 mm. Hg or more associated with a rise in right atrial pressure of 1 mm. Hg or less.

It would be ideal if left atrial pressure could be monitored in critically ill patients, but technical difficulties make this impractical for most patients. The baseline left atrial pressure and right atrial pressure are poorly correlated; significant differences btween these pressures may occur in 20% of the cases. Rapid changes in left atrial pressure induced by various means may not be reflected in right atrial or pulmonary artery pressure changes. The baseline mean pulmonary artery pressure may be useful in predicting left atrial pressure. If the mean pulmonary pressure is not elevated, left atrial pressure is probably normal or only slightly elevated.

▶ [The limitations of central venous pressure monitoring are well documented here.—Eds.]

Aid to Central Venous Pressure Measurement is described by M. J. Notaras[7] (London). The most difficult problem in measuring the central venous pressure serially is ensuring that the baseline on the scale of the saline manometer is at the same level as the reference point on the patient. A horizontal "gun sight" or carpenter's spirit level is not always available. The author has used a simple, inexpensive apparatus consisting of an 8-ft. length of plastic tubing held in a U-tube fashion and filled with colored alcohol for about a third of its length (Fig. 16). By making a ring of tubing, the device can be used at any time without spilling the fluid. One part of the loop is held parallel to the manometer and its opposite to the reference point on the patient (Fig. 17). By raising and lowering the loops, the fluid level is brought to the reference point, and the baseline on the manometer scale is established. To save further adjustments when making serial readings, the tubing may be fixed to the patient and the manometer.

This system is a simple, portable one that is easily readjusted

(7)   Lancet 1:214, Jan. 30, 1971.

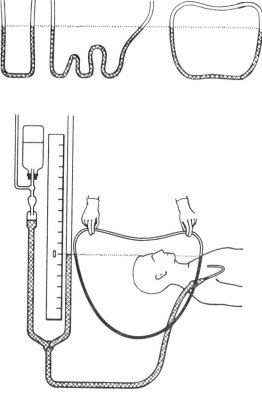

Fig. 16 (top).—Hydrostatic characteristics of tubes.
Fig. 17 (bottom).—Tube in use.
(Courtesy of Notaras, M. J.: Lancet 1:214, Jan. 30, 1971.)

with changes in patient posture and provides calibration of a central venous pressure manometer.

► [The constancy of the reference is an important point.—Eds.]

Dangers of Catheterization of Superior Vena Cava with Particular Consideration of Infraclavicular Entry. A. Fassolt, U. Braun and M. Graber[8] observe that despite the inherent danger of complications, the overriding value of caval catheterization determines its increasing popularity. A survey of 6,000 catheterizations (reported by 20 authors) revealed a mean rate of serious complications of 1.35%, with 7 fatalities. The most fre-

(8)   Helvet. chir. acta 37:18-22, April, 1970.

quent complications of superior vena cava catheterization are consequences of faulty puncture, air embolism, break-off and incorrect intravenous position of the catheter, and phlebitis, thrombosis or thromboembolism. To lessen significantly the possibility of complications, precise puncture technic with tangential orientation toward the pleural apex must be used. A cannula no more than 5 cm. long should be used to avoid accidental penetration of the lung. Correct intravenous positioning must be verified by aspiration of blood. Radiologic control should be used for each inserted catheter and after futile attempts at puncture. Critically diminished Quick prothrombin times are considered a relative contraindication to the procedure. Meticulous airtight closure of the catheter should effectively lessen the danger of air embolism. If the catheter becomes blocked, the infection potential of the adjoining area makes operative removal of the catheter advisable. Incorrect intravenous positioning will occur in about 20% of all catheterizations and increases the thrombotic tendency. However, phlebitis and thrombophlebitis (occasionally with a septic course and danger of infected emboli) are the major complications of the caval catheter with cubital entry, whereas caval catheters introduced via the subclavian route rarely give rise to phlebitic symptoms. Premature removal becomes unnecessary, and the adequate thickness of the covering tissue layer seems successfully to guard against infections, permitting better tolerance of the catheter. Nevertheless, phlebography of 50 patients on the 7th day after infraclavicular catheterization revealed thrombus formation in 35%. Aside from the mechanical effects of endothelial lesions and catheter-determined flow disturbances, a severe disease and consequent worsening of the circulatory status increase the thrombotic potential. Undetected thrombus formation may lead to extensive thrombotic conglomeration and occasionally complete vascular obstruction; infection with eventual spread of bacterially caused basic disease; and massive thromboembolism, fortunately a rare occurrence.

An entirely satisfactory point of entry has yet to be found. For the present, exclusive use of the subclavian route is thought to be justified.

▶ [This does not convince us that the exclusive use of the subclavian route is justified.—Eds.]

Electronic Equipment in Critical Care Areas: Status of Devices Currently in Use in eleven major hospitals was investigated by Henry L. Green, Gregory E. Hieb and Irwin J. Schatz[9] (Wayne State Univ.). There is no general acceptance of design standards by the more than 20 leading manufacturers of monitors, defibrillators, pacemakers and related devices; there also are no recommendations for routine preventive maintenance. Personnel generally consider the devices safe and accurate until an obvious malfunction is noted.

All cardiac electronic equipment was inspected and assessed with a portable electronic testing laboratory. Particular models

DEFECTS IN 71 CARDIAC MONITORS OF
9 DIFFERENT BRANDS

Defect	No. of monitors
Power cord damage: loose or open ground connection, or damage to insulation, plug, or strain relief	11
Rate meter malfunction: counting error greater than 10%, failure to count when sweep not centered on cathode ray tube, inconsistent meter function, jammed meter	6
Cathode ray tube malfunction: sweep speed not uniform, prolonged blanking, wandering base line, distorted tracing, malfunction of vertical position control, inoperative brightness control, burned phosphor	17
Poor high frequency response: under 20 Hz 7, 20–29 Hz 10, 30–49 Hz 20	37
Inadequate gain (only 63 monitors tested)	22
1 mv calibration pulse more than 10% off	17
Excessive leakage current (floating): 10–20 microamperes 4, 21–50 '' 9, over 50 '' 11, Not abolished by grounding in 1 instrument	24
Current spike when monitor switched on or off	6
Faulty internal connection	5
Defective internal component	**4**

(9)   Circulation 43: A101-A122, January, 1971.

of cardiac monitor were found to have characteristic shortcomings. Electric faults are summarized in the table. Many problems were found relating to utilization of monitors by hospital personnel. Six of 44 direct writers and electrocardiographs tested had control knob malfunction, and 33 leaked current in excess of 10 μamp.

Defibrillators showed several unfavorable design features. Thirteen of 33 units examined lacked automatic discharge. Electric malfunction was common. Misutilization was a greater problem than with monitors.

Most hospitals had a poor system for managing cardiac arrest on the general wards. In many of the pacemakers tested, current output was not in direct proportion to the dial setting. Wall receptacles were sometimes insufficient or poorly located. Portable x-ray equipment, electrocardiographs and bed lamps sometimes showed dangerous current leakage.

There should be minimum standards of training for persons engaged in repairing medical electronic equipment. Specialized tasks require an engineering agency or a highly trained manufacturer's service representative. All devices must be inspected periodically, and new equipment should be tested before installation. Output testing of pacemakers and defibrillators and frequency response calibration of monitors and electrocardiographs should be done at least yearly.

▶ [This investigation, which was conducted by physicians and an engineer, emphasizes four important points regarding the use of electronic equipment. They are the hazards related to poorly designed equipment, poorly maintained equipment, poorly trained personnel and poorly designed hospitals. Any of these can be life-threatening from the electric hazard or misdiagnosis.—Eds.]

Pseudomonas Cepacia (Multivorans) Septicemia in an Intensive Care Unit. Pseudomonas cepacia, previously known as P. multivorans, is occasionally isolated from clinical specimens, although it is usually a saprophyte or plant pathogen. Its pathogenicity for man is low; it has most often been found as a superficial contaminant of wounds, although true infection is occasionally seen. Ian Phillips, Susannah Eykyn, M. A. Curtis and J. J. S. Snell[1] (London) report 3 cases of P. cepacia bacteremia due to contaminated blood pressure-monitoring equipment, associated with clinical evidence of infection.

Man, 56, had an aortic valve prosthesis inserted and was given cephaloridine postoperatively as a prophylactic measure. Rigor occurred on the 4th postoperative day, with intense dyspnea and

---

(1) Lancet 1:375-377, Feb. 20, 1971.

hypotension. Blood cultures 4 and 8 days postoperatively yielded the same gram-negative bacillus, resistant to cephaloridine. Oral trimethoprim and sulfamethoxazole were given for 6 weeks. Temperature returned to normal after 8 days of treatment, and the patient was well when last seen about 10 weeks postoperatively.

All 3 patients were nursed postoperatively in an intensive care unit, where gram-negative infections were being surveyed. Motile gram-negative bacilli that metabolized glucose oxidatively were isolated from the patients. All were sensitive to sulfonamide, with and without trimethoprim, and to carbenicillin but resistant to gentamicin and polymyxin. Subcultures revealed P. cepacia in each case. Review of all pseudomonads isolated from patients and ventilators in the intensive care unit over more than a year indicated that P. cepacia was isolated from two other sources, both ventilators in use on 2 patients and in the saline inside syringes used for the blood pressure monitoring equipment. The detergicide was not contaminated.

Pseudomonas cepacia appears to be only a rare cause of human infection. Outbreaks have resulted from contamination of detergicide, chlorhexidine and a chlorhexidine-cetrimide mixture. The organism has definite if limited pathogenicity for man. Two of the present patients had clinical septicemia after catheters were removed. All 3 were treated as for endocarditis, with carbenicillin and then trimethoprim-sulfamethoxazole. All recovered. It is generally dangerous to use apparatus that cannot be properly heat sterilized. No infections have occurred since glutaraldehyde was introduced for disinfecting the pressure-monitoring apparatus.

▶ [Monitoring equipment often is cared for by technicians who may not appreciate the risks involved.—Eds.]

Reliability of Blood Pco₂ Measurements by the CO₂ Electrode, the Whole-Blood Cco₂-pH Method and the Astrup Method were assessed by F. Bärtschi, P. Haab and D. R. Held[2] (Univ. of Fribourg). The technics were tested on blood equilibrated in vitro at known gas tensions, with Pco_2 levels in the physiologic region and Po_2 levels covering nearly the whole range of oxygen saturation.

The results are given in the table. The dispersion of F (measured Pco_2-actual Pco_2) was smallest for the CO_2 electrode and largest for the whole-blood Cco_2-pH method; the Astrup micromethod values were intermediate. At all saturation levels, mean F values were within 3% from unity for the CO_2 electrode and

(2) Resp. Physiol. 10:121-131, July, 1970.

CO$_2$-electrode				Whole-blood C$_{CO_2}$/pH method				Astrup			
n	P$_{CO_2}$ mm Hg	S$_{O_2}$ %	F	n	P$_{CO_2}$ mm Hg	S$_{O_2}$ %	F	n	P$_{CO_2}$ mm Hg	S$_{O_2}$ %	F
9	43	92	1.000 ± 0.009	13	40	92.6	0.996 ± 0.047	22	40	92.6	1.024 ± 0.023
9	53	3	0.997 ± 0.009	14	41	59.3	1.020 ± 0.049	15	44	59.7	1.052 ± 0.027
				14	38	29.5	1.000 ± 0.019	19	38	16.2	1.081 ± 0.017

F, measured P$_{CO_2}$-actual P$_{CO_2}$; n, number of measurements.

within 1.5% from unity for the whole-blood C$_{CO_2}$-pH method; none of the differences was significant. Mean F values yielded by the Astrup method were significantly larger than unity at all saturation levels; the deviation was more marked at low than at high saturation.

The CO$_2$ electrode gave the best performance under the test conditions, with minimal scatter of the values and no directional error regardless of the oxygen saturation level. The method is a comparatively direct one and not dependent on any correction or calculation involving additional parameters. A systematic saturation-dependent error is superimposed on the moderate scatter of the Astrup method, and this error appears to be large enough to be of practical significance. The error could be attributed to two factors affecting the desaturation correction, the presence of small amounts of nonoxygenable hemoglobin in the samples and an overestimation of the Haldane effect.

Blood Pressure Measurement by Doppler Ultrasonic Detection of Arterial Wall Motion. William T. Kemmerer, Ray W. Ware, Hugh F. Stegall, John L. Morgan and Robert Kirby[3] describe clinical situations in which Doppler ultrasonic measurements are useful. Various ultrasound devices for measuring blood flow velocity were evaluated. The transducer is placed over the brachial or other superficial artery, and a pneumatic cuff is placed over the transducer and around the arm. During cuff deflation, Doppler signals generated by the opening snap of the arterial wall appear and disappear in a manner similar to that of Korotkoff's sounds. Study was made of 10 patients requiring direct arterial catheterization for blood pressure monitoring, of 3 patients in clinical shock, of South Vietnamese

(3) Surg., Gynec. & Obst. 131:1141-1147, December, 1970.

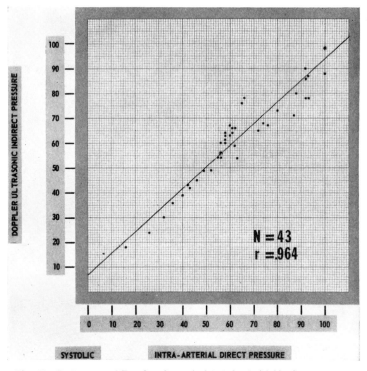

Fig. 18.—Scattergram of Doppler ultrasonic-detected arterial blood pressures compared with direct arterial blood pressures in patients in shock (systolic). (Courtesy of Kemmerer, W. T., *et al.*: Surg., Gynec. & Obst. 131:1141-1147, December, 1970.)

civilians with multiple war wounds, of all ages, and of 25 infants in the 1st month, weighing 2-5 kg.

Mean systolic pressures in the first group of patients differed by 2.6 mm. Hg and diastolic values by 1.2, both showing a high degree of correlation. Comparison of the measuring technics in shock patients is illustrated in Figure 18. Diastolic pressures were always easily discernible with the Doppler system in the civilian injury cases. The equipment tolerated considerable rough handling. The ultrasonic technic gave reproducible values in infants, with sharp systolic and diastolic end points, compared with Korotkoff and oscillometric values.

The accuracy of blood pressure determinations using the Doppler shift ultrasonic detection technic appears to be good in normotensive adults and in patients in shock. The technic appears to be promising for use in infants. The equipment available is still experimental in design and fabrication.

▶ [If this system is so good, why is it so slow in appearing on the commercial market?—Eds.]

Clinical Evaluation of Transthoracic Electric Impedance as a Guide to Intrathoracic Fluid Volumes. According to Marvin Pomerantz, Frank Delgado and Ben Eiseman[4] (Denver Gen'l Hosp.), a sensitive clinical measure is needed to detect intrapulmonary fluid accumulation. Studies in animals with transthoracic electric impedance used as a measurement of changes in intrathoracic fluid volumes showed impedance changes as long as 45 minutes before there were detectable changes in central venous pressure, lung compliance, arterial pressure or blood gases.

Transthoracic electric impedance as a measure of intrathoracic fluid changes was evaluated in 52 patients, 46 considered likely to have subsequent intrapulmonary fluid changes. Six patients were studied acutely; 3 had chest fluid removed by thoracentesis and 3 had total body fluid reduced by membrane dialysis. The Minnesota Impedance Cardiograph was used to measure impedance, electrodes being placed on the neck and upper abdomen. Impedance was usually monitored at least daily. Evaluation of 44 patients lasted 5-25 days.

Impedance reliability reflected fluid loss in all 6 patients who underwent acute removal of fluid. A linear relation between amount of fluid removal and increase in impedance was evident in the patients having thoracentesis for pleural effusion. Impedance paralleled blood gas, venous pressure and chest radiographic changes and often preceded them in patients who had pulmonary insufficiency after trauma. Impedance remained low in 2 patients who died of "respiratory distress syndrome" after nonthoracic trauma. Impedance rose as patients with pulmonary insufficiency after thoracic trauma improved. Measurements accurately reflected intrathoracic fluid volumes in cardiac surgical patients and in patients with systemic illness in whom respiratory insufficiency developed. The hospital course of an emphysematous man, aged 73, in whom pulmonary infiltrates developed after cholecystectomy is shown in Figure 19; changes in impedance reflected x-ray evidence of development of infiltrates.

A problem with use of the technic is that changes in imped-

---

(4)   Ann. Surg. 171:686-694, May, 1970.

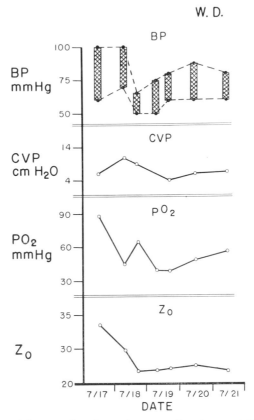

Fig. 19.—Hospital course of emphysematous man with pulmonary infiltrates after cholecystectomy. (Courtesy of Pomerantz, M., *et al.:* Ann. Surg. 171:686-694, May, 1970.)

ance in hyperventilating patients must exceed 1.5 ohms to be significant. However, the technic consistently shows changes from baseline measurements in seriously ill patients with significant intrathoracic fluid accumulation. An important potential use is in early detection of intrapulmonary fluid accumulation such as sometimes follows trauma.

▶ [If this proves to be accurate, it will be an important diagnostic tool.— Eds.]

Pneumocardiogram: Potential Monitor for Operating Room. The pneumocardiogram is familiar to all anesthesiologists as pulsations in the breathing bag, most readily apparent during apnea. N. Ty Smith and John A. Reitan[5] (Stanford Univ.) evaluated the physiologic validity of the pneumocardiogram by comparing it with a standard index of cardiac function—peak ascending aortic blood acceleration. Studies were done in 4 large baboons and 5 mongrel dogs. Baboons were anesthetized with phencyclidine-halothane-oxygen, with ultrasonic flow transducers implanted about vessels. The pneumocardiogram was recorded during 20 seconds of apnea with the use of a Fleisch pneumotachograph, as cardioactive drugs were administered. The dogs were anesthetized with methohexital-halothane and oxygen. The pneumocardiogram and aortic flow were differentiated to obtain acceleration records.

The acceleration pneumocardiogram and peak ascending aortic blood acceleration correlated very closely over inotropic changes as much as eightfold in a single animal. The onset of the pneumocardiographic H wave corresponded closely to that of left ventricular ejection, but the H wave lagged behind the start of aortic flow as the heart rate increased. Positive inotropic agents increased both parameters, and myocardial depressant drugs reduced the amplitude of both.

The pneumocardiogram, a noninvasive measurement, correlates very closely with ascending aortic blood acceleration. It is relatively inexpensive and can be applied rapidly and easily, without discomfort to the patient. Operations should not interfere grossly with the measurement and vice versa. Most of the problems with pneumocardiography can potentially be solved. The findings are reproducible; cardiac depression is evident early in its course. The genesis of the pneumocardiogram is unknown. Its close relation to the ballistocardiogram suggests an analogous origin, i.e., movement of air in and out of the airway caused by movement of blood in the chest. The influence of the conducting airways on the signal is unknown.

▶ [This is interesting. Let us hope it becomes more useful than has the ballistocardiogram.—Eds.]

Postoperative Changes of Ornithine Carbamoyl Transferase Activity in Serum (S-OCT) Related to Oxygen Saturation in Hepatic Vein Blood during Operations in Man. Serum OCT activity has been found to increase postoperatively after a large loss of blood or a fall in blood pressure, especially in aged pa-

(5) Anesth. & Analg. 40:781-790, Sept.-Oct., 1970.

tients. It is reasonable to ascribe this to an effect of hepatic ischemia. Jan Gillquist, Lennart Kaijser and Sten-Otto Lilje-dahl[6] (Karolinska Inst., Stockholm) attempted to relate post-operative S-OCT changes to changes in oxygen saturation of the hepatic vein blood. The subjects were 10 male and 9 female patients, aged 20-89 years, operated on for lower limb fracture; none had a history of liver disease or was receiving cortisone or insulin. The S-OCT was determined with use of citrulline-carbamoyl-[14] C.

Patients were operated on about a week after injury. Premedication was usually with a narcotic and scopolamine. The inspiratory oxygen concentration was always at least 30%. Succinylcholine was used for muscle relaxation. Most elderly patients were ventilated with an Engstrom respirator. Blood for analysis of oxygen saturation was sampled from the hepatic vein at 15 minute intervals during operation.

Fig 20.—Correlation between maximum rise of S-OCT in nanomoles $^{14}CO_2$/(ml. $\times$ hr.) within the first 72 hours postoperatively and lowest value in oxygen saturation of hepatic vein blood ($S_{O2}\%$). Equation of the regression line: $\log y = 1.3558 - 0.0179x$, $r = -0.79$, $P < 0.001$. (Courtesy of Gillquist, J., et al.: Acta chir. scandinav. 136:9-16, 1970.)

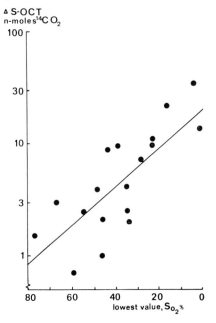

(6)   Acta chir. scandinav. 136:9-16, 1970.

The mean duration of operation was 95 minutes. Mean blood loss was 13% of the initial volume. Three patients had marked transient decreases in blood pressure. Blood loss was usually replaced by Ringer's lactate and albumin. Hepatic vein oxygen saturation decreased only slightly during uncomplicated operations, but it fell markedly when large blood loss or pronounced hypotension occurred. The S-OCT often decreased in the first 48 hours in uncomplicated cases but when the hepatic vein oxygen saturation fell below 45%, a rise in S-OCT occurred within 24 hours, reaching a peak within 72 hours after operation. The rise to the peak level was statistically significant. A subsequent peak occurred in some cases. The rise in S-OCT was negatively correlated with the lowest oxygen saturation (Fig. 20). Even moderate blood loss could be followed by a rise in S-OCT if the hepatic vein oxygen saturation fell. In patients over age 40, rise in S-OCT was also correlated with percentage of blood volume deficit.

The S-OCT activity increases after operation when a large blood loss or circulatory failure occurs. This may be due to reduced elimination of OCT activity from the blood. Increased S-OCT could reflect mitochondrial damage or altered mitochondrial function. A rise in S-OCT appears to represent a reversible effect of hepatic ischemia, provided adequate treatment is given. If circulatory failure impends, immediate substitution is necessary to avoid hepatic ischemia.

▶ [We are doubtful if this will ever be a very useful clinical measurement.—Eds.]

Complications of Brachial Arteriotomy. Brachial arteriotomy is an important avenue for arterial catheterization, but there has been considerable concern regarding morbidity from the procedure. Paul W. Armstrong and John O. Parker[7] (Queen's Univ., Kingston, Ont.) conducted a prospective study of brachial arteriotomy in 70 patients over 6 months. Eleven had atrial fibrillation. Brachial and radial pulse volumes and auscultatory and palpable blood pressures in both arms were determined before and 5-50 days after catheterization. Most patients were assessed within 2 weeks after catheterization. Arteriotomy was done through a vertical antecubital incision. A longitudinal incision was made in a 2-cm. segment of artery, and heparin was instilled before catheter insertion. The artery was probed in both directions before closure, and if flow was impaired, a

(7)   J. Thoracic & Cardiovas. Surg. 61:424-429, March, 1971.

Fogarty catheter was passed in both directions. Arteries were closed with a 5-0 Tevdek everting horizontal mattress stitch. Re-exploration was done immediately if the pulse volume was significantly reduced after arterial closure.

Ten patients had a significant decrease in pulse volume. Four patients with primary occlusion were not re-explored, and in 1 the pulse was not adequately restored with a Fogarty catheter. Five patients had normal pulses when they left the catheterization laboratory and represent cases of secondary occlusion. Four had re-exploration within 48 hours after the procedure. Three had clots removed by the Fogarty catheter; the 1 with a low pulse afterward was the only patient with a major late complication. No clot was found in 1 patient. All 4 patients received heparin and low molecular weight dextran. One patient with a complication was not given heparin until the end of the study. Two others underwent lengthy diagnostic procedures with use of a guided catheter. Two were women with small brachial arteries. A catheter was used in 7 other patients at the time of arteriotomy closure. Clots were removed from 5 of them, and normal pulse volume returned. Brachial artery bruits were audible over the arteriotomy site in 18 patients without a decreased pulse volume on follow-up. No aneurysm, neurologic deficit or significant infection was observed. The over-all rate of complications, including 1 case of bleeding, was 16%.

Brachial arteriotomy for catheterization has inherent risks, which can be minimized. Prompt recognition and treatment of immediate complications can prevent much long-term occlusive morbidity. A Fogarty catheter should not be used routinely but should be reserved for patients exhibiting poor flow after probing in both directions. Brachial artery bruits at the arteriotomy site are probably related to luminal narrowing but are not functionally significant.

▶ [Although these arteriotomies were for cardiac catheterization, the anesthetist should be mindful of the complications since arterial puncture for blood gas determination is now a common anesthetic monitoring procedure.—Eds.]

Anesthetic Requirements in Patient Monitoring are discussed by J. P. Payne[8] (London). The main limitation to monitoring patients in the operating room is the availability or otherwise of suitable equipment. A single-channel oscilloscope is suitable for most ECG monitoring purposes; some form of print-out is useful if a permanent record is needed. Arterial catheterization is

(8)   Postgrad. M. J. 46:388-391, June, 1970.

justified to monitor the blood pressure in critically ill patients. Indirect pressure measurements are least effective when most needed. Deliberate hypotension during anesthesia makes other circulatory criteria more significant. Central venous pressure is useful when patients have severe blood loss or otherwise disturbed fluid balance. Arterial and venous catheters make measurements of circulating blood volume and cardiac output easy; repeated determinations can be made at no risk to the patient. Such access also simplifies the assessment of respiratory and acid-base disturbances through blood analysis. A computer program can be devised to remove interference from EEG recordings and thus enable the anesthetist to follow patterns associated with different depths of anesthesia, hypotension and hypothermia on a single channel. Temperature measurements are important under hypothermic conditions.

Monitoring is more difficult in the recovery room since patients may be restless, semiconscious and uncooperative. Most monitoring equipment involves some interference at a time when the patient can least well tolerate it. Data-handling procedures too often obtrude on the patient's awareness. Special harnesses for leads have been developed, but none has proved entirely satisfactory. Warning systems must work properly to avoid imposing too great a burden on the nurses in attendance. The cathode ray oscilloscope provides a satisfactory visual display unit and does not in itself draw attention to abnormalities. Print-out data sheets must be scanned to detect any deterioration. The best compromise is probably an oscilloscope with a warning light. The basic need in monitoring systems is to combine freedom of patient movement with intimate contact of instruments with blood and tissue.

► [Don't overlook the point, "Warning systems must work properly to avoid imposing too great a burden on the nurses in attendance." In other words, we need monitors to monitor the monitors!—Eds.]

CARDIAC ARRHYTHMIAS AND THEIR TREATMENT

Chest Thump for Reverting Ventricular Tachycardia is discussed by James E. Pennington, Jack Taylor and Bernard Lown[9] (Harvard Univ.). Many texts today recommend a precordial blow for asystole, but none suggests that it is effective

---

(9)   New England J. Med. 283:1192-1195, Nov. 26, 1970.

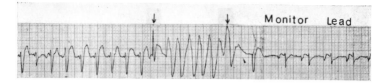

Fig. 21.—Ventricular tachycardia at rate of 150 (note that second complex is captured beat). Chest thump (*left arrow*) evokes ectopic beat of different morphology and results in more rapid tachycardia at rate of 220 per minute. Immediate repetition of thump (*right arrow*) reverts arrhythmia to sinus rhythm. Note single ectopic beat before normal mechanism supervenes. (Courtesy of Pennington, J. E., *et al.*: New England J. Med. 283:1192-1195, Nov. 26, 1970.)

in ventricular arrhythmias. Cardioversion is used for sustained ventricular tachycardia if intravenous lidocaine is unsuccessful, but a sharp blow to the chest is often sufficient to restore normal rhythm, as is a discharge of much lower energy.

Twelve episodes of ventricular tachycardia in 5 patients were ended in the past year by a sharp blow to the lower chest. All the patients were men with ischemic heart disease. Three had acute infarction and required a blow to the midsternum or left precordial area. One patient who did not respond to lidocaine had 6 episodes of tachycardia reverted by a thump on the chest and 12 subsequent ones reverted by cardioversion with a low-energy discharge. The mechanical stimulus evoked a premature depolarization sometimes identical in morphology with the QRS of the tachycardia. In 1 case, tachycardia at a more rapid rate resulted from an initial thump, and a second blow restored sinus rhythm (Fig. 21). Fourteen patients with 32 episodes of ventricular tachycardia had cardioversion. The initial energy used was 10 watt-seconds or less in 27 episodes in 11 patients after intravenous lidocaine had been unsuccessful. Six of these patients had acute infarction. An energy of 10 watt-seconds or less was effective in 93% of the episodes. A number of episodes might have responded to 1 watt-second.

Chest thumping is an important maneuver in cardiac resuscitation. Most arrests are probably due to ventricular fibrillation, preceded by tachycardia that can likely be ended by a single ectopic depolarization of the heart. This requires a small energy and can be induced by a blow to the chest wall. Chest thump is immediately available and will do no harm in cases of asystole. Low-energy cardioversion is more predictable and less traumatic and is preferred when ventricular tachycardia is well tolerated and a cardioverter is available.

▶ [As pointed out in an editorial, we have had electroversion and cardioversion and now we have thumpversion.—Eds.]

Comparative Antiarrhythmic Effects of Mepivacaine and Lignocaine. R. B. Boettner, R. W. Dunbar, J. V. Haley and D. H. Morrow[1] (Univ. of Kentucky) compared the antiarrhythmic effects of mepivacaine and lignocaine in unpremedicated open chest dogs anesthetized with pentobarbitone, as measured by their ability to protect the heart from electrically induced premature ventricular contractions. Ventilation was controlled with an air-oxygen mixture, with the use of a volume-limited ventilator. The end-diastolic ventricular stimulation threshold was estimated with current applied directly to the ventricle through epicardial electrodes at various intervals in the cardiac cycle. The local anesthetics were injected rapidly.

Both mepivacaine and lignocaine significantly elevated the end-diastolic ventricular stimulation threshold. Mepivacaine raised the threshold 0.016 ma. at 1 minute, 0.013 ma. at 2 minutes, 0.012 ma. at 3 minutes and 0.011 ma. at 4 minutes. The respective increases produced by lignocaine were 0.017, 0.022, 0.021 and 0.012. Beyond 4 minutes, the rate of decreasing effect was about 0.001 ma. per minute for both drugs. The greater early response to lignocaine was significant.

This study confirms the antiarrhythmic property of mepivacaine. The findings warrant the continued study of realted local anesthetics for their potential use in the management of cardiac arrhythmias that may occur during anesthesia or outside the operating room. Currently, the effects of mepivacaine on digitalis-induced arrhythmias and those resulting from acute coronary artery occlusion are being evaluated.

▶ [Despite the antiarrhythmic properties of mepivacaine, lidocaine appeared to be superior.—Eds.]

Use of Propranolol in Arrhythmias Complicating Acute Myocardial Infarction. Louis Lemberg, Agustin Castellanos, Jr., and Azucena G. Arcebal[2] (Miami, Fla.) report clinical evidence of the beneficial effects of propranolol on acute tachyarrhythmias which complicate acute myocardial infarction. Study was made of 34 patients with acute infarction who received propranolol. Sixteen had mild and 18 moderate left ventricular failure. Nine had frank pulmonary edema. The 43 arrhythmic episodes included 18 of atrial fibrillation, 6 of atrial flutter, 8 of atrial or A-V junctional tachycardia and 11 of

(1) Brit. J. Anaesth. 42:685-689, August, 1970.
(2) Am. Heart J. 80:479-487, October, 1970.

ventricular tachycardia. No patient had cardiogenic shock, and all had normal electrolytes. A number of patients had been treated conventionally without success. Digitalis was incriminated in only one instance. All episodes occurred within 3 days of infarction. Propranolol was given intravenously at a rate of 0.5-0.75 mg./2 minutes until sinus rhythm returned or the rate slowed to 80, as lead II of the ECG was monitored.

No patient showed an increase in the clinical degree of heart failure, and 37 patients improved when the ventricular rate was slowed to below 100. No significant blood pressure reductions occurred. Fourteen episodes of atrial fibrillation were reverted to sinus rhythm with 2-5 mg. propranolol. Only 1 patient had marked ventricular slowing. All six episodes of flutter were reverted to sinus rhythm with 3.5-15 mg. propranolol. A slow isorhythmic A-V dissociation, developed in 1 patient, which responded to 1 mg. atropine. Eight episodes of supraventricular tachycardia converted to sinus rhythm. A-V dissociation in 1 of these cases responded to atropine. Three patients with ventricular tachycardia had recurrent ventricular fibrillation requiring electric conversion. One episode of A-V dissociation after propranolol was abolished by atropine.

This study showed propranolol to be useful in the treatment of acute tachyarrhythmias following myocardial infarction. The hemodynamic properties of propranolol are as important as its negative inotropic effect in these cases. An excessive chronotropic effect occurred in several cases. When atropine was ineffective in this circumstance, isoproterenol was effective.

▶ [The need, occasionally, to use propranolol, then atropine, then isoproterenol, attests to the need for constant monitoring and extreme care in treating arrhythmias with β-blockers.—Eds.]

Artificial Cardiac Pacemakers. Bernard Lown and Bernard D. Kosowsky[3] (Harvard Univ.) observe that despite nearly a decade of experience with pacemaker systems, failures and complications are the rule rather than the exception. Pacers in current use are inadequate and unreliable. Insertion of a pacemaker carries some surgical risk. Transvenous insertion of endocardial electrodes avoids many of the problems of thoracotomy. Improper positioning can result in pulmonary air embolism, and thrombi at the electrode tip can have the same effect. Pacemaker failure characterizes all present implanted pacing systems. It is basically due to component failure. Cessation of

(3)   New England J. Med. 283:1023-1031, Nov. 5, 1970.

pacing may result from failure of the generator, electrode breakage or displacement or an increase in pacing threshold. Intermittent pacing can result in sporadic pacer failure with symptoms of asystole. Extraneous electric signals can affect pacemaker function and cause intermittent pacing. Battery depletion changes the pacing rate. Special function can be lost despite a normally functioning pacing system. Aberrant stimulation can occur.

Simple tests are available to determine the basis of pacemaker failure. An ECG tracing is important and a portable amplitude-modulation radio can provide valuable information on pacing rate and function. The wave form of a pacer stimulus can be examined by using a high-speed, calibrated oscilloscope. Special radiofrequency stimulators can help in analyzing function. When electrodes are accessible, changes in cardiac threshold can be readily determined. Patients should be seen every 4-6 months in the 1st year, every 2 or 3 months at 12-18 months and every 1 or 2 months thereafter. Follow-up can best be done in special pacer clinics. When pacer failure is documented, replacement should be undertaken without delay.

Provocative cardiac pacing has been used in angina and in A-V block. Pacing has been used to help diagnose puzzling arrhythmias. Atrial pacing may help in recognizing Wolff-Parkinson-White syndrome. Pacing of the atrium can convert or control atrial arrhythmias. Paired pacing can be used for postextrasystolic potentiation, for altering the rate or for atrial stimulation. Prophylactic pacing has been suggested for use during coronary angiography.

▶ [Unfortunately, adequate standards for pacemaker function do not exist. Frequently it is difficult to obtain information on the type of device implanted when the patient appears for operation unrelated to his myocardial problem. Extraneous electric currents (e.g., cautery and monitors) offer additional hazards at the time of subsequent anesthesia.—Eds.]

Ventricular Arrhythmias Associated with Use of Diazepam for Cardioversion are reported by John S. Barrett and E. Berry Hey, Jr.[4] (Reading Hosp., West Reading, Pa.). Diazepam anesthesia has recently been recommended for cardioversion, but light thiopental anesthesia has proved safe and convenient in over 100 patients. The authors' first 2 patients given diazepam anesthesia displayed dangerous ventricular arrhythmias. Both patients, a woman aged 59 and a man aged 67, were prepared with quinidine and cessation of digitalis for at least 24 hours.

(4)   J.A.M.A. 214:1323-1324, Nov. 16, 1970.

A dose of 2.5 mg. diazepam was given intravenously, followed by doses of 2.5 mg. at 2-minute intervals until the patient stopped counting and did not respond to commands. Pure oxygen was given for four or five breaths before d-c cardioversion was carried out. One patient had chronic bronchitis and some ECG evidence of left ventricular abnormality as well as atrial fibrillation. The other had coronary artery disease, an intraventricular conduction defect and ventricular premature beats even off digitalis therapy.

These patients had ventricular fibrillation before countershock and a short run of ventricular tachycardia after a 100 watt-second shock, respectively, under diazepam anesthesia. The only difficulties encountered in over 100 previous cardioversions were an episode of pulmonary edema and 1 of asystole. It is unlikely that the use of diazepam will permit cardioversion to be done without risk of occasional catastrophic arrhythmias. Potentially fatal arrhythmias may occur in patients given diazepam intravenously for other reasons. This drug should probably not be given intravenously if a cardioverter is not available.

▶ [Although these complications may not strictly be due to diazepam, they should place the anesthesiologist on guard.—Eds.]

Digoxin: Immunologic Approaches to Measurement and Reversal of Toxicity. Vincent P. Butler, Jr.[5] (Columbia Univ.) states that there is a distressingly high prevalence of toxic manifestations of digitalis use. The most important factor may be accumulation of excessive amounts of digitalis in the body and particularly in the myocardium. Excessive accumulation sometimes reflects excessive dosage, but it is more often due to reduced excretion. Digoxin is not appreciably metabolized in man. The kidney is the principal route of digoxin excretion. Daily maintenance doses given subjects with normal renal function might elevate serum and tissue digoxin levels in patients with renal failure. Elderly patients are considered to have an increased susceptibility to digitalis toxicity. Factors that increase myocardial sensitivity to the toxic effects of digitalis, such as myocardial ischemia and hypokalemia, are also important.

A double-isotope derivative technic for serum digoxin determinations is precise and specific but requires several days. The author has used an immunoassay to measure digoxin directly in

(5)   New England J. Med. 283:1150-1156, Nov. 19, 1970.

serum. Highly specific antidigoxin antibody is formed in rabbits. The coated charcoal technic is used. The method is sensitive to 0.2 mμg./ml., well below the therapeutic serum level. Patients on maintenance digoxin therapy without toxicity generaly have serum levels below 2-2.5 mμg./ml. Levels of 2 or greater were found in 85% of toxic patients studied and lower levels in 85% of nontoxic patients. A serum level exceeding 0.5 mμg./ml. indicates that the patient is taking digoxin and is absorbing it.

Circulating antibody can prevent some or all of an administered dose of digoxin from reaching myocardial cells in an active form in rabbits. Digoxin-specific antibodies can remove essentially all intracellular glycoside from slices of rat kidney or from human red blood cells. Digoxin-binding antibody can reverse the toxic cellular effect of excessive myocardial digoxin in nonimmunized dogs. Clinical use of antibody can only be considered at present in the most serious, life-threatening forms of digoxin toxicity. The safest course in most patients with digoxin intoxication still lies in withholding digitalis and treating toxic manifestations symptomatically.

▶ [It has been estimated that 60% of patients on digitalis therapy manifest toxic symptoms. A simple radioimmunologic technic is now available for direct assay of serum drug levels. Moreover, the antiserum used in the test may provide a mechanism for treating patients critically ill from high serum digoxin levels.—Eds.]

Factors in Arrhythmia during Dental Outpatient General Anesthesia. Previous studies have shown frequent arrhythmias occurring after general anesthesia for oral surgical procedures. Jerry R. Miller, Charles H. Redish, C. Fisch and R. C. Oehler[6] (Indiana Univ.) attempted to better delineate factors leading to cardiovascular complications in oral surgical outpatients. Study was made of 102 A.S.A. class 1 patients aged 10-69 years, including 75 females. Anesthetics used included methohexital and halothane-nitrous oxide-oxygen. The patients were not premedicated. The initial dose of methohexital, given to semireclining patients, was 1 mg./kg. Supplementary doses of methohexital were given in 30-40-mg. increments. The patients breathed spontaneously. Halothane was given after loss of the lid reflex in 75:25 nitrous oxide-oxygen.

Complications other than cardiovascular were few and minor in this series. Arrhythmias, mainly sinoatrial, were most frequent during anesthetic induction. Junctional and His-Purkinje

(6)   Anesth. & Analg. 49:701-706, Sept.-Oct., 1970.

arrhythmias appeared at the onset of operation and again at the end of anesthesia. Sinus tachycardia occurred in 76 patients, in 47 with a rate above 130; it occurred most often in younger patients. No patients over age 40 had ventricular arrhythmias. Methohexital was not important in the occurrence of arrhythmias. Blood halothane levels ranged from 3 to 20 mg./100 ml. Arrhythmias increased with longer anesthetic periods. Mean blood pressure and pulse increased during anesthesia and operation. Five patients with a Pao_2 below 100 mm. Hg developed His-Purkinje arrhythmias, as did 9 patients with higher oxygen tensions. Ventricular bigeminy occurred 12 times; chaotic ventricular arrhythmia, 3 times; and ventricular tachycardia, twice. All arrhythmias subsided spontaneously without treatment.

A majority of dental outpatients anesthetized with methohexital and halothane-nitrous oxide in this study had cardiac arrhythmias, all subsiding spontaneously. Ventilation appeared to be the most important factor. Arrhythmias were most frequent in younger patients and in females. Attention to CO_2 elimination and adequate maintenance of acid-base balance are essential to the stability of the cardiac rhythm in dental outpatients.

▶ [We doubt if this is any different than the response seen in the average surgical patient.—Eds.]

NEUROSURGERY AND CAROTID ENDARTERECTOMY

Carotid Endarterectomy for Cerebrovascular Insufficiency: Long-Term Results in 592 Patients Followed up to 13 Years. Jesse E. Thompson, Dale J. Austin and R. Don Patman[7] (Baylor Univ.) reviewed the results of 748 carotid artery operations done on 592 patients during 13 years, starting in 1957. The average age of the 373 men and 219 women was 63.1 and 66.5 years, respectively. Bilateral operations were done on 156 patients (26.4%). All patients had significant cervical carotid occlusive lesions demonstrated by arteriography on the basis of at least 50% reduction of the lumen or an appearance suggesting deposition of platelet thrombi or debris. All patients underwent endarterectomy.

METHOD.—Halothane anesthesia is used. A temporary inlying by-

(7) Ann. Surg. 172:663-679, October, 1970.

pass shunt is used for all partially occlusive lesions. A vertical arteriotomy is made and closed with Dacron sutures. A patch graft is used only when the artery is small. Extreme gentleness in manipulation of the artery is emphasized. Blood pressure is maintained with lactated Ringer's solution or small doses of vasopressors.

Complications have been few. Three patients were reoperated for thrombosis of the segment operated on resulting from intimal flap dissection. Wound hematomas occurred in 8 cases and false aneurysms in 6. There were no wound infections. Bilateral operations were done in separate stages at least a week apart.

Cerebral blood flow was restored in all 630 partly occluded arteries treated in 480 patients. Flow was restored in 40.7% of 118 totally occluded arteries in 112 patients. Operative mortality ranged from 1.1% in patients with transient ischemia to 6.1% in those with frank strokes. No deaths have occurred in patients with chronic ischemia and asymptomatic bruits. The over-all mortality in the past 6 years has been 1.47% in 476 endarterectomies. The over-all incidence of permanent deficits related to operation was 2.7%; 8 of the 20 were severe. The incidence in patients in whom a temporary inlying shunt was used is shown in the table. Only 13.4% of long-term deaths were due to strokes, representing 3.9% of the entire series. Improvement occurred in 88.9% of the 126 survivors in the frank stroke group, 96.7% of the 200 in the transient ischemia group and 92.7% of the 55 in the asymptomatic bruit group. Three of 9 survivors with chronic cerebral ischemia are normal, but mental improvement has been limited in this group.

Some patients require cerebral protection during carotid surgery to prevent strokes and aggravation of neurologic deficits. A shunt has been used nearly routinely with general anesthesia, without other adjuncts than adequate hydration and satisfac-

OPERATION-RELATED NEUROLOGIC DEFICITS IN 358 PATIENTS WITH
TRANSIENT CEREBRAL ISCHEMIA AND ASYMPTOMATIC BRUITS UNDERGOING
465 OPERATIONS USING A TEMPORARY INLYING SHUNT

SEVERITY OF DEFICIT	No.	PATIENT INCIDENCE %	PROCEDURE INCIDENCE %
Permanent, severe; not related to operative technic	3	0.84	0.65
Permanent, severe; related to operative technic	1	0.3	0.2
Permanent, mild	5	1.4	1.1
Transient, mild	4	1.1	0.86

tory levels of blood pressure. The operative mortality has been
1%. The shunt had been used nearly routinely because of lack
of precise knowledge as to which patients require it. It adds
very little to the operating time and, along with gentle dissection, affords reliable temporary cerebral support.

▶ [The results of this series without use of added carbon dioxide or elevated blood pressure are impressive. Comparative mortality figures from
several quoted series where the authors do use CO_2 or elevated blood pressure are all 3-4 times higher!—Eds.]

**Effects of CO_2 and Systemic Hypertension of Cerebral Per-
fusion Pressure during Carotid Endarterectomy** were examined
by Henry E. Fourcade, C. Philip Larson, Jr., William K. Ehren-
feld, Robert F. Hickey and Thomas H. Newton[8] (Univ. of California). The stump pressure transmitted to the occluded side by
collateral vessels at carotid endarterectomy has been shown to
increase during hypocarbia and induced hypertension, and it
was predicted that this would result in a rise in flow through
any region of vasomotor paralysis resulting from ischemia. Cerebral perfusion, however, is determined by cerebral venous
pressure as well as by anastomotic arterial pressure and an increase in $Paco_2$ may increase the cerebral venous pressure. In
the present study, 10 patients were examined during 12 carotid
endarterectomies done without internal shunts. Two had staged
bilateral procedures. The patients, aged 57-80 years, had various degrees of atherosclerosis of the extracranial cerebral vessels. Anesthesia was with halothane and oxygen, with ventilation controlled at $Paco_2$ of 15-20 torr. The alveolar halothane
level was kept at 0.55-0.8%. Clamp occlusion time of the carotid
vessels averaged 26 minutes. The lateral cerebral sinus was
catheterized in three of nine attempts. Systemic pressure was
varied with phenylephrine.

Stump pressures were highest at low $Paco_2$ levels. The mean
stump pressure was 22% higher at an average $Paco_2$ of 27 torr
than at 41 torr, and 16% higher than at 58.4 torr; the difference
between pressures at low and normal $Paco_2$ levels was significant. Lateral sinus pressures averaged 31% lower in hypocarbia
than in normocarbia. Calculated cerebral flow equivalents increased as the $Paco_2$ rose, increasing from 15 ml. cerebral flow
per ml. oxygen consumed in hypocarbia to 50 ml. in hypercarbia. Stump pressures fell as phenylephrine support was withdrawn while the $Paco_2$ was held constant. The absolute change
in lateral sinus pressure was much less than that in stump pres-

(8)   Anesthesiology 33:383-390, October, 1970.

sure. Stump pressures did not change at constant systemic arterial pressure as the Paco$_2$ was kept constant during carotid occlusion.

The findings indicate that an area of ischemia may exist in the ipsilateral cerebral hemisphere as a result of vascular occlusion. The ischemia results in vasomotor paralysis. Perfusion pressure and thus flow to the area are increased under conditions of hypocarbia and induced systemic hypertension.

▶ [Hypocapnia—hypercapnia! Normotension—hypertension! Yet look at the preceding article.—Eds.]

Effects of Subclavian Steal and Compromised Cephalic Blood Flow on Cerebral Circulation. Bo Eklöf and Seymour I. Schwartz[9] attempted directly to evaluate the effects of subclavian steal on cerebral blood flow at rest and during augmented flow through the involved limb. Tapes were placed around the carotid, vertebral and left subclavian vessels of 7 adult dogs and 1 baboon. A flowmeter was used to measure extracranial vessel flow, and regional cerebral flow was determined with radioxenon. The external carotid arteries were ligated as the EEG was monitored. The left subclavian artery was occluded proximal to the vertebral artery, followed by production of critical stenoses (15-20% drop in carotid arterial flow) of the carotid and vertebral vessels. The effects of augmented flow to the involved limb, produced by electric muscle stimulation, were examined in 7 other dogs.

Occlusion of the left subclavian artery reversed vertebral flow from 52 ml. per minute cephalad to 44.6 brachiad, with a rise in right carotid flow and a temporary rise in mean aortic pressure. With added stenosis of the right carotid artery, brachiad vertebral flow dropped to 22.8 ml. per minute. Brachiad vertebral flow was 33.8 ml. per minute with left carotid occlusion and 8.5 with right vertebral occlusion added to left subclavian occlusion. Superimposed right carotid stenosis further reduced brachiad flow and sometimes resulted in cephalad vertebral flow. Cerebral blood flow and the EEG remained unchanged in all these circumstances. Cortical oxygen tension decreased and the EEG sometimes slowed when right vertebral occlusion was superimposed on bilateral carotid occlusion. The EEG sometimes slowed with bilateral carotid, right vertebral and left subclavian occlusion. Blood gases were unchanged during these studies. With augmented ipsilateral limb flow, the vertebral

(9) Surgery 68:431-441, September, 1970.

steal increased but the cerebral blood flow and EEG were unchanged.

The findings emphasize the autoregulatory capabilities and
dominant demands of the cerebral circulation. A subclavian
steal per se may not result in critical cerebral ischemia.

► [There is ample clinical confirmation for the conclusions drawn in this
study—Eds.]

Neuroanesthetic Adjuncts for Surgery in Sitting Position.—
I. Introduction and basic equipment.—John T. Martin[1] (Mayo
Clinic and Found.) reviewed the mechanical technics used at
the Mayo Clinic to support the physiologic functions of patients anesthetized and placed in the sitting position for operations on the lateral and posterior cranial fossas or the cervi-
codorsal spine. The sitting position permits better access to
these sites from directly behind the wound. Blood drains away
from the operative site. Resuscitative measures can be rapidly
instituted because of freer access to the anterior chest wall in
the sitting position. Less intrathoracic positive pressure is
needed for intermittent ventilation than in the prone position.
Much of the superior caval drainage system, however, is at sub-
atmospheric pressures, and transected vessels can entrain air.
Resilience of the walls of the inferior caval circuit may be depressed by anesthetic agents, resulting in pooling of blood in the
legs and abdominal viscera. The legs are elevated to facilitate
venous return to the heart.

The Massa type of needle is preferred for indwelling intravascular therapy. Heated blood is administered. A cutdown is
done if accessible peripheral vessels are absent. The Sorensen
central arterial pressure infusor is acceptable for sustained arterial pressure readings. An endotracheal tube with walls rein-
forced with a wire spiral is used. The esophageal stethoscope
is used to monitor sitting patients. A skull-pin head holder is
used. The ECG is monitored continuously during the operation.
The ECG is used as the major guide to the integrity of the hind
brain.

II. The antigravity suit.—Martin[2] discusses the effects of
the antigravity suit in neurosurgical procedures performed in
the sitting position. Vascular support by external compression
was introduced to neurosurgery by Crile in 1903. Gardner and
Dohn revived the external pressure technic in 1956, using a
plastic sheath on cordotomy patients treated in the sitting posi-

(1)   Anesth. & Analg. 49:577-587, July-Aug., 1970.
(2)   Ibid., pp. 588-593.

tion. The Gardner G-suit consists of two layers of heavy plastic sealed around the edges, with a filling tube and manometer tube lead between the layers. The suit is inflated by metered nitrogen, CO_2 or compressed air, but not with oxygen. The patient is placed on the suit after it is placed on the operating table.

A G-suit was applied to 32 neurosurgical patients during 1968-69, and pressure changes were evaluated in 24 cases. The suit was applied before anesthetic induction or just after tracheal intubation and inflated after the sitting position was assumed. Intubation was with an armored latex tube. Anesthesia was with nitrous oxide, oxygen and halothane. Hyperventilation was performed by controlled manual ventilation or with a Bird ventilator. No relaxants were given during maintenance. Venous pressure changes occurred rapidly when the suit was rapidly inflated to 30 mm. Hg and deflated rapidly to zero or inflated in a stepwise manner and similarly deflated. The most marked changes occurred at suit pressures of 20-30 mm. Hg. The venous pressure fell below baseline after deflation. With rapid compression of the suit sustained for 30 minutes, and then a reduction in pressure in 10-mm. Hg steps, a sharp rise to a sustained pressure occurred, with a continued rise in pressure in one instance. Six patients did not maintain an elevated pressure during the high suit pressure phase, apparently because of vascular compensation. One patient had several episodes of hypotension treated with the G-suit.

The Gardner-Dohn G-suit is effective in treating hypotension occurring in anesthetized patients in the sitting position. It is not predictably effective in maintaining venous pressure if inflated to 30 mm. Hg and allowed to remain there for long periods. It probably has minimal value as prophylaxis against embolization of air from an operative site above the heart. The antigravity suit has now been used in over 150 patients anesthetized for neurosurgical procedures in the sitting position. It has been effective in supporting venous return to the heart.

III. Intravascular electrocardiography.—Martin[3] reports the results of right atrial catheterization monitored by the intravascular ECG, undertaken in 132 neurosurgical patients during 1967-1970. Catheters could not be placed in the atrium in 6 cases. No deaths have occurred. Air embolism occurred in 7% of cases. A Cavacath was used in all but a few cases, consisting of a 13-gauge plastic needle and a 36-in. styletted sheathed cath-

(3) Anesth. & Analg. 49:793-808, Sept.-Oct., 1970.

eter. The antecubital system is preferred to direct subclavian puncture for introduction of the catheter. The ECG was monitored oscilloscopically. An isolation amplifier grounded to the patient cable is inserted between the catheter hub and the chest lead. The ECG extremity leads and a chest lead are applied before the catheter is introduced, and all other electrical equipment is removed from the patient.

Intravascular electrocardiography is a useful means of accurately locating a catheter tip in the right midatrium for the subsequent treatment of embolized air. The technic is easily learned and applicable to neuroanesthetic procedures. A composite map of intravascular P wave changes has been prepared. Biphasic P waves can be found at the root of the inferior vena cava, but their amplitude is much less than that of the huge midatrial biphasic P waves. Differentiation of these wave forms and of a W-type of P wave found at the superior cavoatrial junction is important for accurate catheter placement.

▶ [Details of original articles are often lost in abstracting, often to the advantage of the reader. However, in this series of articles, the details are important and they should be read by all resident anesthesiologists and by those who practice neurosurgical anesthesia. Not that one needs to agree with everything written, but at least one should read the arguments.—Eds.]

Report of 10 Operations under Local Cerebral Hypothermia. The ability of the brain to withstand complete circulatory arrest for over 30 minutes at low temperatures was used in the treatment of difficult aneurysms or arteriovenous malformations by Bernard N. Williams and Eric A. Turner[4] (Birmingham, England). An attempt was made to achieve a local temperature of about 15 C. without direct interference with the heart.

Arterial blood was cooled and perfused distally into one carotid artery at a pressure above systemic arterial pressure. With overflow into the opposite carotid territory and cooling by conduction, the other hemisphere was cooled to the point where the opposite carotid could be safely occluded, followed by occlusion of the vertebral arteries in succession. The cerebral oxygen requirements were thus met through one artery that was under direct surgical control. Studies in dogs indicated that regional cerebral hypothermia to a temperature below 12 C. could be obtained with reasonable safety and sometimes without histologic damage. Dextran markedly increased the blood flow to the cerebral tissues. A polyvinyl chloride coil immersed in an

---

(4) J. Neurol., Neurosurg. & Psychiat. 33:647-655, October, 1970.

ice and brine bath was used for heat exchange. Perfusion was at a constant pressure rather than at a constant flow rate.

The technic increased the operating time. Four postoperative deaths occurred; in 1 case the technic appeared to have protected the perfused part of the brain from anoxic damage. In 1 case the method caused bad operating conditions, and the patient eventually died. One survivor had a postoperative intracerebral thrombosis which developed at closure, and another had a clot that required removal after 24 hours. Another patient had a delay in returning to full mental function.

The method is not satisfactory for general use at present. A more effective means of neutralizing anticoagulants or a way of dispensing with them altogether must be found. A method must be developed to monitor parts of the brain distant from those directly perfused, to give warning of threatened anoxia. Presently, one type of case in which the method would be most helpful, an extremely vascular lesion or a lesion that had recently bled, is made riskier by the use of the technic.

Further Studies on Cerebrospinal Fluid Acid-Base Status in Patients with Brain Lesions. E. Gordon (Karolinska Inst., Stockholm) and M. Rossanda[5] (Milan) attempted to reaffirm the relationship previously found between severity of brain damage and the cerebrospinal fluid acid-base status. Study was made of 21 conscious patients having diagnostic procedures or extradural operations, without clinical evidence of brain lesions (group I); 28 with mild symptoms of cerebral disturbance (group II); and 28 who were unconscious with severe brain lesions (group III), including 5 with total areflexia. Some patients were studied during general anesthesia under constant artificial ventilation.

Among spontaneously breathing patients, mean cerebrospinal fluid pH levels were significantly low in group III. Only group II patients had a high pH among ventilated patients. The mean cerebrospinal fluid bicarbonate in group I patients was 23.6 mEq./L. during spontaneous breathing and 22.8 mEq./L. on artificial ventilation. Values were slightly lower in group II patients, but ventricular samples showed near-normal values. Bicarbonate was significantly reduced in group III patients, in both respiratory groups, the mean value being 20.4 mEq./L. Mean juguloarterial ΔPco_2 difference was significantly lower in

(5) Acta anaesth. scandinav. 14:97-109, 1970.

group III cases, and the cerebrospinal fluid-arterial ΔPco_2 change was significantly high in this group, as was the cerebrospinal fluid-jugular ΔPco_2 difference. Ventricular samples showed a greater cerebrospinal fluid-arterial ΔPco_2 difference than lumbar samples in group III patients. Both cerebrospinal fluid-arterial and juguloarterial ΔPco_2 differences were slightly increased with artificial ventilation, but the difference was significant only for the cerebrospinal fluid-arterial difference in groups I and II, considered together.

This study confirmed a cerebrospinal fluid acidosis and an abnormally high Pco_2 gradient between blood and cerebrospinal fluid in unconscious patients with brain lesions. The finding of a high Pco_2 gradient in severely diseased brains supports the use of hyperventilation as a therapeutic measure. It may explain the beneficial effects of respirator treatment carried out early and with adequate volumes. Moderate hyperventilation may be considered a valuable tool in the management of patients with severe brain lesions. Such patients appear to have an intracerebral acidosis due to accumulation of acid metabolites and also CO_2 and hyperventilate spontaneously in an effort to compensate for the acidosis. Arterial Pco_2 levels of about 25 mm. Hg must be attained for effective compensation.

▶ [The patient with a severe brain lesion who is breathing rapidly and deeply needs help. Use a ventilator and keep the $Paco_2$ at about 25 mm. Hg.—Eds.]

PEDIATRIC ANESTHESIA

Some Controversial Aspects of Fluids for the Anesthetized Neonate. Edward J. Bennett, Michael J. Daughety and M. T. Jenkins[6] (Dallas) attempted to determine whether the fluid requirements of anesthetized neonates are similar to those of adults and whether the neonate can handle sodium and water when administered.

After tracheal intubation, neonates were anesthetized with nitrous oxide, oxygen and tubocurarine or halothane, in either instance with controlled ventilation using a Rees modification of the T piece. Operative maintenance was with 5% dextrose in lactated Ringer's solution, 8 ml./kg./hour, and lavage and suction losses were replaced with isotonic saline. A 20% or greater blood loss was replaced. Acidosis was managed with sodium

---

(6) Anesth. & Analg. 49:478-486, May-June, 1970.

bicarbonate, and albumin was given when large intracellular water and sodium shifts occurred. Postoperatively, fluid volume of 5% dextrose in water approximated 100 ml./kg./24 hours, with one fifth of the daily volume given as 5% dextrose in lactated Ringer's solution; two-fifths was given with various conditions such as those associated with increased fluid and electrolyte losses. Study was made of 25 consecutive neonates having operation (group A), including 9 premature infants, and of 11 selected neonates whose only problem required surgery (group B), including 4 premature infants.

In group A, the mean weight was 5.7 lb. Four patients received over 200 ml. fluid during operation, and 4 received 20 mEq. sodium. The mean group B weight was 6.16 lb. Operative fluids averaged 55 ml. water containing 8 mEq. sodium. Only 4 patients received blood. The average intravenous load in the first 4 postoperative days was 250 ml. with 11 mEq. sodium for group A and 240 ml. with 10.5 ml. sodium for group B. Mean weights decreased 0.7 lb. in group A and 1.65 lb. in group B during this period. Sodium fell from 135 to 132 mEq./L. in group A, and a similar mean drop occurred in group B cases. The mean daily output was 151 ml. for group A and 140 ml. for group B; in group B the sodium output was 7.3 mEq. Definite hyponatremia below 130 mEq./L. occurred in 7 group A and 2 group B cases. The maximum rise in the serum sodium level was 6 mEq./L.

The neonate undergoing operation will not show sodium or water retention if adequately hydrated within wide limits. Apparent sodium retention is a matter of interpretation. Neonates require increased amounts of balanced salt solution for surgical operations and increased amounts of sodium in the postoperative period.

▶ [The neonate in this regard appears more as the "small adult."—Eds.]

EXTRACORPOREAL CIRCULATION: TECHNICS, EFFECTS AND RESULTS

Morphine Anesthesia for Open Heart Surgery. Jan D. Hasbrouck[7] (Univ. of Kentucky) used morphine as the sole anesthetic in a group of 37 high-risk patients, aged 17-71 years, with acquired valvular heart disease. The functional rating was class

(7) Ann. Thoracic Surg. 10:364-369, October, 1970.

IV, and the cardiac index was 2 L./minute/sq. m. or less. Morphine and atropine were given about an hour before operation, and an intravenous dose equivalent to twice the premedicating dose of morphine was then given rapidly as the patient breathed oxygen. If consciousness and blood pressure were unaltered in 5 minutes, an infusion of 1 mg. morphine per ml. in lactated Ringer's solution was begun, with manual support of respiration. A dose of 1 mg./kg. was given in 15-20 minutes; succinylcholine was then given for tracheal intubation, followed by infusion of morphine to a level of 2 mg./kg. in 15 minutes. More morphine was given if pain perception was evident, and small doses of curare were given as needed. The P_{CO_2} was kept at 30-40 mm. Hg and the P_{O_2} above 100. The total dose of morphine given ranged from 65 to 595 mg.; the end point was loss of consciousness or a report of patient comfort. Mechanical ventilation was continued for 8-12 hours postoperatively. If the patient did not respond to commands during this period, levallorphan was used to determine whether he was neurologically intact.

Cardiac output and stroke volume increased after morphine anesthesia. A rise in blood pressure and pulse was noted in all cases (Fig. 22), in contrast to the changes ordinarily seen with inhalation anesthesia. Plasma catecholamines were increased from preoperative levels at morphine doses of 1 and 2 mg./kg.

Fig. 22.—Changes in blood pressure (*solid line*) and pulse (*broken line*) with administration of morphine. (Courtesy of Hasbrouck, J. D.: Ann. Thoracic Surg. 10:364-369, October, 1970.)

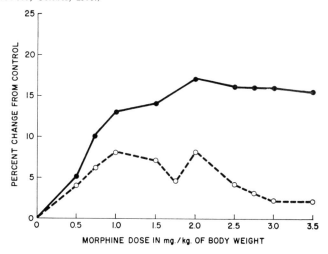

and were positively correlated with the rises in pulse and blood pressure. No patient had recall of events during operation, although they often opened their eyes on command. The EEGs occasionaly showed apparent sleep spindles as well as some toxic changes.

Morphine used alone is an attractive alternative to inhalation technics. Ventricular performance is enhanced and cardiovascular depression is avoided before extracorporeal support is established, through augmentation of adrenergic stimulation of the heart. No depressant effect on cardiovascular function is evident so long as ventilation is maintained. Morphine anesthesia has become the author's technic of choice in patients critically ill with cardiac disease.

▶ [This is reminiscent of the earlier technic for ether analgesia for open heart surgery, where the patient also was able to respond to commands, had no recall of pain and undoubtedly mobilized endogenous catecholamines for cardiovascular support. How well would these technics work in the patient receiving β-blockers preoperatively to control arrhythmias?— Eds.]

Constancy of Myocardial Digoxin Concentration during Experimental Cardiopulmonary Bypass. It is unclear whether digitalis should be given routinely to patients having cardiac operations in the absence of congestive failure or tachyarrhythmias. The situation is more complex with cardiopulmonary bypass, where perfusion and hemodilution may affect the usual pattern of digitalis distribution. Farouk A. Molokhia, George A. Beller, Thomas W. Smith, Panayiotis J. Asimacopoulos, William B. Hood, Jr., and John C. Norman[8] (Harvard Med. School) studied the effects of 2-hour total cardiopulmonary bypass on myocardial, blood and perfusate concentrations of digoxin in dogs, using tritiated digoxin of high specific activity. Eight adult male dogs were given labeled digoxin, anesthetized and ventilated and subjected to total bypass with partial hemodilution for 2 hours. Priming was with whole canine blood, Hartmann's solution, 5% dextrose in 0.9% saline, tromethamine buffer and 10% calcium chloride. The flow rate during bypass was 85 ml./minute/kg. Blood and perfusate were sampled for digoxin concentration at intervals after start of bypass, and right ventricular biopsy specimens were taken at the end of the study.

Initial serum digoxin levels of 28.6 ng./ml. dropped gradually to a plateau of 7.8. A drop of 14.1% occurred to a stable level

(8) Ann. Thoracic Surg. 11:222-228, March, 1971.

of 6.4-6.9 ng./ml. after the start of bypass. Right ventricular tissue digoxin levels did not change significantly. Perfusate levels increased significantly to a mean of 5.9 ng./ml. after 2 hours of bypass. Plasma potassium fell from 4.7 to 3.7 mEq./L. at the end of bypass and hematocrit from 43 to 32%. The fall in serum and perfusate digoxin levels paralleled the decrease in hematocrit and potassium, suggesting hemodilution as the common cause of all these changes. Arterial pH fell from 7.44 to 7.30 after bypass. Hemodynamic variables did not change significantly and oxygen saturation remained at 100%.

The finding of a constant myocardial digoxin level during cardiopulmonary bypass does not necessarily imply a constant dose requirement for patients after bypass. The sensitivity of the myocardium to digoxin depends on many other factors in the postoperative period, including hypoxia, changes in acid-base and electrolyte balances, surgical manipulation and a reduced glomerular filtration rate secondary to decreased cardiac output.

▶ [Although bypass appeared not to alter the myocardial digoxin content, digitalis requirements of cardiac patients remain a highly individual problem requiring careful management of each subject.—Eds.]

Effect of Glucose-Insulin-Potassium Solution on Ketosis Following Cardiac Surgery. Emerson A. Moffitt, John W. Rosevear, George D. Molnar and Dwight C. McGoon[9] (Mayo Clinic and Found.) report the results of treating 10 patients with supplemental glucose, insulin and potassium in the first 48 hours after cardiac surgery (study group). The results were compared with those in 20 patients who underwent similar operations but had no such treatment. All patients but 1 had at least one cardiac valve replaced.

Arterial flows at 30 C. averaged 2.25 L./minute/sq. m. Both coronary arteries were perfused during aortic or multiple valve replacement. A prime of acid-citrate dextrose blood (60%) diluted with 5% dextrose in 0.45% saline and THAM (40%) was used. Assisted ventilation for at least overnight was given to 13 patients. The study patients received 500 ml. of 10% dextrose in water containing 20 units of regular insulin and 40 mEq. KCl each 24 hours. Thus they received 50 Gm. dextrose with insulin compared with 25 Gm. without insulin for the other patients as part of the daily fluid allotment.

---

(9)   Anesth. & Analg. 50:291-297, Mar.-Apr., 1971.

In the study patients, compared with the other patients, the oxygen content of the coronary sinus blood was higher for several hours after operation, blood Pco_2 and buffer base values were higher during operation and on the 1st postoperative day, and arterial potassium levels were higher. Differences in blood glucose between the groups were not apparent. Ketone bodies were lower in study patients. Mean cardiac indexes for the groups were not significantly different.

Administration of glucose-insulin-potassium after cardiac surgery strikingly reduced total ketone bodies and significantly increased plasma potassium levels. Blood levels of glucose, insulin and fatty acids were not different from those in patients given standard treatment.

▶ [It is difficult to find any advantage to using the proposed solution but the idea was worth trying.—Eds.]

Effect of Hypothermia on Lung Compliance. Total body hypothermia is often used as an adjunct to medical and surgical treatment, but no reports of lung function during and after hypothermia could be found. Cedric W. Deal, John C. Warden and Ian Monk[1] (Sydney) correlated changes in pulmonary compliance with varying levels of hypothermia in sheep. Nineteen healthy adult sheep were anesthetized and ventilated mechanically with manual hyperinflation at intervals, and lung compliance was measured in sheep with the chest opened or in excised lungs. Intact sheep were studied over 3 hours of anesthesia alone or at temperatures of 20 or 23 C. over 60-90 minutes, using a femorofemoral arteriovenous shunt. Body temperature was maintained at 35 C. in some sheep for 80 minutes of total heart bypass, followed by ventricular fibrillation and defibrillation 20 minutes later. In other sheep, body temperature was reduced to 15 C. and then raised to 37 C.

Little change in lung compliance occurred over 3 hours with anesthesia alone. On cooling by femorofemoral bypass, lung elasticity decreased steadily with a temperature fall; blood pressure also fell steadily until ventricular fibrillation occurred. The pulmonary artery pressure changed little throughout the procedure. Compliance decreased slightly in some sheep having biventricular bypass without cooling and a period of fibrillation. With cooling in other sheep, the lungs became less elastic, and rewarming produced a steady rise in compliance up to 24-30

(1) Thorax 25:105-109, January, 1970.

C., when the lungs rapidly decreased in compliance. The lungs appeared histologically normal after this procedure. Excised lungs showed little change in compliance at 37 and at 15 C.

The persistent and severe nature of the compliance changes noted following profound hypothermia with perfusion in sheep indicates that the findings be considered before this technic is used either as a medical procedure or in preserving lung tissue for transplantation in man.

Ventilatory Requirements after Open Heart Operations. It is difficult to predict the extent of cardiorespiratory derangement that may follow open heart surgery in spontaneously breathing patients, and almost all adults are now ventilated mechanically in the immediate postoperative period to ensure adequate blood-gas exchange and reduce the work of breathing. Deryck Duncalf, Narendra K. Shah, Elliott Jacobson and Hideo Nagashima[2] (Bronx, N. Y.) describe a procedure that was developed for the ventilatory management of open heart patients. Study was made of 28 males and 52 females (mean age, 47.1 years). Anesthesia consisted of nitrous oxide-oxygen and d-tubocurarine chloride supplemented by thiopental sodium and meperidine hydrochloride (30 cases), droperidol and fentanyl citrate (36 cases) and thiopental and halothane (14 cases). Metabolic acidosis was corrected by intravenous tromethamine. No attempt was made to reverse residual curarization after operation. Ventilation was with an Engström respirator at a rate of 16 for those aged 16 and over, or 20 for younger patients. Air and oxygen were delivered at 150% of the volume requirement predicted from the Engström-Herzog nomogram. Minute volume was increased by 20% if the Pa_{CO_2} was over 45 torr after 10 minutes of ventilation and reduced by 20% if it was below 25 torr or outside the range 35-45 torr at 40 minutes.

Ventilation was increased at 10 minutes to reduce the Pa_{CO_2} below 45 torr in 6 cases and decreased in 3. At 40 minutes, it was increased in 1 case and reduced in 13. The Pa_{O_2} was below 100 torr in 5 cases, in 4 of them at 10 minutes. Reducing the fractional inspired P_{O_2} from 0.6 significantly decreased the Pa_{O_2}. Six patients had spontaneous respiration not in phase with the ventilator at 10 minutes, and in 2 of these patients, asynchronous breathing was present at 40 minutes and in 1, at 100 minutes. They were treated with droperidol or manual hyperventilation. Consciousness generally returned soon after anes-

(2)   Anesth. & Analg. 49:518-522, July-Aug., 1970.

thesia was stopped. Three patients were apprehensive and restless at 10 minutes, and 1 at 40 minutes. Two of these patients breathed asynchronously. Cyanosis was observed in 2 patients, neither of whom breathed asynchronously.

This regimen facilitates blood-gas transport and thus tissue-gas exchange by maintaining an adequate Pao_2 and $Paco_2$ in most instances. The patient is relieved of the work of breathing at a time when myocardial reserve may not suffice to compensate for increased ventilatory effort. This approach has now been used in over 400 open heart cases without respiratory complications occurring.

► [Despite widespread use of ventilators in postpump patients, it should not be assumed that all cardiac surgical units subscribe to this philosophy. There are many exceptions.—Eds.]

Production of Microemboli by Various Blood Oxygenators. Jack Kessler and Russel H. Patterson, Jr.[3] (New York Hosp.-Cornell Med. Center) used an ultrasonic detection chamber to count blood particles larger than 50 μ, and determine the relative concentrations of microemboli produced by disk and membrane oxygenators and two types of disposable bubble oxygenator. The system consists of a detection chamber, transducer, sonarscope and electronic counter. Its sensitivity was determined in studies using plastic microspheres of known diameter.

Heparinized mongrel dogs were put on cardiopulmonary bypass. The extracorporeal circuit was primed with two parts of electrolyte solution and one part low molecular weight dextran. The Temptrol Q110, the Travenol 5MO311, a silicone-coated 18-in. disk oxygenator and the Medical Monitors membrane oxygenator with two double sacs were compared at a blood flow rate of 2 L. per minute and an oxygen flow rate of 6 L. per minute. The Travenol 5MO310 and Temptrol Q100 oxygenators were compared at flow rates of 3 L. per minute for blood and 6 and 9 L. per minute for oxygen. Perfusate volumes were maintained at levels usual during clinical perfusions.

The pediatric disposable bubble oxygenators produced about equal concentrations of microemboli. The 18-in. disk oxygenator released fewer emboli than any of the other oxygenators, about 80 times less than the pediatric oxygenators in the 1st hour of perfusion and 200 times less thereafter. The Medical Monitors membrane oxygenator generated fewer emboli than the bubble oxygenators, but more than the 18-in. disk oxygenator, even

(3)   Ann. Thoracic Surg. 9:221-228, March, 1970.

when the blood flowed without foaming. The Temptrol Q100 and Travenol 5MO310 produced emboli in about equal concentrations at an oxygen flow rate of 6 L. per minute. At a flow of 9 L., however, more emboli were generated, especially by the Temptrol Q100, which thereafter produced 2-13 times the concentration of emboli as the Travenol 5MO310.

The bubble oxygenators produced the fewest emboli when a large volume of blood was kept in the settling compartment and when the oxygen flow was reduced. Microemboli appeared to be increased by an increase in the ratio of gas mixing with blood, a decrease in the volume of blood in the oxygenator and any agitation of the oxygenator.

▶ [Makes us appreciate the human heart-lung pump more.—Eds.]

Total Cardiopulmonary Bypass, Myocardial Contractility and the Administration of Protamine Sulfate. Protamine administered intravenously may be followed by hypotension, bradycardia and dyspnea. Anatole Gourin, Robert L. Streisand and Jackson H. Stuckey[4] (Brooklyn, N. Y.) studied the effects of protamine on myocardial contractility in the isovolumic left ventricle during total cardiopulmonary bypass.

Bypass was instituted in 7 healthy anesthetized, heparinized mongrel dogs; the perfusion rate was 100 ml./kg./minute and body temperature, 37 C. Complete heart block was created by ligating the bundle of His, and the coronary sinus was cannulated. Ventricular fibrillation was induced electrically, and a balloon catheter was placed in the left ventricle. The heart was then driven at a specified rate by an epicardial electrode. Femoral arterial blood flow was measured in 5 dogs. A bolus of protamine sulfate, 10 mg./kg., was given into the blood reservoir, and a second dose was given after 30 minutes. The heparin titer was raised to about 90 μg./ml. before each dose of protamine.

Heparin caused a transient drop in myocardial contractility in all 7 dogs. The average drop in left ventricular pressure was 12% with a 10 mg./kg. dose of heparin and 17% with 20 mg./kg. Contractility returned to preinjection levels within 15 minutes. Transient arrhythmia occurred in 2 dogs. All animals had transient arrhythmia on protamine injection, with a slight augmentation of contractility and a transient elevation of mean arterial blood pressure. The second dose had a delayed, less marked effect. Five minutes postinjection, the average rise in left ventricular pressure was 10.9% with the first dose of pro-

(4)   J. Thoracic & Cardiovas. Surg. 61: 160-166, January, 1971.

tamine and 7.4% with the second. The respective figures 10 minutes after injection were 3.4 and 9.8%.

Coronary sinus blood flow increased in 5 animals after protamine was given; the increase averaged 55% after the first dose and 29% after the second. Blood flow rates were increased with essentially unchanged mean arterial pressures; peripheral resistance decreased. The average drop in peripheral resistance was 33% after the first dose of protamine and 26% after the second.

Protamine did not significantly depress myocardial contractility during total cardiopulmonary bypass in the isovolumic canine left ventricle. After protamine administration, a transient inotropic effect on contractility and an increase in coronary sinus blood flow were shown in most animals. Protamine increased femoral arterial blood flow at a constant perfusion rate during bypass, indicating a decrease in peripheral resistance in the intact extremity.

Sustained Hypotension Secondary to Protamine Sulfate. David R. Jackson[5] (VA Hosp., Northampton, Mass.) reports sustained hypotension occurring after protamine sulfate was used to nullify the effects of heparin after vascular reconstructive surgery. Protamine was given intravenously after lower extremity surgery done under light general anesthesia. Some patients had sustained hypotension requiring vasopressor administration to keep the reconstructed vasculature safely patent. Blood volume deficit or incipient heart failure or infarction was never evident. The condition was spontaneously corrected in 3-5 days, but some graft closures occurred during this period. Generally, prompt reoperation led to salvage of the graft and extremity. Patients rarely had difficulty maintaining their blood pressure at operation, no matter how long the operation lasted. The hypotension occurred at the end of operation or in the recovery room. The problem became less evident when low spinal or local anesthesia was used rather than general anesthesia. Protamine often was omitted at this time.

Woman, 78, had claudication and ischemic rest pain of the right foot and underwent right femoropopliteal vein bypass grafting using local lidocaine anesthesia. When 30 mg. protamine sulfate was given intravenously in 2-3 minutes, the patient became stuporous, with a drop in blood pressure from 140 to 80 mm. Hg systolic. Vasopressors were necessary. Blood volume and electrolyte studies, a hemogram and serial EEGs showed no abnormality. Only after 4 days could

(5)   Angiology 21:295-298, May, 1970.

the blood pressure be maintained without vasopressors. The reconstruction remained patent.

Protamine sulfate is an extremely basic, positively charged protein used intravenously to counteract heparin. It was used topically on the fibrillating epicardium to reduce the heartbeat during early open heart surgery. In susceptible persons it may cause a profound, long-lasting hypotensive effect. The effect may be exerted on the heart itself, making it less sensitive to peripheral stimuli and lasting until the protamine molecular linkages could be broken down. Some complications of early open heart procedures might have been related to this phenomenon.

Protamine sulfate is no longer used or is given in Ringer's solution over 10-30 minutes. No hypotensive problems have occurred on this regimen. The hypotensive declamping effect during abdominal aneurysmectomy has also not occurred, but grafts are preclotted so that protamine does not have to be instilled just before or after declamping.

▶ [Seems as if a good pharmacology laboratory could nail this problem down rather quickly.—Eds.]

MEASUREMENT OF BLOOD LOSS

Method of Control of Bleeding in Prostate Surgery: Review of 20 Cases. V. H. Marwah, P. V. Ginde and S. R. Vaidya[6] (Aurangabad, India) used local hypothermia in 20 cases of suprapubic transvesical prostatectomy, irrigating the "prostatic fossa" with refrigerated sterile water as the chief method of hemostasis. The bladder was evacuated and filled with 200-300 ml. refrigerated water before enucleating the prostate. The fossa was then loosely packed with gauze soaked in refrigerated water and digital pressure maintained for about 5 minutes. The pack was removed, and the fossa irrigated with water through the incision and also the urethral catheter. Cold water was then left in the bladder for 2-3 minutes. The procedure was repeated if necessary. A good operative field was available, and the fossa contracted quickly. Drainage was maintained for about a week postoperatively, and a drain was left in the retropubic space.

No patient in this series died. Three had bladder congestion. None had postoperative shock, and 10 did not receive blood during or after operation. The urine output averaged 750 ml. on the 1st day and was normal on the 2d day in all cases. Drain-

(6) Indian J. Surg. 32:352-357, July, 1970.

age was satisfactory throughout. Clots did not block the urethral catheters, and the bladder did not have to be washed or reopened in any instance. Blood loss was moderate in 17 cases, and major in 3. Six patients had infection postoperatively. Seven had a major leak of urine from the suprapubic incision, and 6 had minor leakage.

This method of irrigating the bladder and prostatic fossa with cold water is a simple means of controlling bleeding at prostatic surgery. Local hypothermia helps in contraction of the prostatic fossa and provides an optimal operative field.

▶ [A control series would be interesting, as would more data on the patients composing the reported series.—Eds.]

Use of Cautery in "Bloodless" Radical Mastectomy. Blood loss during skin flap formation has been a problem in radical mastectomy for breast carcinoma. Gerard S. Kakos and Arthur G. James[7] (Ohio State Univ. Hosp.) evaluated electrocautery for thin skin flap development at mastectomy in regard to blood loss and wound healing. Fifty consecutive patients having radical mastectomy for breast carcinoma were studied. Half had flaps developed by sharp dissection, and half had thin skin flaps elevated by electrocautery dissection. The rest of the procedure was the same in the two groups. The groups were comparable in age and pathology, as well as mean pre- and postoperative hemoglobin and hematocrit levels.

Transfusions were given at operation or in the operating room to 24 patients having sharp dissection and 6 having electrocautery. The respective average blood replacements were 940 and 144 ml. Five patients having sharp dissection and 4 having electrocautery had marginal wound necrosis. One patient in the electrocautery group had a positive wound culture and a clinical infection. Wound healing was not adversely affected by electrocautery.

Three large dogs each had three pairs of standard skin flaps made. One of each pair of skin flaps was raised by sharp dissection and 1 by cautery dissection. All flaps were sutured with nylon. Biopsy specimens were taken after 1, 2, 4, 6 and 12 weeks. No difference in healing was noted between the paired skin flaps. No skin loss or infection occurred. Microscopy showed no difference in scarring, although 1- and 2-week cautery specimens showed a minimal increase in fibrosis and hemosiderin deposition. There was practically no difference at 4 weeks.

(7)   Cancer 26:666-668, September, 1970.

Electrocautery for raising thin skin flaps at radical mastecto-my appears to be valuable for preventing blood loss and reduc-ing the need for transfusion.

▶ [It is not necessary to lose large amounts of blood during radical mas-tectomy. The anesthesiologist can help by properly positioning the patient and controlling the blood pressure. The surgeon can help by proper hemo-stasis, with or without cautery.—Eds.]

BLOOD, PLASMA EXPANDERS AND BLOOD SUBSTITUTES

Commercially Obtained Blood and Serum Hepatitis is dis-cussed by J. Garrott Allen[8] (Stanford Univ.) Posttransfusion or serum hepatitis from infected blood or improperly treated plasma or its products creates a serious clinical problem. It ap-pears that at least two immunologically distinct agents can pro-duce hepatitis from transfusion of blood or blood products and that both can be transmitted orally or parenterally. Both are probably viruses, with some immunization being possible.

An Au-positive carrier is found in about 1,200-1,500 donors by present screening methods. This antigen appears to be hepatitis-associated rather than causal. Susceptibility rates are functions of amount of live virus given in relation to degree of immunity present in the patient. Of 100 recipients of commer-cially obtained blood, 5 are exposed to affected donors. The chance of encountering a carrier donor, assuming a 20% sus-ceptibility rate in recipients of single-unit transfusions, is 1 carrier among 20 commercial blood donors and about 1 among 200 volunteer blood donors.

It seems unwise at present to place much value on the Au antigen test as a screening device for blood donor selection. Commercially obtained blood and that taken from prisoners should not be used, except for that used as albumin and γ-glob-ulin. Other products, with the possible exception of washed red cells, are highly icterogenic. The risk of a unit of blood ob-tained commercially is 10-25 times that of a unit obtained from a volunteer, and there are no regulations at present governing these practices. Commercial blood banks will continue to thrive unless the economic stimulus to their donors is removed. A vol-unteer and a commercial blood program can probably not co-exist without eventual destruction of the volunteer program.

(8)   Surg., Gynec. & Obst. 131:277-281, August, 1970.

Commercial Blood in Our National Blood Program. J. Garrott Allen[9] (Stanford Univ.) points out that an effective national blood program does not exist in the United States. Rather there is a patchwork series of enterprises, the largest being the American Red Cross with 59 blood stations in 42 states, which claims to draw about half the blood collected in the country. Community-oriented blood banks account for about a fourth of the 7,000,000 units of blood collected annually. Commercial blood banks depend on donors who need the payment of $4 to $10, largely Skid Row residents and hippie addicts as well as prison donors. This blood accounts for almost 90% of cases of serum icteric hepatitis. The commercial donor lends quantity rather than quality to the present program. A dependable test to identify Au antigen would be helpful. A second antigen may also be involved in hepatitis. The risks of hepatitis from volunteer and commercial blood are presented in the table. An increasing number of commercial blood banks is being developed throughout the country, and volunteer blood banks find it easier to depend on commercial blood sources to replenish their supplies than to make an effort to sustain a good volunteer program.

A blood bank may operate within a single state without federal sanction, and federal inspection is minimal at best. An increasing number of health insurance plans includes the cost of purchasing blood, making it unnecessary to recruit volunteer

COMPARISON OF RISK OF SERUM HEPATITIS FROM VOLUNTEER AND
COMMERCIAL BLOOD INCLUDING FIBRINOGEN

Study	Patients	Hepatitis Cases	Occurrence Rate, %
Boeve et al[12] (limited to open-heart surgery cases)			
All volunteer blood; no fibrinogen	40	0	0
All volunteer blood plus fibrinogen (commercial)	32	10	31
Walsh et al[13] (limited to open-heart surgery cases)			
All volunteer blood	28	0	0
All commercial blood	82	42	51
Allen[14] (all patients, excluding open-heart surgery patients)			
All volunteer blood	7,497	27	0.3
All commercial blood	1,854	62	3.2

(9) Arch. Surg. 102:122-126, February, 1971.

donors. It may be difficult in the United States to adapt present thinking toward a not-for-profit national blood program. Only 3.5% of persons would need to contribute blood to supply present needs, and many donors give on more than one occasion. The nation's needs could be met if 7% of the eligible population contributed blood annually, preferably not the same persons each year. Volunteer donors should be assured that they will receive volunteer blood in any state. Collecting stations would best be located in areas of cities that are often visited by acceptable donors. The donor should be a treasured person. A program of blood assurance accredited at the national level would represent a significant contribution to community medical care. When the Au antigen or a similar test is proved to be dependable for screening, infectious blood can be discarded. Until then, the most crucial screening device available is whether a donor is paid or not.

▶ [The plea being made by J. Garrott Allen is reasonable and important. Other countries that utilize an all-donor system do not appear to have the hepatitis problem we have in the United States. When did you donate your last pint of blood?—Eds.]

Australia Antigen and Blood Transfusion. Previous studies indicate a highly significant relation between the presence of Australia antigen in donor blood and the subsequent development of hepatitis in recipients, but some problems remain to be settled. D. J. Gocke[1] (Columbia Univ.) tested donor specimens for Australia antigen and followed the recipients of positive blood at 1- or 2-week intervals for 6 months after transfusion. Antigen was detected by the two-dimensional immunodiffusion method and also by counterimmunoelectrophoresis. Observations were made in 2,885 transfused patients, including 108 recipients of Australia antigen-positive blood.

Of 78 evaluable recipients who received positive blood and survived, 39 (50%) acquired hepatitis or Australia antigenemia. Most of those in whom hepatitis developed had the antigen during their acute illness. Antibody developed in 24% of recipients of positive blood. Hepatitis was observed in 16% of 41 recipients of antigen-negative blood who were followed for 6 months. These patients had no antigen during their acute illness. One control acquired antibody to Australia antigen but on retesting was found to have received a positive unit of blood. The counterelectrophoresis method was more effective than gel diffusion in detecting positive donors, but the gain was not proportional

(1)   Vox sang. 19:327-331, Sept.-Oct., 1970.

to the difference in absolute sensitivity between the two methods.

Transfusion of blood containing Australia antigen is clearly hazardous and should be avoided where possible. Elimination of all antigen-positive units, however, will not completely solve the problem of posttransfusion hepatitis. Widespread screening of donor blood for Australia antigen is warranted on present evidence. Test procedures must be standardized. There can be no implied guarantee that antigen-negative blood will not produce hepatitis.

▶ [Screening of donor blood for Australia antigen will markedly reduce posttransfusion hepatitis but will not eliminate it entirely. This is a major advance in blood banking, for which we must be grateful.—Eds.]

Basis of Defective Oxygen Delivery from Stored Blood. Harvey J. Sugerman, Douglas T. Davidson, Santi Vibul, Maria Delivoria-Papadopoulos, Leonard D. Miller and Frank A. Oski[2] (Philadelphia) re-examined the rate of decline of 2,3-diphosphoglycerate (2,3-DPG) in stored blood and determined the effects of massive transfusions of phosphate-deficient blood and the value of various methods of restoring 2,3-DPG levels in stored blood. Five patients given 9-33 units of blood in 14-36 hours were studied. Central venous blood was sampled after administration of every third unit. The levels of 2,3-DPG were determined in each unit of blood. Reconstitution of 2,3-DPG was studied in serum obtained from banked blood stored in acid-citrate-dextrose solution for 21-28 days. Inosine, pyruvate and bisodium phosphate were added in various combinations, to final concentrations of 0.01M each.

The 2,3-DPG level fell rapidly during the first 10 days of blood storage. An average fall of 50% occurred in 3 days, a 75% fall in 6 days and a 95% fall in 10 days. All 5 patients had a positive correlation of the 2,3-DPG level with central venous Po_2. Neither parameter correlated with pH. The 2,3-DPG level in blood stored for 28 days rose from 285 to 1,438 $m\mu M./ml.$ red blood cells in 4 hours when incubated with 0.01M inosine. Incubation with inosine and inorganic phosphate produced a rise to 1,626 in 4 hours. The addition of both agents and pyruvate produced a rise to 6,140 in 4 hours. The buffering of blood to pH 7.4 with THAM did not alter the results.

Massive transfusions of blood low in 2,3-DPG result in a shift to the left in the oxyhemoglobin dissociation curve and a

(2) Surg., Gynec. & Obst. 131:733-741, October, 1970.

fall in central venous oxygen tension, which may critically impair tissue oxygenation in an elderly or hypoxemic patient. Such patients should be given blood stored for less than 5 days. Incubation of stored blood with inosine, pyruvate and phosphate will restore 2,3-DPG levels.

► [This article suggests that orders for banked blood should specify the condition of the patient to receive the blood.—Eds.]

pH and Acidity of Intravenous Infusion Solutions. The pH of commonly used intravenous infusion solutions is 4.0-6.5; some have criticized the infusion of such "acid" solutions. Martin H. Lebowitz, John Y. Masuda and Joseph H. Beckerman[3] (Univ. of California, Los Angeles) compared the pH of commonly used infusion solutions with their total acidity, defined as the reservoir of hydrogen ion titratable with NaOH to a pH of 7.4. Seven commercially available solutions and solutions freshly prepared in the authors' laboratory were examined.

The findings are summarized in the table. Heat-sterilized dextrose solutions had the lowest pH values, ranging from 4.3 to 5.7; commercial dextrose-containing solutions had similar values. Solutions sterilized by ultrafiltration without heat had higher pH values. Heat-sterilized solutions had higher titratable acidity than non-heat-sterilized dextrose solutions. Commercial 5% dextrose in lactated Ringer's solution contained about 1 mEq. acid per L., whereas commercial 5% dextrose in acetated Ringer's solution had a considerably higher acid content. Ringer's solutions had higher pH values than other solutions. Heat-sterilized dextrose-Ringer's solution had a slightly higher

pH AND ACIDITY OF DEXTROSE SOLUTIONS

Solution		Abbott	McGaw	Cutter	Travenol	UCLA (Ultrafiltration)	(Heat)
5% dextrose in water	pH	4.80	4.55	4.85	4.20	5.50	4.40
	mEq of acid/liter	0.142	0.153	0.150	0.233	0.092	0.147
5% dextrose in ½ normal saline	pH	4.80	4.65	4.80	4.35	5.40	4.30
	mEq of acid/liter	0.142	0.180	0.188	0.184	0.105	0.158
5% dextrose in lactated Ringer's	pH	5.10	5.95	4.80	5.20	6.35	5.05*
	mEq of acid/liter	1.480	1.420	3.360	1.270	0.138	1.380
5% dextrose in acetated Ringer's	pH	5.5	5.4	4.9	5.3	6.9	5.8*
	mEq of acid/liter	4.580	3.690	9.480	5.790	0.138	1.460

*One mEq. of hydrochloric acid added for pH adjustment before sterilization. If no hydrochloric acid is added, average pH is 5.7, mEq. acid per L. is 0.363.

(3) J.A.M.A. 215: 1937-1940, Mar. 22, 1971.

acid content than other solutions, whereas commercial dextrose-Ringer's solutions had at least 10 times the acid content of other solutions. Acetated and lactated Ringer's solutions were quite similar in titratable acidity. The pH of normal saline, averaging 5.66, was unaffected by heat, and addition of dextrose did not affect pH if sterilization was done without heat. Neither dextrose nor buffer ions nor the method of sterilization affected the titratable acidity of these solutions as much as they affected the pH.

Sterilization of intravenous infusion solutions without heat would result in solutions with a generally higher pH and a lower acid content. Solutions of pH 7.4 without dextrose might be made more readily available; these can be sterilized at physiologic pH. Lactic acid is less desirable than hydrochloric acid for pH adjustments.

▶ [These quantities of acid are trivial when compared with the buffer capacity of the blood into which they are infused. The acid pH sounds bad but signifies very little.—Eds.]

Experimental Polycythemia and Hemodilution: Physiologic and Rheologic Effects. Robert L. Replogle (Univ. of Chicago) and Edward W. Merrill[4] (Massachusetts Inst. of Technology) wished to determine the hemodynamic, metabolic and rheologic effects of acute normovolemic polycythemia and the influence of subsequent hemodilution in dogs. Flowmeter probes were placed in 20 adult dogs, and polycythemia was induced in the lightly anesthetized animals by continuous exchange of 500 ml. homologous packed red blood cells for 500 ml. whole blood over 60 minutes. Blood was taken from an external jugular vein, and cells were infused into a femoral vein with a roller pump. Hemodilution was then carried out by exchange of 500 ml. of one of four solutions for whole blood over 60 minutes: 10% human serum albumin, 10% dextran (molecular weight 40,000) in saline, 10% dextran (molecular weight 80,000) in saline or fresh homologous dog plasma.

The results are shown in the table, in which Δ^1 refers to statistical comparison of control and polycythemia, Δ^2 to statistical comparison of polycythemia and hemodilution and Δ^3 to statistical comparison of control and hemodilution. Cardiac output and peripheral oxygen consumption were reduced in the polycythemic stage but increased after hemodilution to greater than control levels. The lactate-pyruvate ratio and A-V oxygen

(4) J. Thoracic & Cardiovas. Surg. 60:582-588, October, 1970.

POLYCYTHEMIA AND HEMODILUTION (20 DOGS)

	Control	Δ^1	Polycythemia	Δ^2	Hemodilution	Δ^3
Cardiac output (ml./min.)	1457 ± 338	†	502 ± 240	†	1793 ± 404	‡
Arterial pressure (mean) (mm. Hg)	121 ± 18	§	120 ± 25	||	138 ± 23	||
Hematocrit (per cent)	38 ± 5.3	†	60.5 ± 6.1	†	33 ± 5.2	||
Fibrinogen (mg. per cent)	616 ± 205	§	492 ± 204	‡	284 ± 153	†
Lactate/pyruvate ratio	15.3 ± 3.3	†	25 ± 9.2	†	13.3 ± 2.2	||
Arteriovenous O_2 difference (ml. per cent)	4.29 ± 1.2	‡	7.15 ± 2.13	†	4.01 ± 1.22	§
Peripheral qO_2 (ml./min.)	58.7 ± 16.8	†	36.3 ± 12.0	†	68.3 ± 13.3	||
Yield stress* (dynes/cm.²)	0.0452 ± 0.0032	||	0.2209 ± 0.0038	||	0.0445 ± 0.0247	§
Viscosity at 0.1^{sec-1}* (centipoise)	69.1 ± 36.8	‡	244 ± 105	‡	66.1 ± 29.7	§
Weight average (kilogram)	17.5 ± 1.59					

*Fifteen dogs.
†0.001 > P (highly significant).
‡0.01 > P > 0.001 (very significant).
§P > 0.05 (not significant).
\|\|0.05 > P > 0.01 (significant).

difference were increased after polycythemia and decreased after hemodilution to control levels. Blood viscosity and yield shear stress increased with polycythemia and decreased after hemodilution. Plasma fibrinogen was altered significantly only by hemodilution. Arterial pressure rose slightly after hemodilution. Cardiac output did not return to control level after hemodilution with plasma, but there were no other differences between the control and hemodilution periods in the plasma group.

The physiologic effects of normovolemic polycythemia and subsequent hemodilution correlate well with in vitro measurements of blood viscosity and yield shear stress. The rheologic abnormalities are primarily responsible for the hemodynamic and metabolic changes observed. The rheologic disadvantages of polycythemia outweigh the advantages of increased oxygen-carrying capacity. Acute polycythemia reduces tissue perfusion and oxygen availability significantly, causing a shift in cellular metabolism toward anaerobic paths.

▶ [Data that, in a negative way, add support to the concept of volume replacement with colloidal solutions rather than worrying so much about hemoglobin levels per se.—Eds.]

Physiology of Synthetic Blood was investigated by Leland C. Clark, Jr., Samuel Kaplan and Fernando Becattini[5] (Univ. of Cincinnati). Fluorocarbon liquids dissolve enough oxygen and CO_2 to support the respiration of entire animals. Fluorocarbon particles prepared by sonication with surfactants remain in the circulation if small enough. In the dog, attempts were made to increase intravascular oxygen transport, mainly as measured by mixed venous Po_2, with the infusion of fluorocarbon emulsions. Studies were done on inbred beagle dogs. Toxicity studies were done in mice.

The half-life of fluorocarbon in the blood was about 2 days and that of fluorocarbon oxygen transport, about 20 minutes. Oxygen transport ability lasted longer if the blood of the animal was largely replaced by Ringer's lactate solution and dextran. Albumin-fluorocarbon emulsions were rapidly transported to the liver. Opalescent emulsions were not deposited in the liver. Toxic materials in the emulsion could be removed by filtration through micropore filters, passage through ion-exchange columns or dialysis. A transient drop in arterial pressure followed emulsion infusion. There was a high mixed venous Po_2, and there were no disturbing physiologic events. Animals survived in apparent good health. Normal clotting times were found after intravenous administration of fluorochemical surfactants, but nonpurified emulsions could cause massive hemorrhagic diathesis.

Fluorocarbon emulsions may prove valuable in transporting enzymes or enzyme systems, to substitute for congenitally deficient ones or for other reasons in specific organs or cells.

Erythrocyte Substitutes are discussed by Henry A. Sloviter[6] (Univ. of Pennsylvania). A substitute for whole blood must transport oxygen and metabolic substrates to the tissues and carry away carbon dioxide and other metabolic products as well as maintain the exchange of water, ions and other solutes with extracellular fluid. The presence of hemoglobin outside the red blood cells is not physiologic. Microcapsules of hemoglobin solution have not yet been shown to remain in the circulation of living animals, and oxidation to methemoglobin may rapidly occur. Both silicones (polysiloxanes) and perfluoro compounds are chemically inert and have a high solubility for oxygen and

(5) J. Thoracic & Cardiovas. Surg. 60:757-773, December, 1970.
(6) M. Clin. North America 54:787-795, May, 1970.

carbon dioxide. Ultrasonic dispersion of liquid fluorochemical in blood plasma or other protein solution has been used to form stable particles which are about the size of erythrocytes. Perfusion has been done successfully with FX-80, a liquid fluorochemical composed mainly of perfluorobutyltetrahydrofuran, dispersed into 2-μ particles in simulated blood plasma composed of 8% bovine albumin in Krebs-Ringer bicarbonate buffer solution. Liquid FX-80 saturated with oxygen at atmospheric pressure contains about 0.6 ml. dissolved gas per milliliter, a greater capacity than that of human red blood cells. The oxygen is chemically unbound.

Studies were done with FX-80 in an isolated perfused rat brain preparation, using electric activity as a sensitive functional measure. Perfusions were done at 25 C. with 5% carbon dioxide-95% oxygen for oxygenation. About 20% of the total volume was FX-80, with an initial glucose concentration of 200 mg./100 ml. The EEG activity persisted as long with FX-80 as with perfusion fluid containing blood. Lactate concentration curves were similar, as were arteriovenous Po_2 and Pco_2 differences and pH. Infusion of FX-80 into intact animals (rats, cats, rabbits, hamsters, dogs and chickens) led to death in several hours due to marked resistance to flow through the pulmonary vascular bed. Administration to frogs and mice, however, did not have this result. Total red blood cell replacement by fluorochemical was not feasible in frogs or mice. Fluorochemical-treated frogs and mice, however, had prolonged survival in a carbon monoxide environment.

These results indicate that the synthetic fluorochemicals in dispersed form can serve in intact animals as functioning substitutes for erythrocytes. Dispersed fluorochemical particles would probably be useful as transporters of oxygen under conditions in which red blood cells cannot survive, as with toxic agents, detergents and other hemolytic substances. The fluorochemical, however, cannot provide the buffering and the enzymatic activities that the erythrocyte has, but absence of enzyme activity may be useful in certain experimental situations.

▶ [We're still a long way from having a clinically useful blood substitute.—Eds.]

Study of Intraoperative Plasma Expansion with a Balanced Electrolyte Solution. Replacement of operative blood loss by plasma expansion with balanced electrolyte solutions has been reported to be effective and well tolerated. W. A. Tweed and John G. Wade[7] (Univ. of Manitoba) attempted to quantitate the plasma volume expansion produced by intraoperative infusion of an isotonic electrolyte, Normosol, in 11 surgical patients. Seven patients received electrolyte solution intraoperatively equal to about 3 times the measured blood loss; 4 received no electrolyte solution intraoperatively. The patients were in good general health and had no evidence of a fluid deficit or excess. Blood loss was comparable in the two groups; the mean gravimetric loss was 766 ml. Patients were given 5% dextrose in water preoperatively. Anesthesia was with thiopental and halothane or halothane-nitrous oxide, with respiration controlled. No patient became hypotensive during anesthesia. In the study group, 27% of the total electrolyte solution on the operative day was given intraoperatively. Blood volume was measured with ^{51}Cr or radioiodinated albumin.

Control patients had a mean blood loss of 760 ml., 21% of their preoperative blood volume. No plasma volume expansion was evident at the end of operation. Study patients had a mean loss of 920 ml., 24% of their blood volume, and received an average of 2,500 ml. electrolyte solution, 2.7 times the blood loss. The mean change in plasma volume was 430 ml., replacing 46% of the blood lost. Of the electrolyte solution infused, 16% remained intravascular. The difference in plasma volume change between the two groups was significant. At 24 hours the study patients had received an average total of 3,500 ml. electrolyte solution, with a change in plasma volume of 840 ml., replacing 84% of the blood loss. There was 24% intravascular retention of electrolyte solution at 24 hours. No significant change in serum electrolytes was found postoperatively in either group. The lowest hematocrits found in the study group were near 30%. Study patients excreted more than twice as much urine on the day of operation than controls. The net fluid balance was −730 ml. at 48 hours in the control group and +2,450 ml. in the study group. The interstitial fluid excess in the study group amounted to about 1.5 L.

Plasma expansion with balanced electrolyte solution is a useful means of avoiding intraoperative whole blood replacement in patients with moderate operative blood loss. Use of the

(7)   Canad. Anaesth. Soc. J. 17:213-220, May, 1970.

technic has been limited to reasonably healthy patients without cardiopulmonary disease.

▶ [This supports what most of us do daily. But why only for the healthy? —Eds.]

Clinical Physiologic Study of Hydroxyethyl Starch. Hydroxyethyl starch has been reported to be nontoxic and nonallergenic and as effective as dextran or more so as a plasma expander in dogs. Few clinical studies have been reported. William Metcalf, Aristotle Papadopoulos, Rachel Tufaro and Alexander Barth[8] (New York) studied the physiologic effects of hydroxyethyl starch in patients with relatively minor surgical conditions. Two lots of starch were available as 6% solution in 0.9% saline. Twenty patients received 500 ml. by infusion and were observed for local or systemic effects. Sixteen received 1 L. and were studied for 72 hours; blood was sampled at 10 minutes and 1, 3, 6, 12, 24, 48 and 72 hours after the end of the infusion.

Volume expansion averaged 900 ml. 10 minutes after completion of the 1-L. infusion of hydroxyethyl starch and 660 ml. over the first 6 hours; at 24 hours, it was 285 ml., but at 48 and 72 hours, the plasma volume had returned to its original level. At 24 hours, there was 38% in the circulation, with 39.3% excreted and 22.7% unaccounted for. About half had been excreted at 72 hours. The plasma level was 13.5 mg./ml. just after the infusion and 4.5 mg./ml. at 72 hours. Clearance of the starch was 9.1 ml. per minute initially and 0.67 ml. per minute at 12-24 hours. Of the starch given, 30% was excreted slowly with a half-time of 67 hours, 17.1% with a half-time of 8.5 hours and 18% with a half-time of 2 hours. The molecular weight of the material excreted averaged 58,200.

The sedimentation rate increased fourfold to fivefold soon after the infusion. The white blood cell count just after the infusion was 74.2% of the initial count. Total circulating hemoglobin showed little change. Two patients had chills and fever with headache 4 days after operation. Two others had patchy urticaria after being given starch from the other lot. No local reactions of any kind occurred.

Hydroxyethyl starch appeared to be relatively nontoxic in this study. It was an effective plasma expander and potentially as effective as dextran. It is biologically more compatible than dextran.

▶ [Seems as if it should be rather cheap, too!—Eds.]

(8)   Surg., Gynec. & Obst. 131:255-267, August, 1970.

POSTOPERATIVE COMPLICATIONS

Postoperative Myocardial Infarction: Study of Predisposing Factors, Diagnosis and Mortality in a High-Risk Group of Surgical Patients. In an attempt to improve understanding of postoperative ECG changes and cardiac complications, F. Maxton Mauney, Jr., Paul A. Ebert and David C. Sabiston, Jr.[9] (Duke Univ.) prospectively studied 365 selected patients over age 50 who underwent major operation during 1968-69. All had abnormal preoperative ECGs with one or more of the following: signs of previous infarction (no clinical symptoms within 24 months); bundle-branch block; left ventricular strain or hypertrophy; ST-segment signs of subendocardial injury. Most operations lasted 2 hours or longer. ECGs were routinely recorded 3 and 7 days postoperatively.

No changes between pre- and postoperative ECGs were noted in 301 patients. Nine of them died, 2 with suspected silent infarction. Changes of new or additive myocardial ischemia appeared in 64 patients (18%), of whom 34 had T-wave inversion or ST-segment changes but no clinical evidence of myocardial injury; 2 of the 34 patients died, and autopsy showed infarction in both. Of all 365 patients, 30 (8%) had acute myocardial infarction. Serial ECG tracings were diagnostic of infarction in 28 of these. Sixteen died of infarction.

Analysis of the anesthesia records showed that 118 patients had an intraoperative fall in systolic pressure of 30% or more for 10 minutes or longer. Infarction developed in 15% of these compared with 3.5% of 247 patients with no such pressure reduction. Thus risk of myocardial infarction was increased fourfold if there was significant hypotension during operation. Factors such as diabetes and previous infarction did not significantly increase the incidence of postoperative ECG changes of ischemia or of infarction. The average anesthesia time was 165 minutes for patients with no postoperative ECG change, 190 minutes for those with ST and T changes and 222 minutes for those with actual infarction. Time of onset of hypotension was not related to ECG evidence of ischemia or to infarction. Hypertensive cardiovascular disease was present in 56% of patients with infarction and 40% of those with unaltered postoperative ECGs.

(9) Ann. Surg. 172:497-503, September, 1970.

The mortality with documented myocardial infarction was 53% in this study, compared with 15-20% mortality in non-surgical patients reported from coronary care units. Mortality appeared to be mainly related to a low cardiac output and associated "power failure." Persistence of hypotension in the anesthetized patient may result in a larger area of infarction, since angina is not recognized and reflex mechanisms to elevated blood pressure are less reactive.

▶ [This study is incomplete and the conclusion drawn not necessarily valid. Hypotension from what cause? Hypotension from blood loss, from hypovolemia or during hypoxia is one thing. Hypotension in the presence of an adequate blood volume and in the well-oxygenated is another. The two groups cannot be lumped together.—Eds.]

Pulmonary Edema in Operative and Postoperative Period: Review of 40 Cases was made by Lee H. Cooperman and Henry L. Price[1] (Univ. of Pennsylvania). The diagnosis was made by roentgenography or by recovery of frothy blood-tinged secretions from the trachea. The incidence was 1 in 4,500 anesthetic administrations.

The mean age of the 21 females and 19 males was 53. Seven patients were in ASA physical status I, 10 in status II, 12 in status III and 11 in status IV or V. One third of the patients had emergency operations. Nineteen had pre-existing cardiovascular disease, usually hypertension or coronary arteriosclerosis. Two had bronchiectasis, 1 each had peritonitis and upper gastrointestinal bleeding and 4 were in septic shock. Laparotomy was done in 21 patients and thoracotomy in 5; no neurosurgical procedures were performed. All the common general anesthetics and muscle relaxants were represented.

The mean blood loss at operation was 2.1 L. and the average replacement volume was 3.7 L. The mean duration of surgery was 3.5 hours. About half the patients had overinfusion of fluids. Edema developed in 2 patients during anesthesia and in 8 at operation; 33 instances occurred within 30 minutes after anesthesia and 28 in the 1st hour.

Wheezing was the first sign in 11 patients, followed by rales and frothy secretions. Tachypnea, tachycardia and hypertension usually occurred. The Pa_{O_2} was 60 torr or below where measured. Nineteen patients had a tidal volume below 100 ml. with cyanosis or prolonged airway obstruction. Negative airway pressure was a factor in 1 patient and aspiration in another. In recent patients, ethacrynic acid has been used rather than

(1) Ann. Surg. 172:883-891, November, 1970.

mercurial diuretics, along with oxygen, positive-pressure ventilation, morphine, aminophylline, tourniquets and digitalis.

Seven patients died within a day of operation and 1 after 3 days; all had intractable heart failure or septic shock along with pulmonary edema. The other 32 patients recovered from pulmonary edema.

Tachypnea and reduced tidal volume were frequent findings in these patients. Several patients who had received myoneural blocking drugs were given additional Prostigmin. Another error was not to consider pulmonary edema because rales could not be heard. A normal measured central venous pressure delayed the diagnosis in 7 patients or half of those in whom the pressure was estimated. Half the patients had arterial hypertension just before pulmonary edema developed and 2 others were in septic shock. Immediate postoperative pulmonary edema is explicable in physiologic terms.

Pulmonary Complications after Tonsillectomy in Children are discussed by W. Falk[2] (Univ. of Graz). The pulmonary process triggered by tonsillectomy proceeds through several distinct phases. After an average postoperative interval of about 10 days, the temperature rises; pulmonary involvement is evident on x-rays as a shadow extending from the hilus to the periphery. Although only one lobe is usually affected, 1 patient in the present series of 19 had right upper and lower lobe abscesses on the 19th postoperative day, considered attributable to particularly massive aspiration.

The possibility of bronchiectatic alterations after aspiration occurred when bronchial stenosis or obturation had existed for several months. Only thorough anamnestic data revealed a temporal coincidence of the onset of chronic pulmonary disease and preceding tonsillectomy.

The pathogenesis of pulmonary disease may involve a hemogenic etiology, with spread of infectious material from the operation site via hematologic pathways and settling in the lung. It may also be a consequence of aspiration of blood, pus, mucus or even tonsillar residual. Most investigators favor the second etiologic possibility because of the rapid remission of at least the atelectatic alterations on prompt elimination of the obturation by bronchoscopy or suction.

Aspiration of larger amounts of mucus and pus is a result of too deep and too long a general anesthesia; recent preoperative

(2) Ztschr. Kinderchir. 8:30-39, January, 1970.

upper respiratory infection certainly increases vulnerability. Because of pulmonary complications, indications for tonsillectomy should be carefully weighed. A preoperative infection-free period of 4 weeks is strongly advised or a prophylactic broadband antibiotic regimen should be started 1-2 days before operation and continued 2-3 weeks postoperatively. Intubation narcosis is suggested, particularly because of the absolute clearance of respiratory pathways, avoidance of intraoperative aspiration, lack of temporal pressure and control of eventual respiratory disturbance by the closed respiratory system.

► [With endotracheal anesthesia for tonsillectomy, the incidence of such complications should be negligible in the next study on this subject.—Eds.]

Hypoxemia Immediately after Operation. Reduced blood oxygenation has been noted after anesthesia for major and minor surgery when patients resume breathing room air. Dola S. Thompson and Carol N. Eason[3] (VA Hosp., Little Rock, Ark.) studied the degree and trend of hypoxemia occurring in the early period after anesthesia in patients given general or spinal anesthesia for various operations. None of the patients, men aged 45-55, had severe lung disease.

In 98 patients, arterial blood gas analyses were made in the immediate postoperative period using radial arterial samples. General anesthesia was with nitrous oxide-oxygen and halothane and spinal anesthesia with tetracaine. Lung disease, mainly pulmonary fibrosis, was present without severe functional impairment in 28 patients. Preoperative measurements were made in 32 patients.

In the recovery room immediately after operation, the mean $Paco_2$ was 48.7 mm. Hg, the Pao_2 69.5 mm. Hg and the pH 7.34. The mean oxygen saturation was 89.8%. The values for blood gases after 30 minutes were 46.8 and 72.3 mm. Hg, respectively, with a pH of 7.36 and an oxygen saturation of 91.7%. All the differences were significant.

Oxygen levels were related to length of operation but not to patient temperature in the recovery room. Oxygen tensions were significantly higher in patients who had spinal anesthesia. Patients without lung disease had slightly higher oxygen tensions and lower CO_2 tensions but the differences were not significant. No significant differences were found between patients who had upper abdominal operations compared with those who had operations at other sites.

---

(3) Am. J. Surg. 120:649-651, November, 1970.

Hypoxemia characterizes the early postoperative period, making this a time when cardiac irregularities and even cardiac arrest may occur. Oxygenation can be enhanced postoperatively by encouraging coughing and deep breathing and administering oxygen.

▶ [One would hope that all first year anesthesia residents were well aware of these facts.—Eds.]

Postoperative Brachial Plexus Palsy: Study on the Mechanism. Jack H. M. Kwaan and Irving Rappaport[4] (Univ. of California, Irvine) defined the causal factors in postoperative brachial plexus palsy in studies on 9 fresh cadavers, aged 40-85, with a mean age of 61. None had antemortem symptoms of thoracic outlet syndrome or a cervical rib.

Stretch on the brachial plexus was measured by a spring gauge with the arm in full adduction and then in various degrees of abduction in relation to the shoulder. The movements were combined with extension and side-to-side head rotation, simulating operative postures. Compression was estimated digitally with the arm in various degrees of motion. Three cadavers weighed 110-121 lb., 3 weighed 132-143 lb. and 3, 165-198 lb.

Tension or stretch on the brachial plexus increased with the degree of arm abduction. Abduction with rotation of the head to the contralateral side increased tension on the nerve. Maximal nerve stretch occurred with 90 degrees of arm abduction combined with 30 degrees of extension. Simultaneous abduction of both arms exerted an additive effect on nerve tension on either side. Nerve tension was less in heavier cadavers. Compression was not a significant factor.

Examination of patients with brachial plexus palsy after operation confirms these findings. The duration of the procedure probably does not in itself cause the lesion or influence its outcome. Early management includes support of the limb and with loss of hand function, immobilization in a position of optimal function. Dynamic splinting may be useful in the later stages of recovery.

The early phase probably represents traumatic neuritis and massage or stretching may be harmful although steroid therapy may enhance recovery. Late management should include serial electromyographic studies and physical therapy. Surgical exploration is not necessary. The prognosis of postoperative

(4) Arch. Surg. 101:612-615, November, 1970.

brachial palsy is excellent; recovery is the rule. No permanent injury has been reported in the English language literature.

▶ [This article should be required reading for all anesthesia and surgical residents.—Eds.]

Postoperative Changes in Fibrinogen and Its Fractions. Many coagulation factor changes have been observed in the 1st week or 2 after extensive surgery, when thromboembolic complications appear. Among these is an increase in plasma fibrinogen and a qualitative change in the fibrinogen molecule; fibrinogen B, an intermediate between fibrinogen and fibrin, appears in the plasma. The heparin-precipitable fraction of fibrinogen has been reported to be increased; this probably reflects in vivo thrombin activity. R. C. Cotton and J. L. Craven[5] studied total fibrinogen and the heparin-precipitable fraction in 25 patients, aged 31-81 years, before and after operation. There were 17 males and 8 females. The series included 16 laparotomies done for various conditions. Plasma fibrinogen was determined by the tyrosine method.

All parameters were increased preoperatively in the study patients, compared with healthy males with an average age of 38 years. A further significant rise followed operation, but serum cholesterol was significantly reduced. Plasma fibrinogen increased from 470 to 631 mg./100 ml. 1 or 2 days postoperatively, the heparin-precipitable fraction from 159.8 to 203.1 mg./100 ml., the euglobulin lysis time from 269.5 to 303.5 minutes and the erythrocyte sedimentation rate from 22.2 to 46.6 mm. in the 1st hour. Plasma fibrinogen and the sedimentation rate were still significantly elevated 8-10 days postoperatively, but the heparin-precipitable fraction and the euglobulin lysis time were not. Correlation between fibrinogen and sedimentation rate decreased postoperatively and was not significant after 8-10 days. There was a high correlation at this time, however, between the sedimentation rate and the heparin-precipitable fraction of fibrinogen.

The changes seen after operation in this study may result from increased in vivo thrombin activity coupled with a decrease in plasminogen activator activity. These alterations may result in a postoperative hypercoagulable state.

▶ [Suppose hypercoagulability were combined with hypovolemia. Would this predispose even more?—Eds.]

(5)   Surg., Gynec. & Obst. 131:1073-1076, December, 1970.

Prevention of Fatal Postoperative Thromboembolism by Heparin Prophylaxis. J. George Sharnoff and Guido DeBlasio[6] (Mount Vernon, N. Y., Hosp.) reviewed results of attempted heparin prophylaxis of thromboembolism in 750 patients aged 60 and over. They were generally at risk because of their age or were cardiac patients, or both, often with diabetes, obesity, hypertension, past coronary thrombosis, embolism, etc. Operation during general or spinal anesthesia was predominantly for abdominal conditions. Comparison was made with 18,729 non-heparinized, average-risk patients having similar operations. Patients received 10,000 units of heparin subcutaneously the night before operation. More heparin was given if necessary, in a dose not usually exceeding 2,500 units, and this dose was given subcutaneously every 6 hours after operation until the patient was fully active or discharged. Both Lee-White and Dale-Laidlaw coagulation times were used for control. The goal was to keep coagulation time normal, preferably at 2 minutes by the Dale-Laidlaw estimation. Excessive bleeding occurred only twice when heparin was given incorrectly.

There were 23 deaths in the study group. One of 9 autopsies showed pulmonary thromboembolism, and this might have been averted had prophylaxis been started earlier. The autopsy rate was similar in the control group, about 40%. There were 84 deaths attributed to pulmonary thromboembolism in this group, and coronary thrombosis or acute myocardial infarction, or both, was noted in 15 other patients. There was 1 thromboembolic death in 285 study cases and 1 in 90 control cases or, including coronary thrombosis, 1 in 70 control cases.

The results suggest that thrombosis may be averted in high-risk surgical patients by giving heparin prophylactically to prevent hypercoagulation. Heparin was given merely in sufficient quantity to maintain normocoagulation in this trial. The increased risk of thrombosis at operation is probably related to pulmonary megakaryocytes and to a sudden release of coagulation material to the blood with increased heart action during operation. The ease of administering and controlling heparin therapy and its freedom from complications make it a distinct advance in the prevention of fatal thromboembolism.

▶ [The critical point appears to be that patients with short coagulation times present an increased risk of thromboembolism and that this risk is decreased when the coagulation times are returned to normal.—Eds.]

(6) Lancet 2:1006-1007, Nov. 14, 1970.

Cardiac Herniation after Pneumonectomy. The first case of herniation after pneumonectomy was reported by Bettman and Tannenbaum in 1951. Subsequently, similar cases were reported, each occurring immediately after operation and associated with profound shock. Paul D. Levin, L. Penfield Faber and Richard A. Carleton[7] (Presbyterian-St. Luke's Hosp., Chicago) describe a similar patient who had severe hypotension and systemic venous congestion due to extreme dextroposition and dextrorotation of the heart after right pneumonectomy.

Woman, 53, had a cough 1 month before admission. Biopsy at bronchoscopy demonstrated bronchogenic carcinoma of the right lung and irradiation with a total dose of 4,000 R was given.

Rales were present. Respiratory function was normal. At operation tumor invaded the pericardium at the level of the right inferior pulmonary vein, and right radical pneumonectomy and partial pericardiectomy were performed. The right pericardium was excised widely. Hypotension and systemic venous congestion were evident postoperatively. An x-ray 1 day after operation showed marked mediastinal shift to the right; heart tones were audible only in the right chest. The venous pressure was over 25 cm. blood. Emergency angiocardiography showed the heart to be entirely to the right of the midline, with torsion at the inferior vena cava-superior vena cava-right atrial junction to the right.

Exploration showed 90-degree rotation of the heart to the right. The heart was returned to its normal position and pericardiopexy done with use of fascia lata. Postoperatively, peripheral vasoconstriction, reduced urine output and a temperature of 103 F. were noted. Copious bronchial secretions were aspirated. The response to tracheal aspiration and increased fluids was excellent, but the patient suddenly became hypotensive 48 hours later and died. Autopsy showed atelectasis, bronchopneumonia and thrombosis of small arteries in the left lower lobe.

This patient's poor postoperative course was due to compromised return of blood to the right heart caused by torsion of the vena cava-right atrial junction. Incarceration was probably due to inadequate anterior pericardial excision; at exploration, the left ventricle seemed to be held back by a shelf of pericardium. All of the anterior pericardium must be excised to prevent incarceration. Closure of the pericardial defect with a pleural flap is a safer approach. A fascia lata graft can be used if necessary. If wide excision is elected, possibility of cardiac herniation in the postoperative period must be considered.

Effects of Anesthesia and General Surgery on Geriatric Patients. The increase in the aged population and advances in medical care have increased the number of geriatric patients

(7)   J. Thoracic & Cardiovas. Surg. 61:104-106, January, 1971.

having surgical procedures. P. Brander, M. Kjellberg and T. Tammisto[8] (Univ. of Helsinki) reviewed data on 174 patients, aged 70-92 years, including 92 males and 82 females, operated on during 1966, representing 10.6% of procedures done during this period. A total of 206 operations was done. About half the patients were aged 70-74. Complications were about equally frequent in these and in older patients, but mortality was higher in those aged 75 and over. Abdominal operations comprised almost half the series and carried the highest incidence of complications. Mortality after bowel resection was 71% in the older group and 20% in the younger. About two thirds of deaths after abdominal operations occurred in the older group. The outcome of urologic operations was fairly good. Emergency operations constituted 18% of the series. Complications and mortality were higher after emergency operations, especially in the older patients. Correlation of complications with duration of operation was clearer in the older group.

Nitrous oxide-oxygen-relaxant anesthesia with controlled respiration was used in 92% of the operations. Pethidine or halothane, or both, was used when needed for supplementation. Coexisting disease increased postoperative complications and mortality. Circulatory problems occurred preoperatively in 97 patients and ventilatory difficulties in 3. Of the 58 patients who had postoperative complications, 45% had circulatory and 38% had ventilatory difficulties. Oliguria occurred in 26% of patients. Nine of 22 patients with postoperative respiratory difficulty had artificial ventilation after operation. Mortality was 31% among patients having complications in the first 2 postoperative days and 3% among the others. Eleven of 22 deaths were due to the primary disease, and 8 resulted from thromboembolic complications. Older patients had more general derangement after discharge. More mental and physical deterioration followed emergency and abdominal operations. Four of 5 cases of postoperative dementia followed abdominal operations.

Para-anesthetic Headache in Female Patients. S. A. McDowell, J. W. Dundee and S. K. Pandit[9] (Queen's Univ., Belfast) studied the incidence of headache before and after minor gynecologic operations in patients at two hospitals. Data on 635 patients were reviewed. Premedication consisted of drugs other than opiates, small doses of opiates or heavy opiate doses such

(8) Ann. chir. et gynaec. Fenniae 59:138-145, 1970.
(9) Anaesthesia 25:334-340, July, 1970.

as 10-15 mg. morphine and 100 mg. pethidine. Anesthesia was with methohexital and nitrous oxide and oxygen. No volatile agent was used. Patients were seen 1 and 6 hours postoperatively. Para-anesthetic headache included all headaches occurring from the time of awakening until about 6 P.M. the same day, covering a period of 8-10 hours.

Each premedication group contained about 30% headache-prone and 20% migraine-prone patients. The incidence of para-anesthetic headache was 42% in the entire group. It was 83% in the headache-prone group and 22% in those not headache prone; in the migraine-prone group the incidence was 92%. Opiate premedication did not significantly reduce the incidence in any of these groups, but heavy opiate premedication reduced the incidence in headache-prone patients. Headache-prone patients had a high over-all incidence of headache on awakening. The incidence was high at both postoperative intervals in headache-prone patients and low in those not prone to headache. Severe para-anesthetic headache was most frequent in migraine-prone patients. Over one third of headache-free patients who had a headache before operation also had one afterward. A similar relation was found in headache-prone patients. The incidences of pre- and postoperative headache did not differ significantly in any of the groups.

Headache-prone patients and others must be considered separately in studies of para-anesthetic headache. Preoperative sedation is not helpful in preventing para-anesthetic headache. Mild analgesia may be more effective in treating headache than opiates. If headache is as common in general surgical patients as in those having minor gynecologic operations, perhaps it should not continue to be considered a minor sequel.

▶ [Frankly, the thought of being in the hospital gives us a headache!— Eds.]

Physostigmine Treatment of Anticholinergic Drug Depression in Postoperative Patients is described by Lynne T. Greene[1] (Columbia-Presbyterian Med. Center). In 1967, a survey was started on the incidence of delirium in patients on emergence from anesthesia in the recovery room. Of 545 patients studied in 1967, 10.2% had delirum and 5.5% had to be restrained; the respective figures for 619 patients operated on in 1969 were 8.1 and 1.1%. No delirium was due to hypoxia. The decrease in profound delirium was due mainly to early use of intravenous

---

(1)   Anesth. & Analg. 50:222-226, Mar.-Apr., 1971.

narcotics in patients with mild delirium. Over 20% of patients in both series given scopolamine preoperatively had delirium, a significantly increased incidence.

Thirty postoperative patients with delirium and 1 nondelirious depressed patient who was difficult to arouse were given physostigmine. All had received sedatives and/or narcotics as premedicants in addition to an anticholinergic drug. Physostigmine was given intravenously where possible in a dose of 0.16-2 mg. or 6.8-56.5 μg./kg. Delirium was promptly relieved in 18 of 22 patients who had received scopolamine and 2 others had equivocal results. In 4 of 8 delirious patients who had received atropine, delirium was relieved within 5 minutes of intravenous physostigmine administration; 1 patient had equivocal results and 3 were unresponsive to physostigmine. The nondelirious unresponsive patient was immediately aroused by physostigmine. No adverse effects of physostigmine were noted except in 1 patient who experienced a temporary drop in pulse rate and several ectopic beats.

The evidence is strong that physostigmine reverses a toxic side effect of anticholinergic drugs, both scopolamine and atropine. The failures encountered indicate that it is sometimes difficult to differentiate the causes of postanesthesia delirium. Postanesthetic anticholinergic drug depression is probably much more common than is recognized. It should be possible to reduce its incidence by use of anticholinergics with a quaternary ammonium nitrogen rather than those with a tertiary nitrogen. Physostigmine may also be of use in patients with toxic effects of belladonna alkaloids encountered in medical practice outside anesthesiology.

▶ [Postoperative emergence delirium can be relieved by drugs representing many different chemical groups, e.g., narcotics, apomorphine, analeptics and chlorpromazine. Now physostigmine is added. It's getting to be like the numerous therapies for hiccups.—Eds.]

Potential Hazard of Oxygen after Bilateral Cordotomy. Respiratory dysfunction may follow bilateral cervical cordotomy, especially with large lesions resulting in a high level of analgesia. Sleep-induced apnea, or Ondine's curse, may occur in severe cases and is apparently due to a disordered respiratory control system. Abraham S. Kuperman, Rogelio B. Fernandez and Hubert L. Rosomoff[2] (Albert Einstein College of Medicine) studied 2 patients with Ondine's syndrome following cordotomy. A man, aged 45, and a woman, aged 44, acquired

(2) Chest 59:232-235, February, 1971.

respiratory dysfunction after bilateral cervical cordotomy, with no previous evidence of lung disease. Percutaneous radiofrequency cordotomy had produced analgesic levels at C2-3 and C4-5, respectively. There were dyspnea and inability to take a deep breath, hypoventilation, and sleep-induced apnea reversible by arousing the patient. Both patients died from the complication. The ventilatory responses to oxygen and CO_2 are shown in Figure 23. One patient had significant, progressive reductions in maximal breathing capacity and forced vital capacity after cordotomy, and the other had only a minimal reduction in vital capacity and an improvement in maximal breathing capacity. Both patients had a reduced minute ventilation and tidal volume on air breathing and a marked reduction in these parameters on CO_2-air.

Development in hypoventilation and/or an irregular breathing pattern on oxygen administration indicates a dependence on hypoxic stimulation for regulation of ventilation. The findings support the view that central chemosensitivity is, in part, regulated by afferent input from the spinal cord. The interdependence of the aortocarotid reflex and the central chemosensitive mechanisms is such that significant depression of one en-

Fig. 23.—The ventilatory response to CO_2 and O_2 in 2 patients in whom the Ondine syndrome developed after bilateral cervical cordotomy. Note cyclic breathing pattern after cordotomy. *Left,* in the woman, aged 44, this was evident during air breathing and aggravated by O_2 breathing. *Right,* in the man, aged 45, this was evident during O_2 breathing. The cyclic pattern was almost entirely abolished by CO_2-air but was still evident on CO_2-O_2. (Courtesy of Kuperman, A. S., *et al.*: Chest 59:232-235, February, 1971.)

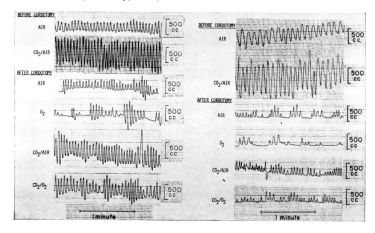

hances the relative importance of the other. The mechanism of the irregular breathing pattern induced or aggravated by oxygen remains obscure. Administration of oxygen to patients who have had bilateral cordotomy may result in serious hypoventilation. This may be especially hazardous during sleep or when sedatives or narcotics have been given.

▶ [Isn't this comparable to the patient with a high spinal anesthesia (T1 or T2) who may stop breathing after he goes to sleep from 50 or 75 mg. thiopental? We never heard of Ondine's curse—sounds like something from *Macbeth*.—Eds.]

Respiratory Causes of "Sudden Unexplained Arrhythmia" in Postthoracotomy Patients were investigated by John J. Osborn, John C. A. Raison, James O. Beaumont, J. Donald Hill, William J. Kerth, Robert W. Popper and Frank Gerbode[3] (San Francisco). Often the development of life-threatening arrhythmias in an intensive care ward is very unexpected. Signs of previous cardiorespiratory deterioration were found in retrospect in 4 of 7 such instances, usually involving respiratory function and starting several hours before the acute episode. Computer monitoring technics are used in patients who have had open heart operations and those with acute coronary occlusion or other cardiopulmonary difficulties. Measurements are made at 10-minute intervals, 24 hours a day. Data were obtained on 150 patients during 16 months, representing about 320 patient-days.

There were six instances of "sudden" ventricular fibrillation and two of sudden ventricular tachycardia with shock in this series. Three patients had no etiologic physiologic changes preceding the episode. Three episodes were associated with unrecognized hypoventilation and hypercarbia resulting from maladjustment or malfunction of a pressure-controlled, patient-triggered respirator. Two occurred in patients on volume-guaranteed respirators with adequate minute ventilation, followed by a change in the respirator setting to reduce mildly the minute volume, causing mild hypercarbia and stimulation of respiratory drive. Increased oxgen uptake and CO_2 output was followed by further hypercarbia, restlessness, extrasystoles and, finally, ventricular fibrillation. There were eleven other instances of potentially serious respiratory abnormalities. Five were due to malfunction of apparatus; two were undetected leaks. Incidence became less frequent as ward personnel became more experienced

(3) Surgery 69:24-28, January, 1971.

with the on-line quantitative measurements. There were often large discrepancies between respirator settings and what was actually delivered in terms of gas volume or concentration.

About 10% of patients in this series had a potentially serious episode of preventable respiratory difficulty. Most incidents involved hypoventilation and hypercarbia. Some abnormalities may be unrecognizable without continuous measurement of respiratory parameters. They may be common causes of "sudden unexplained cardiac arrhythmia." Sophisticated instrumentation and continuous respiratory gas measurements may be needed to prevent catastrophes among patients on respirators.

▶ [There is an important message here. When patients are committed to respirator therapy, they demand the same careful, continuous and knowledgeable observation as does an anesthetized patient.—Eds.]

Effect of Changes in Inspired Oxygen and Carbon Dioxide Tensions on Wound Tensile Strength: Experimental Study. There is abundant evidence that healing processes are oxygen-dependent and that the supply of oxygen at the healing edge is extremely precarious. Frederick O. Stephens and Thomas K. Hunt[4] (Univ. of California) studied the tensile strength of healing wounds in rats in relation to varying partial pressures of oxygen in inspired air and in relation to combinations of normal and increased atmospheric oxygen with normal and increased atmospheric carbon dioxide, then examined the effects of increased atmospheric carbon dioxide on the P_{O_2}, P_{CO_2} and pH of tissue fluid in healing wounds.

Young male Sprague-Dawley rats were anesthetized and subjected to a 6-cm. skin wound in the back. Wounds were closed with continuous 4-0 silk atraumatic sutures. Groups of 12 rats were kept in 10% oxygen with less than 0.5% carbon dioxide and about 89.5% nitrogen; 20% oxygen with less than 0.5% carbon dioxide and 79.5% nitrogen; and 40% oxygen with less than 0.5% carbon dioxide and about 59.5% nitrogen. Groups of 6 rats, slightly younger than the others, were kept in 20% oxygen, less than 0.5% carbon dioxide and approximately 79.5% nitrogen; 20% oxygen with 8% carbon dioxide and 72% nitrogen; 40% oxygen with less than 0.5% carbon dioxide and approximately 50.5% nitrogen; and 40% oxygen with 8% carbon dioxide and 52% nitrogen. Wound tensile strengths were determined after 7 days. A steel wire cylinder, 4 cm. long and 1 cm. in diameter, was inserted subcutaneously into each flank

(4)   Ann. Surg. 173:515-519, April, 1971.

EXPERIMENT 1: ATMOSPHERIC OXYGEN AND WOUND TENSILE STRENGTH

	No. of Animals	Average Wound Tensile Strength (Gm.)	Standard Error	Statistical Significance of Difference with Control Group	Average Change in Weight (Gm.)
Group 1 10% oxygen	12	445.6	27.4	$p < 0.05$	+2
Group 2 (control) 20% oxygen	12	517.3	22.5		+30
Group 3 40% oxygen	12	563.1	31.3	$p < 0.025$	+31

of 12 other rats. Half were kept in 20% oxygen, less than 0.5% carbon dioxide and about 79.5% nitrogen and half in 20% oxygen with 8% carbon dioxide and 72% nitrogen. Wound fluid was aspirated from the cylinders after 7 days.

Rats breathing 10% oxygen exhibited a significant reduction in wound tensile strength after 1 week when compared with control rats breathing 20% oxygen (table). Those exposed to 40% oxygen had a significant increase in wound tensile strength. Those on 10% oxygen gained significantly less weight than the others. The differences in younger rats were greater than in older ones. Exposure to 8% carbon dioxide resulted in significantly reduced tensile strength in rats breathing either 20 or 40% oxygen. The Pco_2 of wound fluid from rats breathing 8% carbon dioxide was significantly elevated, whereas the pH was slightly but significantly increased.

The rate of healing of "normal" wounds depends on the available oxygen supply. Imposition of excessive Pco_2 in inspired air fails to increase and actually reduces wound tensile strength, indicating that the increased healing associated with oxygen is directly due to increased available oxygen and is not a secondary result of an increased Pco_2. The degree of "acceleration" observed is relatively slight, and it is not suggested that oxygen therapy be given to patients with cleanly incised and closed wounds. Oxygen therapy, however, may be beneficial to patients with decreased oxygen availability, extensive wounds, respiratory failure or poor local perfusion.

▶ [This article suggests the early application of inhalational therapy in appropriate patients will decrease the incidence of wound dehiscence.— Eds.]

Risk of Operation in a Patient with Unsuspected Pheochromocytoma is discussed by H. A. Samaan[5] (Edinburgh), with report of a case. Failure to recognize the cause of cardiovascular changes in the patient with undiagnosed pheochromocytoma during anesthesia and operation may lead to circulatory collapse and death. Most of the changes are due to excessive catecholamine secretion. Few patients with pheochromocytoma respond normally to anesthesia and operation. Mortality is high after the tumor is stimulated if the toxic levels of circulating catecholamines are not immediately neutralized, as these usually lead to spasm, tissue anoxia and acidosis, with shock resulting. A history of normal delivery or operation with general anesthesia without complications does not exclude pheochromocytoma.

Woman, 53, was hospitalized with a painless lump in the breast, present for a month. Delivery of a child 20 years before had been uneventful, as had cholecystectomy 10 years later. There were no symptoms suggestive of paroxysmal hypertension. The blood pressure was 160/90 mm. Hg.

The lump in the breast was excised using general anesthesia with halothane-nitrous oxide-oxygen after premedication with pethidine and chlorpromazine. A frozen section diagnosis of adenocarcinoma was made, and radical mastectomy was done. The operation took about 1½ hours. The blood pressure rose to 230/100 mm. Hg after about 45 minutes and then dropped to 160/100 mm. Hg toward the end of the operation. Blood loss was 500 ml.

Postoperatively, the pulse rate was 160 per minute and the blood pressure, 170/100 mm. Hg. Two pints of blood were given, but the hypertension and tachycardia persisted, and the patient collapsed in dyspnea 14 hours after operation. Hydrocortisone and oxygen were given. An ECG showed signs of myocardial ischemia. The patient died a few hours later. Autopsy showed a pheochromocytoma in the right adrenal gland.

Pheochromocytoma was not considered in this case. It should be suspected if otherwise unexplained sudden hypertension, markedly fluctuating arterial pressure, tachycardia or arrhythmia occurs during anesthesia. If hypertension occurs, phentolamine and a β-adrenergic blocking drug should be given until the patient recovers from the anesthetic. If an adrenal tumor is found and removed at abdominal exploration, the patient should be treated as though a pheochromocytoma had been removed, with blood transfusion, cortisone, digitalis and blocking agents, as required. If the hypertensive crisis is rec-

(5) Brit. J. Surg. 57:462-475, June, 1970.

ognized after operation or delivery, phenoxybenzamine can be given, with dextran and electrolytic fluids. Corticoids and chlorpromazine may also be useful.

―――――

OBSTETRIC ANESTHESIA

Cardiovascular Changes in Vaginal Deliveries and Cesarean Sections. How much added load is imposed on the heart by cesarean section compared with vaginal delivery is not known. Jerome W. H. Niswonger and Charles F. Langmade[6] (Los Angeles) made hemodynamic determinations on 44 patients, obtaining adequate data from 20 of them. Eleven had vaginal delivery and 9 underwent cesarean section. All patients were at 36 weeks' gestation or later except 2 undergoing section. In all the cardiovascular system was normal. All had living fetuses.

Section was done with spinal anesthesia in 8 cases and epidural anesthesia in 1, the average level reached being T7. Vaginal delivery was conducted using spinal anesthesia in 8 cases and caudal anesthesia in 2; 1 patient was delivered before a spinal anesthetic could be administered. The average level in this group was T11. Intravenous fluids were given during delivery. Pitocin was given after delivery of the placenta. Three patients received Methergine because of increased blood loss.

The central venous pressure was significantly lower after anesthesia in the section group. In this group, mean blood pressure was also significantly lower after spinal anesthesia. Mean circulation time progressively increased to delivery in the vaginal delivery group and decreased at delivery of the placenta; it changed little in the section group. The greatest rise in cardiac output occurred in the section group immediately after delivery of the placenta when an increase of 2.5 L. per minute was apparent (41%), which is of questionable significance. An increase of 20% occurred in the vaginal delivery group at delivery of the placenta. Central blood volume rose more markedly in the vaginal delivery group, but there was no statistically significant difference between the two groups. Peripheral resistance was lower in the section group after anesthesia. Stroke work and stroke volume were similar in the two groups.

(6)   Am. J. Obst. & Gynec. 107:337-344, June 1, 1970.

The findings indicate that cardiac strain is very similar in vaginal and abdominal delivery. The length and type of labor should therefore be primary considerations in the pregnant cardiac patient.

▶ [The most striking finding was a 2.52 L. per minute increase in cardiac output immediately after delivery of the placenta at cesarean section, but it was only of questionable statistical significance!—Eds.]

Tilt Cesarean Section. Supine hypotension may occur in any pregnant woman at or near term and is more common and more severe in women having cesarean section under spinal anesthesia. It is due to inferior caval compression by the pregnant uterus, resulting in a reduced cardiac output. Vasopressors do not provide a complete solution to the problem nor does temporary left uterine displacement. I. Ansari, G. Wallace, C. A. B. Clemetson, V. R. Mallikarjuneswara and C. D. M. Clemetson[7] (Brooklyn, N. Y.) measured umbilical arterial and venous blood gases and examined infants delivered by section done in a 10-degree left-side-down "tilt" position. A side rail was designed for tilting patients. Analysis was made of 67 patients having spinal or general anesthesia and having the table tilted or not tilted. Most patients having elective section received meperidine and atropine preoperatively. General anesthesia was induced with sodium thiamylal and maintained with nitrous oxide-oxygen, methoxyflurane being added after delivery. Spinal anesthesia was done with 1% tetracaine in 10% dextrose.

Use of the left-tilt position did not prevent hypotension during spinal anesthesia for cesarean section. A 30% fall in systolic pressure occurred with spinal anesthesia in all 13 patients in the left-tilt position and all but one of 22 who were supine, despite the prophylactic use of ephedrine in most cases. Hypotension did not develop in any of the 30 patients given general anesthesia; none received ephedrine. The tilt position was associated with marked improvement in the Po_2 and oxygen saturation of umbilical venous and arterial blood, especially with spinal anesthesia. There was a highly significant difference in oxygen saturation of umbilical venous blood in the tilt and no-tilt groups, considering only uncomplicated cases. A smaller, insignificant difference was found in the group given general anesthesia. The pH, Pco_2 and bicarbonate in cord blood did not differ significantly in tilt and no-tilt cases. Apgar scores in these groups did not differ significantly at 1 or 5 minutes.

(7) J. Obst. & Gynaec. Brit. Commonwealth 77:713-721, August, 1970.

Use of the 10-degree left-tilt position with cesarean section leads to considerable improvement in the oxygenation of infants, especially with spinal block. The improvement in oxygen saturation could make the difference between life and death for a severely distressed fetus. The risk of brain damage from hypoxia should be reduced by using this technic. Hypotension from spinal block may be reducible by elevating the legs.

▶ [Seems reasonable, particularly with a slow surgeon.—Eds.]

Maternal Acid-Base Status during Cesarean Section under Thiopental, N_2O, and Succinylcholine Anesthesia. There is not yet a consensus on the preferred anesthesia for cesarean section. Rukmini Kalappa, Kent Useland, J. M. Hansen, Marlene Eng and J. T. Parers[8] (Univ. of Washington) studied the effects of balanced anesthesia during section on the maternal acid-base status and the fetal outcome. Seventeen normal term pregnant women undergoing repeat section were studied. Catheters were placed in the brachial artery and cephalic vein. No premedication was given. Anesthesia was induced with thiopental in all cases and, after ventilation with 100% oxygen, 0.2% succinylcholine was infused to facilitate tracheal intubation. Anesthesia was with nitrous oxide and oxygen. Maternal arterial blood was sampled nine times during the procedure, and a uterine vein and the cord were also sampled.

No significant differences were found between patients given 2.5 and 4 mg. thiopental per kg. Induction of anesthesia and operation before delivery resulted in a mild acidosis, due to a slight rise in $Paco_2$ and a slight drop in bicarbonate. The arterial pH rose to about 7.40 after delivery and remained there for at least an hour. The lowest mean pH, 7.355, occurred at the time of extubation of the trachea. The Pao_2 with the patient awake and breathing room air was about 10 mm. Hg below the initial control level. Apgar scores at 1 minute were related to the induction-to-delivery interval. Five of 6 patients with intervals greater than 45 minutes had 1-minute Apgar scores of 5 or less. This relationship was not apparent at 5 minutes, when all infants but one had a score of 7 or higher; the exception was delivered of a hypotensive mother. The mean uterine venous blood oxygen tension just after delivery, before removal of the placenta, was 7 mm. Hg higher than just before delivery.

The use of thiopental, nitrous oxide and succinylcholine for cesarean section is associated with only minimal changes in ma-

(8) Am. J. Obst. & Gynec. 109:411-417, Feb. 1, 1971.

ternal acid-base levels. Placental transfer of thiopental is well documented, but neonatal depression does not usually occur with clinical dosages. Succinylcholine does not cross the placenta in significant concentrations with therapeutic dosages, and it is unlikely that this drug contributes to neonatal depression.

▶ [It is not surprising that Apgar scores were related to the induction-to-delivery time. As time progresses there would be more of an uptake of thiopental as well as nitrous oxide in fetal tissues and there is evidence that the two agents are additive in their depressant tendencies.—Eds.]

Placental Transfer and Fetal Metabolism of Diazepam in Early Human Pregnancy. Diazepam has been used extensively as an analgesic adjunct in labor and cesarean section, and measurable levels have been found in cord blood after a single maternal dose given intravenously at parturition. Juhana E. Idänpään-Heikkilä, Pentti I. Jouppila, Jukka O. Puolakka and Martti S. Vorne[9] (Univ. of Oulu) examined placental transfer of diazepam in early pregnancy and the ability of the human placenta and fetal tissues to metabolize diazepam in vitro.

Eight healthy pregnant women received 5 mg. diazepam (1 mg. diazepam-C^{14}) with 4 mg. unlabeled carrier, intramuscularly, before hysterotomy. Premedication was with atropine and meperidine, and anesthesia was induced with thiopental and maintained with 75% nitrous oxide in oxygen. Muscle relaxation was induced with succinylcholine. Diazepam and its metabolites were identified by thin-layer chromatography.

The peak maternal blood diazepam level of 8 ng./ml. was found 30 minutes after intramuscular injection, with a nearly linear decline for up to 6 hours. A considerable amount remained in the blood at 24 hours. Cord blood levels were higher; the mean was 47.5 ng./ml. at 1 hour, compared with 25.6 ng./ml. in maternal blood. The cord blood level at 6 hours was 19 ng./ml.

Peak fetal tissue levels of diazepam occurred an hour after injection, with high uptake in the gut, liver and brain. The placental level was highest at 1 hour and decreased rather rapidly. Amniotic fluid accumulation of the drug was low. Low enzyme activity was noted in premature fetal liver supernatant, metabolizing about 3% of added diazepam into its metabolites. Neither the premature nor the term placenta metabolized diazepam in vitro, and the fetal gut and brain also showed negative results. Adult rat liver supernatant metabolized about 30% of

(9) Am. J. Obst. & Gynec. 109:1011-1016, Apr. 1, 1971.

added diazepam. In 48 hours after diazepam was injected intramuscularly, 86% was recovered in maternal urine.

Considerable diazepam was present in maternal blood 24 hours after injection. Diazepam crossed the human placenta in early pregnancy and accumulated rapidly in the fetus, presumably because of the high solubility of the drug in lipid. Concentrations in fetal blood consistently exceeded those in maternal blood.

▶ [Another drug given for the benefit of the mother, but passing in significant proportion into the infant.—Eds.]

Catheter Subarachnoid Block for Labor and Delivery: Differential Segmental Technic Employing Hyperbaric Lidocaine. James O. Elam[1] (Univ. of Chicago) performed a series of spinal blocks for labor and delivery in 14 patients using low doses of hyperbaric lidocaine, producing insignificant sympathetic blockade. This technic can produce predictable differential sensory block without motor impairment. Inadvertent dural puncture at attempted peridural block is switched to catheter spinal management for labor and delivery. Headache is relieved by injecting lactated Ringer's solution intrathecally. A remarkable reduction in lidocaine dosage was noted during catheter subarachnoid block with a switch from 1 or 2% lidocaine to 5% lidocaine with 7.5% dextrose. Whereas 20-40 mg. hypo- or isobaric solution produced 30-40 minutes of pain relief in early labor, only 2 or 3 mg. hyperbaric solution produced 40-70 minutes of analgesia. The technic was evaluated in 12 primigravidas and 5 multigravidas, aged 12-36, in labor. An injection of 2.5 mg. hyperbaric lidocaine with 7.5% dextrose was made slowly with the patient supine and the catheter tip at T11. The catheter was withdrawn to about 1 cm. within the dura at the end of the 2d stage, and 5-10 mg. lidocaine was injected about 15 minutes before delivery. An intravenous infusion of 5% dextrose in water was given during labor, and 30-70 ml. lactated Ringer's solution was injected into the subarachnoid space about 40 minutes after delivery. Oral tolazoline was given at least every 4 hours for 4 days after delivery.

The average duration of medicated labor was 4½ hours. The average requirement for hyperbaric lidocaine was 6.2 mg. per hour. The total dose for labor and delivery averaged 27.4 mg. (range, 5-80). Three patients given iso- or hypobaric lidocaine

---

(1) Anesth. & Analg. 49:1007-1015, Nov.-Dec., 1970.

had hourly requirements 4-7 times higher than those given hyperbaric lidocaine and a total requirement 8 times greater. Motor function was preserved and hypotension was absent in most of the 1st stage of labor. Profound sacral motor and sensory block often occurred with the predelivery block, without significant lumbar motor block. All infants had adequate Apgar scores. Five patients delivered spontaneously.

Catheter subarachnoid block provides successful obstetric analgesia with a negligible dose of local anesthetic, eliminating maternal and fetal toxicity. The method is flexible; early 2-segment sensory block can be extended to 12-segment sensorimotor block at delivery. A catheter spinal technic with hyperbaric lidocaine has many advantages over other analgesic blocks for parturition.

▶ [It is somewhat surprising to see a revival of continuous spinal anesthesia for vaginal delivery, and even more surprising to learn of the use of tolazoline for prophylaxis and treatment of spinal headache.—Eds.]

Cardiovascular Effects of Oxytocic Drugs Used Post Partum were investigated by Charles H. Hendricks and William E. Brenner[2] (Univ. of North Carolina). Oxytocic drugs, used before delivery, can endanger the fetus and possibly cause uterine rupture. The principal complication from ergot drugs in the early puerperium is hypertension. Oxytocin had marked cardiovascular effects when given in a single intravenous dose but not when infused, even in high doses. However, single doses, sometimes as high as 10 I.U., are still given by many obstetricians.

The present studies were done on gravid and postpartum women and on a healthy male. Two subjects had therapeutic abortion induced by hypertonic saline with postpartum recordings. Intrauterine and arterial pressures and relative uterine blood flow were recorded.

A patient given 5 I.U. oxytocin rapidly 2 hours postpartum had a precipitous fall in blood pressure, with a small "overshoot" following. The heart rate increased rapidly. Contractions were converted to a tetanic type. The extent of the pressure drop and the recovery time were always directly proportional to the dose of oxytocin given.

A healthy male had hypotension after doses as small as 0.003 μg./kg. and with 0.1 ng./kg., the mean arterial pressure was reduced by 46%. The reduction occurred earlier than in pregnant or postpartum women.

A patient with bleeding after twin delivery and a blood pres-

(2)   Am. J. Obst. & Gynec. 108:751-760, Nov. 1, 1970.

sure of 70/42 mm. Hg was given 5 I.U. oxytocin rapidly, intravenously and had a transient drop in pressure to 44/26 mm. Hg within 30 seconds. She became unresponsive until saline was given to raise the pressure. Uterine activity increased in a normotensive postpartum patient when 0.2 mg. ergonovine was given. Arterial pressure rose from 110/50 to 130/70 mm. Hg within 3 minutes after injection. A patient given 10 I.U. oxytocin and 0.2 mg. methylergonovine 2 hours post partum had an initial fall in blood pressure by about 40%, with a rise above baseline about 1½ minutes after injection. Vomiting ensued and the blood pressure returned to near the pre-injection level after about 6 minutes.

These observations confirm those made in previous studies. Both oxytocin and ergot drugs have been implicated in postpartum hypertension. Significant hypertension after oxytocin administration has never been recorded by the authors.

Most patients would do well without any oxytocic after normal delivery but prophylactic oxytocics are indicated post partum in certain patients, such as those with uterine overdistention or long, difficult labor. The most common indication is inadequate postpartum uterine contraction during general anesthesia. Ergot preparations should be used only intramuscularly. Oxytocin should be given intramuscularly or if a prolonged effect is desired, as a dilute intravenous drip.

Used correctly, oxytocin can provide good protection against excessive hemorrhage and can control postpartum hemorrhage due to uterine "atony." Given intravenously in grossly toxic doses, it may have disastrous consequences.

▶ [Yet how often do we see oxytocics given intravenously by the circulating nurse when, in the same hospital, the nurses are forbidden to give other medication intravenously?—Eds.]

Use of Bupivacaine in Labor is discussed by R. A. Browne and D. V. Catton[3] (Hamilton, Ont.). About two thirds of our obstetric patients now have continuous lumbar epidural block for pain relief in the first 2 stages of labor. A block extending from midthigh to the umbilicus is adequate for delivery by episiotomy and forceps. Review was made of 120 patients given a continuous epidural block with Bupivacaine, a new local anesthetic, during labor and delivery. The block was started when the cervix was 5-6 cm. dilated. An initial dose of 5-7 nl. of 0.5% Bupivacaine was injected; 1:200,000 epinephrine was added in

(3) Canad. Anaesth. Soc. J. 18:23-32, January, 1971.

39 cases. Similar doses were repeated when contractions became painful, and a terminal dose of 10-15 ml. was given for perineal analgesia just before delivery, if required. A Syntocin nasal spray or infusion was used if contractions slowed markedly during labor.

Pain relief was excellent in 75% of the patients and satisfactory in 95%. The peak effect occurred in 15-20 minutes. The upper level of analgesia ranged from T8 to T11. Moderate muscle weakness in the legs was usually noted. Contractions progressed satisfactorily in most patients. Nearly half of the patients were in labor for over 12 hours and only 5% for less than 4 hours. All six cesarean sections were done with epidural analgesia. Apgar scores were satisfactory in 96.7% of cases. The maternal blood pressure never fell below 80 mm. Hg, and vasopressors were not required. Over half the patients required three or more injections. Shivering presented no significant problem. Six patients had spotty analgesia for no apparent reason.

Bupivacaine produced efficient analgesia in 95% of patients in this study. No serious complications occurred, and its duration of action was greater than that of lignocaine. The nursing staff was quite impressed with the reduced frequency of injections required compared with lignocaine, and consequently the reduced number of blood pressure readings to be taken. Bupivacaine is a safe, very efficient local anesthetic for continuous epidural analgesia in obstetrics. Its long duration of action is particularly useful in obstetric cases.

▶ [Bupivacaine may be neurologically safer and require less injections and fewer repetitive blood pressure recordings, but one doubts the wisdom of combining longer drug action with less observation of the patient, especially in a casual environment.—Eds.]

Acid-Base Studies in Elective Cesarean Sections during Epidural and General Anesthesia. Gordon S. Fox and Germain L. Houle[4] (Royal Victoria Hosp., Montreal) report observations made on three groups of 13 parturients and their neonates at elective cesarean section. One group had thiopental-nitrous oxide-oxygen-succinylcholine anesthesia and two groups had epidural anesthesia. Half the latter patients breathed pure oxygen via a Magill circuit and face mask for at least 10 minutes before delivery. Premedication was with atropine. Epidural anesthesia was with 2% lidocaine with 1:200,000 epinephrine, with a catheter in the L3-4 interspace. General anesthesia patients were

(4) Canad. Anaesth. Soc. J. 18:60-71, January, 1971.

given 100% oxygen for 3 minutes before induction for tracheal intubation. Respiration was controlled at tidal volumes of about 7.5 ml./kg.

Mean blood pressure declined appreciably in both epidural anesthesia groups. It was easily raised to preoperative levels before delivery by left uterine displacement or intravenous methamphetamine. A hypotensive tendency was not noted in the general anesthesia group. Maternal arterial blood gases were comparable before anesthesia in all three groups. The Po_2 was particularly high at delivery in the epidural-oxygen group, and the Pco_2 was highest in the general anesthesia group at this time. Differences in umbilical vessel carbon dioxide tensions were difficult to explain. The epidural group, with a higher umbilical venous oxygen tension and saturation, had a decreased capacity to combine with carbon dioxide, but, with less fixed acids, combination with more carbon dioxide was possible without a change in carbon dioxide tension. Infants in the general anesthesia group had more fixed acid and a greater base deficit; their umbilical arterial blood had a lesser carbon dioxide capacity for a given oxygen saturation. The general anesthesia group had a relative respiratory and metabolic acidosis. The higher umbilical venous Po_2 in the epidural-oxygen group appeared to be due to an extremely large maternal-fetal oxygen gradient, which substantially aided diffusion of oxygen across the placenta.

Epidural analgesia appears to be the anesthetic of choice for elective cesarean section. Neonates born to mothers given epidural analgesia have less acidosis and better oxygenation than those born to mothers given general anesthesia. Among neonates born to mothers given epidural analgesia, those to whose mothers oxygen is given have a better acid-base state and begin breathing spontaneously sooner after birth than those whose mothers breathe air.

▶ [An interesting study favoring epidural anesthesia. However, what is the end point? Is it fetal salvage, Apgar scores, umbilical gases and pH, or the number of infants who grow up as respectable members of society? What are we really trying to document?—Eds.]

Effect of Maternal Hypercapnia on the Newborn Infant. Maternal hypercapnia is associated with increased oxygen tension and saturation in the lamb fetus. Anthony D. Ivankovic, James O. Elam and John Huffman[5] (Univ. of Chicago) studied 45 healthy term pregnant women, in none of whom were signs of

(5) Am. J. Obst. & Gynec. 107:939-946, July 15, 1970.

fetal distress during labor. Fifteen were denitrogenated for 3-5 minutes with an oxygen flow of 8 L. and then subjected to hypercapnia by removal of the carbon dioxide absorber from the system. The oxygen flow was then reduced to 400-800 ml. per minute. Methoxyflurane was introduced to produce light surgical anesthesia at a respiratory minute volume of 7-10 L. Fifteen other patients received methoxyflurane anesthesia, and 15 had saddle-block anesthesia with heavy dibucaine and received no oxygen. All mothers had lactated Ringer's solution infusions throughout labor. Narcotics were not given in the 3 hours before delivery.

Hypercapnia did not alter the maternal arterial or umbilical arterial methoxyflurane concentrations, but umbilical venous levels were significantly higher in the hypercapnia group. Induction time and induction-delivery interval were significantly shorter in this group. Degrees of metabolic acidosis did not differ importantly among the three groups. Mean umbilical venous Po_2 was 49.5 mm. Hg in the hypercapnia group, 39.7 in the control methoxyflurane group and 32.9 in the saddle-block group; the differences were significant. Maternal Pco_2 and umbilical venous Po_2 were positively correlated in patients given general anesthesia. Umbilical venous oxygen saturation was higher with general than with saddle-block anesthesia. Umbilical arterial Po_2 was highest in the hypercapnia and lowest in the saddle-block group. Umbilical venous-umbilical arterial oxygen saturation difference was 32.6% in the hypercapnia group and 37.3% in the methoxyflurane control group. Apgar scores were highest in the hypercapnia group and lowest in the control methoxyflurane group. All mothers and neonates had uneventful postpartum courses. No respiratory acidosis was evident within an hour after delivery with hypercapnic methoxyflurane anesthesia.

Maternal hypercapnia increases umbilical venous oxygen tension during methoxyflurane anesthesia. No adverse effect of hypercapnia was noted in the present study. Moderate elevation of the Pco_2 can improve the clinical status of newborns. Also, hypercapnic induction of anesthesia may increase maternal safety during general anesthesia by preventing vomiting and possible aspiration.

▶ [Interesting, but not surprising.—Eds.]

Effects of Simulated Maternal Hyperventilation on Umbilical Vein. There is some question about the role of hyperventilation in obstetric anesthesia, since clinical and animal studies suggest that severe hypocapnia and the resulting maternal alkalosis may lead to fetal depression. Frederic A. Berry, Jr., and John S. Mitchell[6] (Univ. of Virginia) conducted an in vitro study to isolate a fetal segment of the human uteroplacental unit and investigate its alterations when subjected to simulated hyperventilation. The umbilical vein, the source of fetal blood, was considered the most important vessel to examine in this regard. Umbilical cords were taken after 22 normal spontaneous deliveries and 1 cesarean section. Anesthesia was with light inhalation technic or regional block. Perfusion of the umbilical vein was begun within 10 minutes of delivery, using a balanced salt solution, at 36.5-38 C. The pH was varied from 7.1 to 7.9, the Pco_2 from 8 to 100 torr, and the Po_2 from 135 to 150 torr. Flow was adjusted to 200-300 ml. per minute with a roller pump to establish a baseline pressure of 25-40 torr.

The umbilical vein dilated with an increase in Pco_2 and the resultant drop in pH and constricted with a drop in Pco_2 and an increase in pH. The vein was quite sensitive to the interval between delivery and initiation of perfusion. Most toxemic umbilical veins exhibited so much vasospasm and unpredictable change as not to be usable in the study. At a constant Pco_2 and pH, the pressure fell slowly after about 30 minutes of stabilization, at a rate of 2-3% over the next 90 minutes.

This model is an appropriate one for studying blood vessels in vitro. A well-oxygenated fetus in good acid-base balance will probably have no difficulty from maternal hyperventilation. With hypoxia or altered acid-base balance, the drop in blood flow with alkalosis might cause further decompensation. With a compromised maternal-fetal relationship, any drop in blood flow from alkalosis might cause a depressed fetus. Dilatation might not lead to increased fetal blood flow because, with acidosis, there is less response to catecholamines, and pooling of blood may occur in the fetus, reducing the effective circulating volume.

▶ [Good evidence that maternal hyperventilation is not likely to be important to the fetus except in the presence of hypoxia or fetal acidosis. The observation that the cord from toxemic patients exhibited so much vasospasm as to be useless for these studies is interesting and should be investigated further.—Eds.]

Fetal Effects of Spinal Hypotension: Observations in the Dog at Term of Pregnancy. Hemorrhage and hypotension are nei-

(6) Am. J. Obst. & Gynec. 109:20-23, Jan. 1, 1971.

ther equivalent nor synonymous. Antonio Boba, Daniel M. Linkie and E. Jurgen Plotz[7] studied the fetal effects of maternal normovolemia-hypotension and of maternal hemorrhage induced under such a condition. Normovolemic hypotension was induced by subarachnoid injection of 1.5 ml. of 1.5% lidocaine into the lumbar area. A total of 21 spinal blocks was performed on 15 pregnant dogs at or near term. A rapid, sustained fall in systolic pressure occurred in all instances. Data were obtained with the fetus in utero and with no loss of amniotic fluid. Aliquots of 1% of maternal body weight of blood were withdrawn at about 20-minute intervals. Three such withdrawals lead to fetal bradycardia and hypoxia. Sequential maternal hemorrhage was induced after subarachnoid block in 4 dogs and before the block in 4 others.

Maternal subarachnoid block produced a rapid fall in blood pressure without appreciable change in the pulse rate. The hypotension did not lead to changes in fetal blood pressure, pulse or Pao_2. Maternal hemorrhage after subarachnoid block led to profound maternal hypotension, with minimal maternal pulse change. The fetal blood pressure, pulse and Pao_2 were altered only after the third withdrawal of blood. Subarachnoid block did not alter the course of events anticipated with sequential hemorrhage. In the hypovolemic mother, subarachnoid block produced the expected fall in blood pressure, but no fetal bradycardia or hypoxia was evident.

It could be inferred that spinal hypotension would reduce blood flow through any circulatory region, including the pregnant uterus, but neither fetal hypoxia nor bradycardia was noted in the present study despite a presumed fall in uterine blood flow. The discrepancy between the effects of hemorrhage and those of spinal block on the fetus may be explicable in terms of "patterns" of flow, as opposed to total flow. Fetal hypoxia and maternal hemorrhage are the only variables that are always associated, and it can be reasonably concluded that the factors limiting oxygen transport across the placenta are the availability of blood in the maternal circulation and the pattern of flow through the placenta as it is influenced by vasoconstrictor responses. Merely increasing the Pao_2 in the mother is not a valid alternative; when maternal vasoconstriction occurs, fetal hypoxia may coexist with maternal hyperoxygenation.

(7) Obst. & Gynec. 37:247-252, February, 1971.

▶ [Hypotension plus vasoconstriction equals fetal hypoxia. Treatment with oxygen alone is not enough. Makes sense.—Eds.]

Vasopressors in Obstetrics: III. Fetal Effects of Metaraminol Infusion during Obstetric Spinal Hypotension were studied by S. M. Shnider, A. A. de Lorimier and J. L. Steffenson[8] (Univ. of California) in 11 term pregnant ewes. The fetal femoral vessels, the umbilical vein and the maternal carotid artery and uterine veins were cannulated using low spinal and local infiltration anesthesia. Blood flows were calculated by the steady-state diffusion method, using antipyrine solution. High spinal anesthesia was induced and rapidly resulted in maternal hypotension. Blood was sampled and, after 45 minutes of hypotension, 0.002% metaraminol was infused and the maternal arterial pressure was maintained at control levels for 45 minutes.

The mean maternal arterial pressure fell about 35% during spinal hypotension and returned to normal after metaraminol was given. Fetal blood pressure did not change significantly throughout the study (Fig. 24). The maternal pulse rate fell about 25% during hypotension and rose toward normal after metaraminol. The fetal pulse rate fell slightly during hypotension and rose with metaraminol. The fetus became acidotic during maternal hypotension, and this became worse after me-

Fig. 24.—Changes in maternal and fetal arterial pressure after maternal spinal hypotension and subsequent correction with metaraminol. (Courtesy of Shnider, S. M., *et al.*: Am. J. Obst. & Gynec. 108:1017-1022, Dec. 1, 1970.)

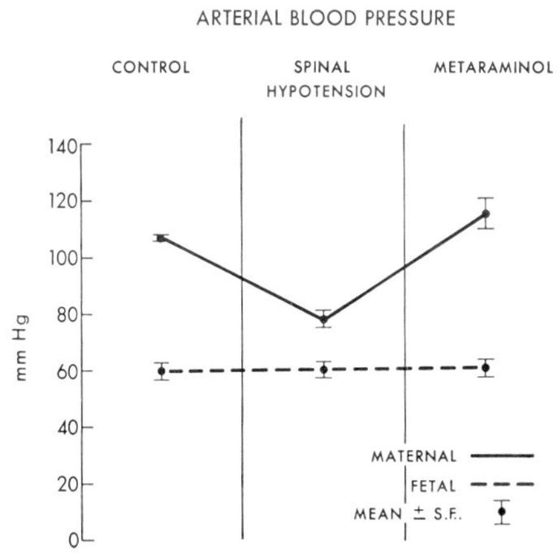

ARTERIAL BLOOD PRESSURE

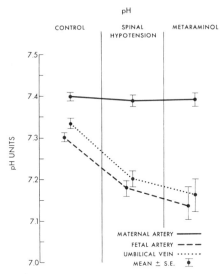

Fig. 25.—Changes in maternal and fetal arterial and umbilical venous pH after maternal spinal hypotension and subsequent correction with metaraminol. (Courtesy of Shnider, S. M., *et al.*: Am. J. Obst. & Gynec. 108:1017-1022, Dec. 1, 1970.)

taraminol. The maternal pH did not change significantly (Fig. 25).

Base excess decreased in the umbilical vein and fetal artery during maternal hypotension and dropped further after vasopressor therapy. The fetal Pco_2 rose significantly during maternal hypotension; it fell significantly after vasopressor therapy. Maternal Po_2 was above normal during hypotension. Fetal hypoxia developed during maternal hypotension, but oxygenation improved when maternal hypotension was corrected with metaraminol. Uterine blood flow fell 45% after spinal hypotension, and umbilical blood flow increased 16%. With metaraminol infusion, the uterine blood flow returned to within 4% of the control level, and the umbilical blood flow fell.

Fetal metabolic and respiratory acidosis and hypoxemia during maternal hypotension are related to reduced uterine blood flow. Metaraminol slightly improves placental gas exchange, but the fetal metabolic acidosis progresses. This may be due to a direct metabolic effect of the vasopressor in the fetus, possibly related to a direct effect of catecholamines on intracellular enzyme systems. Ephedrine is still the vasopressor of choice for correcting maternal spinal hypotension; it corrects both fetal hypoxia and acidosis.

▶ [At what level of blood pressure in the normal healthy parturient does hypotension become sufficient to be of concern?—Eds.]

Effects of Some Vasopressor Drugs on Uterine Contractility in Pregnant Women. Luis Sentíes G., Guillermo Arellano, Arturo Casellas F., Eduardo Ontiveros and Javier Santos[9] (Mexico City) studied the effects of three synthetic vasopressor amines, mephentermine, methoxamine and novadral, on the dynamics of the human pregnant uterus. The first of these drugs acts by releasing norepinephrine; the others act directly on adrenergic nerve receptors.

Amniotic pressure was recorded by the Alvarez-Caldeyro-Barcia technic during 48 drug doses in 26 pregnant women aged 16-39, most at 37-40 weeks' gestation. All had uterine contractility, either prepartum or in the 1st stage of spontaneous labor. All carried either dead ova or acranial fetuses. Five patients had an epidural lumbar anesthetic blockade when studied. Two patients had been on a low-sodium diet with thiazide diuretic therapy. Single injections were given in 5 minutes, or continuous, slow infusions were administered. Single injection doses were 2-6 mg., and infusion doses were 0.05-0.8 mg. per minute. Intramuscular doses were 6-10 mg.

All women showed increased uterine contractility when given the drugs (Fig. 26). The increases were less marked in the patients on diuretic therapy and low-sodium intake. The peak increase in uterine activity was 166 Montevideo units. An oxytocic effect was noted at doses lower than those commonly used to produce local vasoconstriction or raise the arterial pressure. From 1 to 4 minutes were required for labor to begin after intravenous drug injection. The effect on uterine dynamics exceeded that on blood pressure in all cases. Novadral produced the greatest and mephentermine the least contractility response. Polysystole was invariable with a single intravenous dose of 2 mg. or more and with infusion of over 0.4 mg. per minute. Contraction intensity rose moderately after about half the applications except in periods of tachysystole or hypertonia. There was no consistent relation between the increased uterine activity and the rise in blood pressure that occurred. Coordination was produced except where no marked rise in contractility occurred or where hypertonia was produced. Usually the maternal

(9) Am. J. Obst. & Gynec. 107:892-897, July 15, 1970.

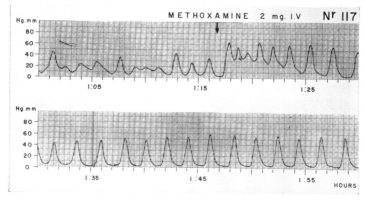

Fig. 26.—Amniotic pressure tracing of woman in the 40th week of pregnancy and early labor. Intravenous administration of 2 mg. methoxamine (*arrow*) produced a considerable increase in uterine contractility, with passing hypertonia that can be easily distinguished in the tracing. Subsequent contractility remained at a higher level than prior to administration of drug. Arterial pressure showed no appreciable change at this dosage. (Courtesy of Sentíes G., L., *et al.*: Am. J. Obst. & Gynec. 107:892-897, July 15, 1970.)

heart rate did not change markedly. Fetal heart rate did not change with low doses in patients with live fetuses.

In some patients, the uterus at term appears to be more sensitive than blood vessel muscle to certain substances. It is assumed that sensitivity to these drugs would increase in the course of pregnancy, as is generally true of oxytocic agents.

▶ [The use of vasopressors with spinal anesthesia for cesarean sections has been frowned upon by many people for years. This study supports this concern.—Eds.]

Awareness during Operative Obstetrics under General Anesthesia. Much concern has been aroused by reports of patients being able to recall events occurring during general anesthesia. The anesthetist wishes to limit the amount of nervous system depressants given to mothers at operative delivery.

J. Selwyn Crawford[1] (Birmingham, England) surveyed 740 preoxygenated patients with general anesthesia induced with thiopentone followed by suxamethonium and maintained with nitrous oxide-oxygen. Awareness tended to be less with hyoscine than with atropine premedication. It was more frequent with 50 than with 67% nitrous oxide in oxygen and greater at elective than at emergency procedures. The incidence of awareness remained at 2.5-4% even when hyoscine was given with 67% nitrous oxide for maintenance.

(1) Brit. J. Anaesth. 43:179-182, February, 1971.

Moir (1970) noted that 0.5% halothane, added to 50% nitrous oxide-oxygen, reduced the incidence of awareness to 0%, but halothane is a powerful myometrial relaxant. Methoxyflurane therefore was evaluated as a maintenance agent; administration was started after delivery of the infant. Elective surgery patients received chlordiazepoxide on the day of operation. After preoxygenation and cricoid pressure, hyoscine was injected, followed by thiopentone and suxamethonium for tracheal intubation. Anesthesia was maintained with nitrous oxide-oxygen in 456 cases; in 34 of them pethidine was given after delivery also. In 424 other cases methoxyflurane was introduced into the anesthetic mixture. Elective section was done in 121 study cases, emergency section in 151, operative vaginal delivery in 40 and postpartum sterilization in 112.

Significant differences in awareness between study and control patients occurred only in the elective section group, but a significant difference was found for all purely obstetric cases; the incidences were 3.14% for control patients and 0.32% for study patients. Unpleasant dreams were always less frequent in study cases. The incidence of awareness in the elective section group was 3.7% in control cases and 0% in study cases.

The introduction of 0.1% methoxyflurane after delivery into a standard general anesthetic technic virtually abolished the risk of awareness in operative obstetrics. This modification cannot affect the infant and does not induce uterine hypotonia. Patients take a little longer to emerge from anesthesia and are drowsy for longer periods postoperatively, but they give no cause for concern with regard to ventilation.

▶ [It all depends what we are after—keep them awake, deliver in the home and practice Lamaze so you will recall everything of delivery—or put them to sleep so they don't (but sometimes do) remember.—Eds.]

Narcotic Addiction in Pregnancy. There are an estimated 25,000 female narcotic addicts in New York City, and pregnant addicts are being seen increasingly often. Martin L. Stone, Louis J. Salerno, Marvin Green and Carl Zelson[2] (New York Med. College-Metropolitan Hosp. Center) reviewed data from 382 pregnant addicts who delivered infants between 1960-69. The ratio of addicted mothers to total deliveries in the East Harlem institution has risen from 1:164 in 1960 to 1:47 in 1969. The average age was 26.7 years; the number of teenagers has increased markedly. The group included 61% Negroes,

(2) Am. J. Obst. & Gynec. 109:716-723, Mar. 1, 1971.

23% Puerto Ricans and 16% Caucasians. About one third of the subjects were married. Parity generally reflected patients' ages. All the subjects were users of heroin; about 20% used barbiturates and tranquilizers as well. The duration of addiction ranged to over 20 years.

The obstetric and medical complications seen could be attributed to absent or inadequate prenatal care. Only one quarter of the patients had registered, and most of them did so in the last trimester. Serious complications were fewer than expected, and there were no maternal deaths. The average length of observed labor was considerably shortened. The cesarean section rate was only 2%. Low birth weight and neonatal addiction were the chief complications. Nearly half of the infants were premature by weight. Addiction and withdrawal symptoms were present in two thirds of the infants. The time of onset and frequency of symptoms were related to the amount of drug taken and the interval before delivery. The symptoms were characteristic, with central nervous system irritability most prominent (table). Treatment was necessary in about half of the total group for the presence of two or more symptoms. Treatment consisted of chlorpromazine 2.2 mg./kg./day in 4 equally divided doses intramuscularly or by dropper for up to 40 days. The mortality rate was 3.6%, deaths being related to respiratory distress syndrome and prematurity. Only 3 of the 14 deaths were of infants weighing over 2,500 Gm. Significant congenital anomalies were not increased.

SYMPTOMS IN ORDER OF FREQUENCY OBSERVED IN NEWBORN INFANTS

SYMPTOM	No.
Irritability	170
Tremors	169
Vomiting	95
High-pitched cry	68
Sneezing	66
Hypertonicity and hyperactivity	53
Respiratory distress	33
Fever	22
Diarrhea	18
Mucus secretion	15
Sweating	14
Convulsions	8
Yawning	7
Scratching face	4
Occasional minor symptoms	10

It is feasible and recommended to withdraw and detoxify patients during pregnancy and in the postpartum period. The significant incidence of low birth weight infants in the present series raises the possibility that maternal narcotics use may lead to intrauterine growth retardation. Prompt treatment of symptomatic patients may be expected to result in an improved perinatal outcome.

▶ [An important series of observations for those who rarely encounter the parturient who is a narcotic addict.—Eds.]

MONITORING AND THE NEONATE

Role of Fetal Heart Rate Patterns in Recognition of Fetal Asphyxia with Metabolic Acidosis. J. A. Low, R. W. Boston and S. R. Pancham[3] (Queen's Univ., Kingston, Ont.) examined the complementary role of continuous monitoring of the fetal heart rate with periodic acid-base assessment of the fetal blood as a means of identifying fetal asphyxia in 100 patients delivered of infants with and without evidence of fetal asphyxia with metabolic acidosis. Acid-base measurements were made on capillary blood sampled in the last 2 hours of labor and on umbilical venous and arterial blood. Fetal acidosis was diagnosed when the umbilical arterial buffer base was under 40 mEq./L. and was considered moderate or severe when the buffer base was under 37 mEq./L. Acidosis was mild in 33 infants and moderate to severe in 21.

Baseline tachycardia occurred in 6% of the 46 infants without metabolic acidosis, 12% of those with mild acidosis and 33% of those with moderate or severe acidosis. Infants with baseline tachycardia may not have metabolic acidosis at delivery (Fig. 27). Decelerations significantly increased in frequency with increasing fetal asphyxia with metabolic acidosis. A marked frequency pattern (more than 30% of contractions associated with a deceleration) was found in 76% of cases of moderate to severe metabolic acidosis. Late deceleration was noted in 37% of the infants; there is a very significant increase in its frequency in relation to increasing degree of asphyxia with metabolic acidosis.

Careful interpretation of fetal heart rate patterns should permit identification of probable presence of fetal asphyxia with

(3)   Am. J. Obst. & Gynec. 109:922-929, Mar. 15, 1971.

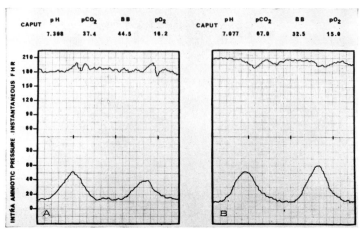

Fig. 27.—Example of baseline tachycardia with no metabolic acidosis (*A*) and with fetal asphyxia with metabolic acidosis (*B*). (Courtesy of Low, J. A., *et al.*: Am. J. Obst. & Gynec. 109:922-929, Mar. 15, 1971.)

moderate or severe metabolic acidosis or possible presence of fetal asphyxia with mild metabolic acidosis. Fetal capillary blood sampling is necessary for acid-base assessment, which is essential for diagnosis of fetal asphyxia with metabolic acidosis. Monitoring of the fetal heart rate should begin early in the intrapartum period and the record should be uninterrupted. Proper interpretation requires continuous supervision by persons capable of accurately assessing the records and of deciding when acid-base assessment of the fetal blood is indicated.

▶ [A sensible complement to fetal acid-base measurements. Since so few obstetric units are equipped to do the fetal blood analyses, and recording fetal heart rate is so simple, wouldn't this alone be better than no continuous monitoring?—Eds.]

Acid-Base Balance in Early Evaluation of Fetal Distress during Labor. M. Sharf, I. Eibschitz, A. Valero and A. Stein[4] (Haifa, Israel) attempted the early diagnosis of fetal distress at the onset of labor in various pathologic states. Amnioscopy was done and blood sampled from 120 fetuses during labor, and acid-base levels were determined in maternal capillary blood. There were 10 cases of diabetes, 18 of maternal hypertension and/or pre-eclamptic toxemia, 44 of acute fetal distress, 36 of prolonged labor and 12 of premature labor. Blood was sampled twice in nearly half the cases, at two fingers' cervical dilatation

(4) Israel J. M. Sc. 6:617-621, Sept.-Oct., 1970.

and when the findings indicated repeat study. When the first estimates were normal, fetal blood was re-examined only if clinical signs of distress appeared.

A pH below 7.20 was found in 43.3% of cases in the fetal blood. Acid-base values were normal in all maternal capillary blood samples. Apgar scores were 7-10 in 61 of 68 cases with a pH of 7.20 or above but low in 46 of 52 cases with a low pH. Scores were 0-2 in 29 cases with an average pH of 7.16, constituting 24.1% of the pathologic cases; another 37% of cases (17) had Apgar scores of 3-6 and an average pH of 7.18. Biochemical findings were abnormal with a good Apgar score in 6 cases and normal with a low Apgar score in 7. The pH was low in half the cases of hypertension or toxemia. The most marked metabolic changes were found in patients with prolonged labor, in 55-60% of whom metabolic acidosis was present, without classic signs of fetal distress. Many cases of clinical distress were due to twisting of the cord about the neck or another part of the body. Only 40% of cases with clinical distress had biochemical disturbances. The findings in premature labor were similar to those of normal labor. Most infants born in severe distress were in the prolonged labor group. Correlation between the pH and Apgar score was quite high. Labor was terminated in all cases with a fetal blood pH below 7.20.

In cases of prolonged labor, pre-eclamptic toxemia or maternal diabetes, in which there are no clinical signs of fetal distress, the fetus seems to be subject to a greater hazard than where there is evidence of fetal distress. Estimation of the acid-base balance may disclose early signs of distress in these pathologic states. Routine examination may help reduce the perinatal morbidity and mortality in these states. The percentage of errors is reduced by examining fetal blood on two occasions at different stages of labor.

▶ [One often hears the statement that monitoring the fetal metabolic state only confirms the clinically obvious condition of the fetus. This article effectively dispels that concept.—Eds.]

Paracervical Block Anesthesia in Obstetrics: II. Etiology of Fetal Bradycardia Following Paracervical Block Anesthesia. J. H. Asling, Sol M. Shnider, A. J. Margolis, G. L. Wilkinson and E. L. Way[5] (Univ. of California) found that high fetal blood mepivacaine levels can be correlated with fetal bradycardia and acidosis and subsequent infant depression. Studies

(5) Am. J. Obst. & Gynec. 107:626-634, June 15, 1970.

were done on 17 healthy women in active labor with single term pregnancies; 8 were primiparas, 9 were multiparas. The fetal heart rate was monitored before and after paracervical injection of 200 mg. mepivacaine (20 ml. of 1% solution). Fetal scalp blood was sampled 5 minutes after the block. Maternal and umbilical vessel samples were taken at birth. No additional anesthesia was given for 30 minutes after the paracervical block.

Fetal bradycardia followed paracervical block in 7 cases, starting 3-16 minutes after drug administration and lasting 2-14 minutes. Tachycardia preceded the bradycardia in 1 instance. One infant without bradycardia and 4 of 7 with bradycardia were depressed at birth. All infants were vigorous at age 5 minutes. The mean maternal mepivacaine blood level reached a peak of 2.08 μg./ml. 5 minutes after the block and fell to 1.42 at 1 hour. Levels were similar in the groups of mothers whose fetuses acquired bradycardia or did not react to the block. The mean fetal mepivacaine blood levels were 1.16 and 4.11 μg./ml., respectively, for the groups without and with bradycardia, a sig-

Fig. 28.—Paracervical area in relation to uteroplacental circulation. Arrows indicate possible routes for mepivacaine absorption. (Courtesy of Asling, J. H., *et al.*: Am. J. Obst. & Gynec. 107:626-634, June 15, 1970.)

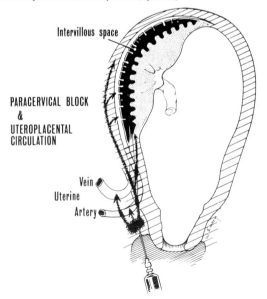

Intervillous space

PARACERVICAL BLOCK
&
UTEROPLACENTAL
CIRCULATION

Vein
Uterine
Artery

nificant difference. The fetal blood level exceeded the peak maternal arterial level in 6 of 7 cases with 2 of 10 cases without fetal bradycardia. Neonatal blood levels were uniformly low. Fetal acid-base changes were independent of maternal changes in at least 4 of the 7 cases with fetal bradycardia.

This study showed a significant relation between bradycardia, decreasing pH and high mepivacaine blood levels in the human fetus after paracervical block. It is proposed that mepivacaine diffuses across the arterial wall to be deposited into the intervillous blood pool (Fig. 28). The intervillous drug level might then well be higher than the maternal brachial arterial level, and a high fetal level could result from direct passive diffusion. Regardless of the fetal level achieved soon after paracervical block, the fetal blood mepivacaine level decreased significantly by the time of birth, indicating drug uptake and/or metabolism by the fetus and/or rapid placental clearance to the mother.

▶ [Bradycardia in 7 of 17 cases suggests this is not a very good technic for obstetric analgesia.—Eds.]

Fetal Heart Rate during Breech Delivery. Nicholas J. Teteris, Andrew W. Botschner, John C. Ullery and Garth F. Essig[6] (Ohio State Univ.) recorded the fetal heart rate during delivery in 12 frank and 3 double footling breech presentations and compared the rate with the fetal heart rate variations occurring during deliveries of cephalic presentations. The series included 7 primiparas. The prenatal course was uncomplicated in all cases, as was the 1st stage of labor. Premedication was with meperidine and an ataractic drug in sufficient dosage to relieve pain. Pudendal block, nitrous oxide and oxygen were used to deliver the buttocks, with ether added for uterine relaxation. Amniotomy was done when the presenting part was on the perineum, and a needle electrode was placed subcutaneously into the fetal buttock. Assisted breech extraction was carried out over a midline episiotomy, using after-coming head forceps. Birth weights ranged from 2,720 to 4,480 Gm.

Bradycardia was a constant finding in this series. Mild tachycardia of 150-170 beats per minute was often noted during uterine contractions in the latter part of the 1st stage of labor. Traction applied to the fetal groin usually resulted in a mild transient deceleration of the fetal heart. The fetal heart rate rarely fell below 100 beats per minute during delivery of the

(6) Am. J. Obst. & Gynec. 107:762-766, July 1, 1970.

buttocks. The lowest rate was noted when the shoulders were delivered, with a similar decline when the head was delivered. The heart rate recovered more quickly in the cephalic group than in breech deliveries. The average delivery times in these groups were 69 and 110 seconds, respectively. The average Apgar score was 5.7 for 15 breech deliveries and 8.7 for 28 cephalic deliveries.

Pearse points out that it is not clear whether the fetal heart slowing noted at delivery is harmful to the fetus or whether it is a physiologic adaptation of no significance or possibly a protective mechanism of some sort. The actual cause of the rate decrease is also unknown. Neither forceps compression of the newborn head nor forceps traction and stimulated delivery materially alter the heart rate of the recently born infant.

▶ [Although fetal heart slowing during breech delivery may not be dangerous, most fetal monitoring systems today would treat this as a genuine cause for alarm.—Eds.]

Reliability of Fetal Blood Sampling: Maternal-Fetal Relationships were determined by E. T. Bowe, R. W. Beard, M. Finster, P. J. Poppers, K. Adamsons and L. S. James[7] (New York). Review was made of 679 blood analyses made in 355 fetuses during labor. All gestations were at term, and all infants were born alive. Most presentations were vertex. Sampling was done after the 2d stage of labor only for specific indications. Serial maternal and fetal samples were obtained in 50 cases.

The incidence of acidosis was 29.8%; it was severe in 5.3% of the infants. The fetal pH was significantly correlated with the 1-minute Apgar score; with a fetal pH below 7.22 a score of 6 or less was highly probable. The incidence of a vigorous fetus with a pH below 7.2 (false abnormal) was 7.6% and that of a depressed fetus with a pH above 7.2 before delivery (false normal) was 10.4%. High correlation existed between the fetal capillary blood pH just before delivery and the umbilical venous or arterial pH at delivery.

Serial studies during labor showed maternal pH fell slightly and base deficit rose. There were 31 mildly acidotic fetuses that scored 7 or higher at birth, 9 which were more acidotic just before delivery but also vigorous and 10 with more severe acidosis who scored 6 or less. The mothers of the second group showed significant metabolic acidosis during labor, but the mothers of

(7)   Am. J. Obst. & Gynec. 107:279-287, May 15, 1970.

the third group had values similar to those in the normal group. Base deficit differences between mother and fetus were significantly correlated to the condition of the infant at birth.

In the entire group, 22 of the fetuses (6.2%) had a pH of 7.2 or lower at birth with no signs of distress; 4 of these 22 were depressed at birth, whereas 18 scored 7 or higher.

The fetal scalp sample is a reliable index of the fetal acid-base status. The fetal pH is predictive of the 1-minute Apgar score. Medication or anesthesia given to the mother is probably the commonest cause of "false normal" values. Maternal acidosis is the commonest cause of "false abnormal" values. Fetal blood pH should be repeated on indication, and the trend noted should be acted on.

▶ [If one is to interpret the "false abnormal" and "false normal" the authors talk about, he had better be concerned with obstetric anesthesia full time. Those of us who spread our wings over all anesthesia administered in a hospital sometimes can't keep up with every single segment.—Eds.]

Chemoreceptor Reflexes in the Newborn Infant: Effect of CO_2 on Ventilatory Response to Hypoxia. In the newborn hypoxia stimulates breathing for only a short time, and it is not clear whether CO_2 augments the response. June P. Brady and P. M. Dunn[8] (Univ. of California) studied this problem with control of the alveolar O_2 tension and the thermal environment in healthy term newborns who breathed spontaneously at birth. Pregnancy and labor had been uncomplicated and sedation had been minimal. Minute ventilation was compared at alveolar O_2 tensions of 110 and 60 mm. Hg, with breathing of 0.2, 2.3 or 4.4% CO_2 for 11 minutes. Thirty satisfactory studies were made on 8 infants. Two infants twice received 4.4% CO_2 and the response was the same in each study. Capillary blood was taken from 12 infants to identify significant pH changes with hypoxia and hypercapnia.

Minute ventilation, respiratory frequency and heart rate were not significantly altered with 0.2% CO_2, but with 2.3% CO_2 there was a 43% rise in breathing and a 3.1-mm. Hg increase in $Paco_2$. With 4.4% CO_2 there was a 151% rise in ventilation, a 7.7 mm. Hg rise in $Paco_2$ and no significant change in breathing frequency or heart rate. Hyperventilation began within 10-20 seconds of CO_2 inhalation and reached a steady state in 3 or 4 minutes. It was almost entirely due to increased tidal volume. Minute volume was usually further increased with hypoxia at all CO_2 levels, with an increase in tidal volume but not respira-

(8) Pediatrics 45:206-215, February, 1970.

tory frequency. A small but significant and sustained increase in heart rate accompanied hypoxia. A small decrease in capillary pH occurred with hypoxia and 4.4% CO_2 inhalation.

Hypercapnia appears to potentiate the initial stimulant effect of hypoxia on ventilation in the newborn. Every effort should be made to keep infants well oxygenated, since even mild hypoxia will depress breathing after 1 or 2 minutes, particularly at low P_{CO_2} levels. Infants with respiratory problems must not be exposed to a cool environment. Failure of hypoxia, with or without hypercapnia, to induce sustained hyperventilation in the newborn appears to convey no benefit.

▶ [A neonate could hardly be expected to sustain a stimulus very long to breathe from either hypoxia or hypercarbia.—Eds.]

RESPIRATORY DISTRESS SYNDROME

Negative-Pressure Artificial Respiration: Use in Treatment of Respiratory Failure of the Newborn. Leo Stern, Angeles D. Ramos, Eugene W. Outerbridge and Pierre H. Beaudry[9] (McGill Univ.) evaluated use of a modified Isolette negative-pressure respirator (Air-Shields) in treating 91 infants with a birth weight of over 1,000 Gm. and with respiratory failure secondary to respiratory distress syndrome (87) or massive meconium aspiration (4) during 1965-68. The table lists arterial blood indicators for respirator therapy, after acidosis and hypoglycemia were maximally stabilized and corrected with intravenous fluids and bicarbonate. Criteria in the left column were used during the first half and those in the right, during the second half of the study period.

Of the 91 infants, 54 survived the respirator episode; 7 of 54 died in the postrespirator period. Of the 54 survivors, 25 were treated according to the early and 29 according to the revised criteria. Autopsy in all 37 who died showed hyaline membranes in confirmation of the antemortem diagnosis of respiratory distress syndrome. Of 57 males, 23 (40.4%) died; of 34 females, 14 (41.2%) died. Whereas all 11 infants whose birth weight was under 1,250 Gm. died, 18 of 19 whose birth weight was 2,500 Gm. or over survived. A similar upward trend occurred with increasing gestational age. The times in hours needed for respirator therapy to improve P_{O_2} to over 80 mm. Hg in 61 infants was

---

(9)   Canad. M. A. J. 102:595-601, Mar. 28, 1970.

CRITERIA OF RESPIRATORY FAILURE (WHILE BREATHING 100% OXYGEN)

Po_2 <40mm.Hg	Po_2 <50mm.Hg
$[H]^+$>80 nEq./l.	$[H]^+$>63 nEq./l.
Pco_2 >75mm.Hg	Pco_2 >70mm.Hg

Survivors	25 (53.2%)	29 (65.8%)
Deaths	22	15
Total	47	44

Fig. 29.—Infant with respiratory distress syndrome. Birth weight was 1,700 Gm. and gestational age, 34 weeks. Initial disordered parameters were corrected when respirator was turned on, only to revert toward previous level when respirator was shut off. Note repeated improvement and deterioration with repeated "on" and "off" periods. Broken line represents level achieved spontaneously when respirator use was no longer necessary. (Courtesy of Stern, L., *et al.*: Canad. M. A. J. 102:595-601, Mar. 28, 1970.)

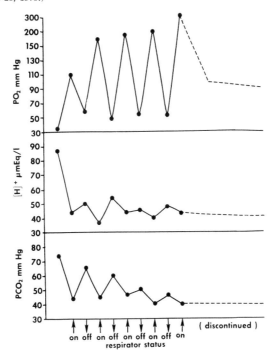

1-112 (mean, 10.5); hydrogen ion concentration to less than 50 nEq./L. in 54 infants was 1-65 (mean, 11.6); and Pco_2 to under 50 mm. Hg in 53 infants was 1.5-136 (mean, 22.6). Average age at entry into the respirator was 40.9 hours for the survivors and 19.2 for the infants who died. For the 37 who died, average prolongation of life was 24.6 hours; for the 54 survivors, the average time of complete dependency on the respirator was 53.7 hours. The child successfully managed in the respirator for over 24 hours had a better than 50% chance of survival. Tension pneumothorax requiring tube insertion and underwater drainage occurred in 11 infants before placement in the respirator and in 9 while they were in the respirator; 3 of the 11 and 6 of the 9 died. Of the 37 who died, 23 had intracranial hemorrhage, the intraventricular location of which suggested anoxic rather than traumatic origin. Figure 29 shows the repeated efficacy of the respirator in correcting disorders of hydrogen ion concentration, Pco_2 and Po_2 in an infant with respiratory failure secondary to respiratory distress syndrome.

▶ [The authors believe that negative-pressure respiration in a tank respirator, as opposed to positive-pressure respiration, has the advantages of better ability to achieve oxygenation, avoidance of tracheal intubation, reduction in high incidence of pulmonary infection (presumably related to the endotracheal tube) and a decrease in the incidence of respirator lung. They claim that respirator lung requires positive pressure and perhaps an endotracheal tube for its development.—Eds.]

Mechanical Ventilation of Newborn Infants: IV. Technic of Controlled Intermittent Positive-Pressure Ventilation. There is no evidence that the type of mechanical ventilation used for neonates with respirator failure affects their survival, but changes in the pattern of intermittent positive-pressure ventilation predictably influence the oxygenation and ventilation of infants with respiratory distress syndrome. Since 1964, Penelope Cave Smith and William J. R. Daily[1] (Stanford Univ.) have mechanically ventilated 204 newborns with respiratory failure who did not respond to conventional treatment.

Maximal oxygenation was given before nasotracheal intubation by manual hyperventilation with 100% oxygen for 3-5 minutes. Foregger plastic tubes 9-11 cm. long are now used; the largest tube possible is placed. The tube is fixed with umbilical tape, and is changed 24 hours after the start of ventilation and thereafter every 48-72 hours. A Bennett PR-2 respirator with a low-dead-space infant circle ("Q-circle") was used in most

(1) Anesthesiology 34:127-131, February, 1971.

instances. Ventilation was controlled by adjusting the respiratory rate and airway pressure until the infant did not attempt to breathe. A Pao_2 of 60-100 mm. Hg, a $Paco_2$ of 25-35 mm. Hg and an arterial pH of 7.4-7.5 were maintained. An 80-100% inspired oxygen concentration was used initially, followed by decrements of 2-5% until an optimal Pao_2 was present without metabolic acidosis; attempts were made to reduce the concentration to below 70% as rapidly as possible. All equipment was washed in Cidex and sterilized with ethylene oxide before use.

Pulmonary physiotherapy, including vibration, percussion and suction in different positions, was done every 2-4 hours. The endotracheal tube and airways were suctioned hourly. Weaning was done by reducing the inspired oxygen concentration while keeping the Pao_2 over 60 mm. Hg, and then separating the infant for 1-3 minutes while it breathed an oxygen concentration 20% higher than that required during mechanical ventilation. Extubation was attempted when the infant could breathe spontaneously for 8 hours or longer. The attempt was dropped when there was inadvertent excessive hypercapnia, hypoxemia or metabolic acidosis during weaning. Initially hydration was maintained by infusing 5-10% dextrose in water. A gastrostomy was done at 72 hours if ventilation was still necessary, and small feedings of 5% aqueous dextrose were given.

This technic has been effective in maintaining prolonged controlled ventilation in newborns. Technic and experience are more important in this treatment than the specific ventilator used.

▶ [It's not the ventilator used but the ventilation achieved!—Eds.]

Gas Embolism in Hyaline Membrane Disease. George A. Gregory and William H. Tooley[2] (Univ. of California) recently encountered an infant with severe hyaline membrane disease who died suddenly during ventilation, presumably of a pulmonary venous gas embolus.

Male infant, weighing 1,700 Gm., was born at 31 weeks' gestation to an Rh-negative woman aged 36. The 1- and 5-minute Apgar scores were 1 and 4, respectively. The trachea was intubated, and controlled positive-pressure ventilation begun. Total lung compliance was about one-fifth the predicted value. Inflation pressures of 40-50 cm. water were needed for normal blood gases to be maintained. A Bird Mark 9 respirator was used. With 70-100% oxygen, the lower abdominal aortic blood Po_2 was 50-70, and the Pco_2 was 40-60 mm. Hg. Reduction of inflation pressure caused a rapid fall in Po_2 and

(2) New England J. Med. 282:1141-1142, May 14, 1970.

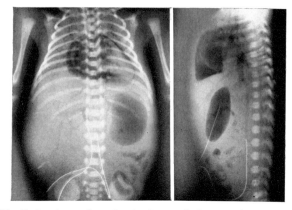

Fig. 30.—Postmortem radiographs showing gas in heart, pericardium, aorta and hepatic and pulmonary vasculature. Both catheters are in pockets of gas. (Courtesy of Gregory, G. A., and Tooley, W. H.: New England J. Med. 282:1141-1142, May 14, 1970.)

a rise in $Paco_2$. Paralyzing doses of d-tubocurarine were given. The chest x-ray was consistent with severe hyaline membrane disease. The pulse pressure narrowed, and a precordial millwheel murmur appeared in the 54th hour of life, during ventilation with 100% oxygen at an inflation pressure of 55 cm. water; the infant died. A total of 8 ml. gas was taken from the umbilical catheters. Postmortem x-rays showed pneumopericardium and gas in the heart, aorta and hepatic vessels (Fig. 30).

This patient, like many premature infants with severe hyaline membrane disease, had stiff lungs that required high inflation pressures to maintain adequate ventilation. Gas could have entered the infant's arterial vasculature from the inferior vena cava through a patent foramen ovale or ductus arteriosus, been drawn into the umbilical vein around the catheter during spontaneous ventilation or injected into a pulmonary vein during ventilation and distributed to both the venous and arterial systems. The latter seems the likeliest explanation. The patient's abnormal lungs might easily have torn with the airway pressures used. Gas embolism may be more common than has been apparent in infants given positive-pressure ventilation. Postmortem x-rays are seldom obtained, and autopsy is usually done many hours after death, by which time intravascular gas, especially oxygen, will have been absorbed.

► [An interesting case, perhaps representing a situation that develops more commonly than we know.—Eds.]

Measurement of Functional Residual Capacity in Distressed Neonates by Helium Rebreathing. Evaluation of treatment for infants with hyaline membrane disease is difficult because of the lack of an accurate means of diagnosing and assessing the severity of the disease. Atelectasis is a major pathologic process in hyaline membrane disease; decreased functional residual capacity (FRC) is an expression of this process. A. N. Krauss and P. A. M. Auld[3] (Cornell Univ.) developed a test for physiologically characterizing these infants. Study was made of 22 infants with retractions, grunting and cyanosis in room air. Sixteen had x-ray changes consistent with hyaline membrane disease; 2 had questionable findings. One meconium-stained infant was felt to have aspiration pneumonia. Two infants died and were found at autopsy to have atelectasis and hyaline membranes. Study was also made of 23 nondistressed infants weighing 794-2,500 Gm. at birth. The closed-circuit rebreathing method was used to determine FRC, with a mixture of 12-14% helium and oxygen. Rebreathing lasted for 30-60 seconds or for at least 30 breaths. The test was repeated if hyperventilation or crying occurred. Repeated values within 5-10 ml. were obtained under proper conditions, when face mask leaks were avoided. A nitrogen plateau was reached within 20 seconds in regularly breathing subjects and within 30 breaths in those with apneic pauses, in both well and sick infants.

Normal infants with birth weights over 1,500 Gm. had a mean FRC of 1.3 ml./cm. in the first 24 hours compared with 0.9 cc./cm. for those with hyaline membrane disease. The respective mean values for lower birth weight infants were 0.8 ml./cm. and 0.4 cc./cm. Two infants had low FRC values on the 1st day and normal values on the 2d day. The infant with meconium aspiration had a larger than expected FRC.

This test can be used diagnostically as well as for an indication of the severity of hyaline membrane disease in premature infants. Longer, more mature infants have larger airways, higher pulmonary compliance and lower chest wall compliance compared with the immature infants.

▶ [The use of this simple, reproducible bedside measurement of functional residual capacity will allow repeated follow-up of changes during treatment.—Eds.]

Starch in Lungs of Newborns Following Positive-Pressure Ventilation. Granulomas and adhesions have been reported in

---

(3)   J. Pediat. 77: 228-232, August, 1970.

wounds and surgical incisions due to starch glove powder, and animal studies have confirmed the ability of the powder to cause these lesions. Common surgical glove powder is composed of cornstarch etherified and treated with 2% magnesium oxide. It appears as round or polyhedral bodies 10-70 μ in diameter and showing a Maltese cross configuration under polarized light. David W. Dain, John L. Randall and James W. Smith[4] (Univ. of Vermont) reviewed lung slides from 16 infants who died in 1967 after positive-pressure respirator treatment. The amount of starch present was quantitated by using polarized light. Granules embedded in exudate, surrounded by neutrophils or present in macrophages were considered to have been present in the lungs before death.

Starch granules were found in bronchial and alevolar exudate or phagocytes in 7 infants. They did not appear to have caused the exudate. Some granules were surrounded by neutrophils. Several in 1 case were present in multinucleated giant cells within alveoli. The pathologic changes of "respirator lung" were present in some cases. Small amounts of starch were found in most controls, who included 6 stillborn infants and 7 not on respirator therapy. Eight adults were also examined after positive-pressure respirator therapy; an occasional adult had small amounts of starch, but these were considered to be of postmortem origin in all instances.

The most likely source of starch in the lungs of these infants was the sterile gloves used to handle the endotracheal catheter during tracheal toilet. Starch granules were presumably deposited on the tracheal wall during suctioning and forced into the lungs when the respirator was reconnected. Evidence of a cell reaction to the starch was seen. Granulomas probably form in surviving infants having positive-pressure ventilation. Foreign material is easily forced into the lungs by respirators. Surgical glove powder should be considered a potentially harmful foreign substance and care taken to exclude it from the lungs. ▶ [How about this! But, is it cause or effect?—Eds.]

Respiratory Distress Syndrome of Newborn Infants: II. Technic of Catheterization of Umbilical Artery and Clinical Results of Treatment of 124 Patients are presented by Dharampuri Vidyasagar, John J. Downes and Thomas R. Boggs, Jr.[5] (Univ. of Pennsylvania). The 124 patients were the first treated

(4) Am. J. Dis. Child. 119:218-220, March, 1970.
(5) Clin. Pediat. 9:332-337, June, 1970.

by catheterization of the umbilical artery, which has been used in management of newborn infants with respiratory distress syndrome for 5 years. A presumptive diagnosis was made within 8 hours after delivery. The mean gestational age was 34 weeks and the mean birth weight, 1690 Gm.

Catheterization was done under sterile conditions with the infant in an incubator or under a warming device and receiving oxygen by a mask and bag. The recommended procedure is shown in the table. Penicillin or nafcillin and kanamycin were given for the duration of catheterization and for 1 day afterward.

Catheters remained in place for an average of 49 hours and a maximum of 8 days. Catheterization was unsuccessful in 16 cases (13%), due to inadvertent periarterial introduction or intense arterial spasm. Seven infants (6%) had arterial spasm in a lower limb, usually within 12 hours of catheterization. Normal circulation returned to the extremity 1-6 hours after removal of the catheter. Two infants had fatal mesenteric thrombosis. One infant had fatal sepsis starting after removal of the catheter. The mortality due to respiratory distress syndrome itself was 30%; that due to definite or possible sequelae of umbilical artery catheterization was 2.4%.

Catheterization of the umbilical artery is the most practical way for frequent assessment of the Pao_2. The catheter also provides a means of continuous monitoring of the aortic pres-

---

RECOMMENDED PROCEDURE FOR UMBILICAL ARTERY CATHETERIZATION IN NEWBORN INFANTS WITH RESPIRATORY DISTRESS SYNDROME

1. Use a molded-tip no. 5 French plastic umbilical artery catheter with an end hole.*
2. Place catheter tip in iliac artery or just above aortic bifurcation (insert a distance equal to 50% of umbilicus-shoulder distance).
3. Keep fluid infusing continuously through the catheter and also flush lumen once an hour with 0.1% heparin solution.
4. Confirm position of catheter with a portable roentgenogram immediately, regardless of all technical difficulties involved.
5. Remove catheter as soon as Pao_2 has remained at or above 70 mm. Hg in 40% oxygen and pH at or above 7.30 for 12 hours without sodium bicarbonate infusion.
6. Apply antibiotic ointment to the umbilicus both at time of catheterization and when catheter is removed.

---

*This does not have a dead space for thrombus formation as found in the closed tip of the side-hole feeding tube.

sure, of use in any critically ill newborn infant. The procedure is easy to perform. The recommended procedure (table) and recent introduction of end-hole, molded-tip plastic catheters with continuous fluid infusion should minimize major thromboembolic difficulties.

▶ [A 3% mortality from a monitoring catheter seems high, but then the mortality from respiratory distress syndrome is high.—Eds.]

INHALATION THERAPY

Investigation of the Nine Most Commonly Used Resuscitator Bags. Edward Carden and Melvyn Bernstein[6] (St. Paul's Hosp., Vancouver) tested the Ambu, Ambu Compact, Hope, Pulmonator, Laerdal, Air-Viva, Aga, Puritan and Ambu (Air Shields) resuscitator bags to see if they were significantly different.

All bags had face masks and could be attached to a 15-mm., 1-degree taper endotracheal tube connector. Ambu bags were tested with both E-2 and Ruben valves. The Laerdal was used with face mask and then with attachments to fit an oxygen reservoir onto the bag. In the tests, the bag was connected to a one-way valve, which led through a Wright respirometer to a 10-L. bag into which was inserted the sampling catheter of an oxygen analyzer. A fixed-size resistance was inserted into the tubing so that pressure during a squeeze of the bag was 15-25 cm. water. The pressures were recorded on a polygraph. The bag was squeezed for 2 seconds, then released for 4 seconds. Each squeeze forced 800 cc. air into the collecting bag; when the bag was full, the oxygen content of the gas mixture was noted. Oxygen to the resuscitator flows were 5, 10 and 15 L. per minute and were delivered from a calibrated, backpressure-compensated flowmeter. The 2 observers tested at least two samples of each bag make and each bag on three occasions. Bags were then tested on a volunteer to see if the valve jammed or stuck.

All bags gave increased oxygen concentration with increased oxygen flow, but none gave 100% oxygen even when the flow was twice the minute ventilation (Fig. 31). In Ambu and Air-Viva bags, air was enriched by oxygen fed directly into the bag. In Air-Viva and Ambu with the E-2 valve, pressure did not build up during the patient's expiration; displaced air leaked

(6) J.A.M.A. 212:589-592, Apr. 27, 1970.

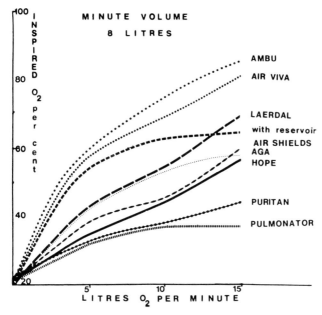

Fig. 31.—Oxygen concentrations delivered with up to 15 L. oxygen flowing to resuscitation bag. Maximum concentrations delivered from Ambu and Pulmonator bags are 87 and 37%, respectively. (Courtesy of Carden, E., and Bernstein, M.: J.A.M.A. 212:589-592, Apr. 27, 1970.)

out around the inflating valve. The longer the pause between respirations, the greater the amount of oxygen delivered. In the Laerdal, oxygen fed directly into the bag, but some escaped through holes around the oxygen input tube. Oxygen entering at 2 or 3 L. per minute raised the internal pressure of the bag enough to jam the valve in the inspiratory position during expiration. This also occurred in the Ambu with a Ruben valve at over 5 L. per minute and in the Pulmonator at 4 L. per minute, so these three bags should be restricted to use with a face mask. The Ambu (Air Shields) tended to jam when wet. The Laerdal with reservoir and Aga had attachments so that oxygen was delivered into a reservoir before entering the bag, and they were tested with a 250-cc. reservoir tube. If this reservoir was a closed bag or of larger volume, up to 100% of oxygen could be delivered. The other bags used a method in which oxygen was blown past the air inlet valve and sucked in as a mixture. Ambu bags were not as easily cleaned as the other bags tested.

The Laerdal was the most portable bag. The Aga or Ambu with an optional extension between bag and inflating valve is convenient when the patient is being transported. Either of the two Ambu bags with the E-2 valve or the Air-Viva valve would be suitable for most people.

▶ [It is important that new medical devices be evaluated by those qualified to do so because of the absence of Federal or other standards regulating their manufacture. What seems like a good idea in the laboratory may function poorly on the ward or in an ambulance. Hopefully, manufacturers will take into consideration poor design and eliminate it in newer models. Physicians and paramedical personnel should be aware of the limitations of the devices they use.—Eds.]

Effect of Compliance and Airway Resistance Change on Oxygen Delivery by Pressure-Cycled Respirator. Pressure-cycled respirators using a Venturi mechanism for air entrainment deliver oxygen concentrations that vary with changes in cycling pressure and manual flow adjustment. William R. Winn and

Fig. 32.—Relationship of oxygen concentration to resistance at four different compliances with nebulizer functioning. Each point represents the mean oxygen concentration delivered at the selected peak inspiratory pressures. Respiratory frequency = 10 breaths per minute. (Courtesy of Winn, W. R., and Hale, F. C.: Am. Rev. Resp. Dis. 102: 107-111, July, 1970.)

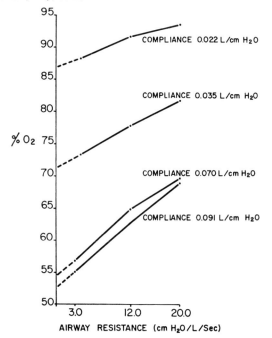

Frank C. Hale[7] (Univ. of California) adjusted three new pressure-cycled, flow-variable Bird Mark VII respirators to ventilate a mechanical test lung system at frequencies of 10 and 15 breaths per minute at peak airway pressures of 20, 25, 30 and 40 cm. water. The ratio of inspiratory to expiratory time was kept constant at 1:2. The respirators were set to "air mix" and powered with 100% oxygen at 55 lb./sq. in. An 0.7-L. reservoir, jet-type nebulizer was included in the system, but no liquid was nebulized. Airway resistances of 3, 12 and 20 cm. water per liter per second were placed just downstream to the main line tubing and attached to a 5-L. anesthesia bag. Compliances of 0.091, 0.070, 0.035 and 0.022 L./cm. water were obtained. Oxygen concentrations were 52-95% with and 41-65% without the nebulizer.

With the nebulizer functioning, oxygen concentration was nearly directly proportional to airway resistance with each compliance (Fig. 32). With normal or near-normal compliance, increasing resistance caused relatively large increases in oxygenation; with markedly reduced compliance, resistance changes had little effect on oxygen concentration. Compliance changes altered oxygen delivery independently of resistance changes. The least ventilation occurred when the compliance was low. More reduction in ventilation occurred with markedly reduced compliances than with the highest resistances. There was a high negative correlation between ventilation (mean inspiratory flow) and observed oxygen concentrations. Increasing the frequency usually increased mean flow. The nebulizer contribution is indicated in the table.

EFFECT OF BIRD JET-TYPE NEBULIZER ON OXYGEN DELIVERY AT
FOUR TOTAL COMPLIANCES AND ONE AIRWAY RESISTANCE*

COMPLIANCE	OXYGEN CONCENTRATION (PER CENT)	
(L./cm. H_2O)	Without Nebulizer	With Nebulizer
Normal 0.091	41	53
Minimally reduced 0.070	44	59
Moderately reduced 0.035	54	74
Markedly reduced 0.022	65	91

*3 cm. H_2O/L./second; peak inspiratory pressure, 25 cm. H_2O.

(7) Am. Rev. Resp. Dis. 102:107-111, July, 1970.

Toxic oxygen concentrations could be delivered by this respirator when used with its nebulizer and functioning normally. It often was observed to provide increasing oxygen concentrations to patients who were difficult to ventilate. Oxygen toxicity might be avoided by not using the jet-type nebulizer when the respirator is used for long periods. Use of the jet-type nebulizer is justified initially while evaluating the patient's oxygenation in acute situations such as pulmonary edema.

Antibacterial Action of Copper in Respiratory Therapy Apparatus was investigated by Robert S. Deane, Ernest L. Mills and Augert J. Hamel[8] (Univ. of Vermont). Pulmonary infection is increased in patients having intermittent positive-pressure breathing (IPPB) or humidity from large reservoir nebulizers. The factors include inadequate cleaning and sterilization of equipment, the duration of continuous use, contamination from the patient or by hand filling and airborne contamination. Cross-infection may also occur. The Emerson postoperative ventilator has copper scrubbing sponges on both the afferent and efferent sides of the heated humidifier. When pathogens were introduced into it and the respirator was used to ventilate a rubber bag for a number of hours, no growth resulted on culturing the humidifier contents. Laboratory studies of the influence of commercial copper sponges were done on the growth of Escherichia coli, enterococci, klebsiella, pseudomonas, paracolons and mimeae. In patients, nebulizers were changed every 48-110 hours, and the tubing, valves, etc., every 24 hours. Nebulizers were filled by a closed system. A total of 108 cultures of tracheal aspirate were taken from patients on continuous IPPB. The nebulizer was sampled at 48 and 72 hours and sometimes later. A group of 100 random samples of nebulizer contents were taken (Fig. 33). Fifty patients with positive tracheal aspirates received IPPB for over a week with a sponge in the nebulizer and a copper sponge-filled trap attached to the expiratory port of the respirator.

Turbidity and growth of test organisms were prevented by a single copper sponge in laboratory studies. Nine of the 108 cultures of tracheal aspirate and nebulizer without a copper sponge were positive, the same organism being cultured from both sites in three instances.

A single copper sponge in the nebulizer significantly reduced growth after continuous use for 48 hours. In 100 random samples

(8)   Chest 58: 373-377, October, 1970.

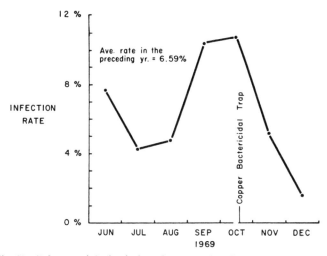

Fig. 33.—Pulmonary infection in intensive care unit. (Courtesy of Deane, R. S., *et al.*: Chest 58:373-377, October, 1970.)

from nebulizers with copper sponge, none was positive. Patients on IPPB with a copper trap attached to the respirator exhalation port had positive tracheal aspirate cultures but negative cultures from the interior of the outlet adaptor. The trap appeared to prevent pathogens from being vented onto the bedclothes and into the surrounding environment. The rate of pulmonary infection dropped from 4-10% to 1.6% when copper traps were introduced, without a substantial change in the number of patients on respirators. Serum copper levels exceeded normal in only one instance.

Addition of a copper bactericidal trap on the exhaled side of an IPPB circuit significantly reduces contamination of air and the patient's environment with pathogens and decreases the risk of cross-infection. The apparent incidence of pulmonary infection is also reduced.

▶ [This seems like a simple expedient for reducing contamination in nebulizers as well as in the exhaled air of patients on respiratory therapy. Although these authors found no important increases in serum copper levels, the possibility of copper toxicity should be recognized.—Eds.]

Sterilization of Pulmonary Ventilators is discussed by J. L. Whitby[9] (Queen Elizabeth Hosp., Birmingham, England). Pulmonary ventilators in current use are of two types, bellows and pressure-cycled. Pressure-cycled ventilators should present lit-

(9) Proc. Roy. Soc. Med. 63:909-910, September, 1970.

tle difficulty in sterilization. Early attempts to sterilize bellows ventilators involved boiling the connecting tubing and water in humidifiers. The practice of cycling the machine while generating a bactericidal vapor has persisted. Low-pressure steam has been combined with formalin in an autoclave chamber. Ethylene oxide in a chamber has been used at greater than atmospheric pressures. Detachable ventilatory parts make this process easier. As ventilators cannot be cycled inside sterilizing chambers, valves have been dismantled to insure that the gas reaches all parts.

Satisfactory results have been reported with use of humidifiers filled with 1:5000 chlorhexidine, which is changed daily. Resiguard, a liquid disinfectant, has also been used in this way, but difficulties may occur with some volume-cycled machines. A nebulizer can be used to create a mist while the machine cycles. Ultrasonically nebulized alcohol has also been used, but there is risk of explosion. Results with hydrogen peroxide used in this way are conflicting. It is technically difficult to use high-efficiency "Williams filters" to isolate the machine from the patient.

The most practical method of sterilizing volume-cycled ventilators at present is by use of a nebulizer to distribute a disinfectant throughout the machine after use. Improved machine design may provide a readily detachable ventilator circuit, which can then be readily sterilized by autoclaving, ethylene oxide or low-temperature steam and formaldehyde, the choice depending on the materials used in the circuit.

▶ [How about a disposable patient circuit or a bacterial filter system?—Eds.]

Mechanism for Water-to-Air Transfer and Concentration of Bacteria. Duncan C. Blanchard and Lawrence Syzdek[1] (State Univ. of New York, Albany) report that bacteria can be carried into the air by drops from bursting bubbles and that the concentration of bacteria in the drops can far exceed that in the water in which the bubbles break.

Bubbles were generated in a glass beaker containing tap water inoculated with Serratia marcescens by forcing filtered air through an immersed capillary tube. The top jet drop, formed when the bubble broke, was collected.

Concentrations of bacteria in the bulk water ranged from 10^3 to 10^6 per ml.; S. marcescens could be concentrated in the

(1) Science 170:626-628, Nov. 6, 1970.

jet drop up to a factor of 1,000 over that of bulk water. The bacteria were apparently concentrated in the surface microlayer and ejected into the air when the bubbles burst. Depending on the drop size, the bacterial concentrations in ejected drops were 10-1,000 times that of the water in which the bubbles burst.

A high concentration of many species of organism could be expected at air-water interfaces, where they find the organic material they need to survive. Such material may become concentrated in air-borne drops.

▶ [The authors' interest is in atmospheric pollution, but their work has obvious applicability to respiratory therapy and serves to emphasize the need for absolute sterility for inhaled aerosols.—Eds.]

Common Misconceptions in Inhalation Therapy.—I. *Humidity.*—D. S. Tysinger, Jr.[2] (Dothan, Ala.) points out that the inhalation therapist deals with water in two simple forms, water vapor or humidity and particulate water produced by one means or another. Water vapor, being a gas, changes in density and volume as the temperature changes. The saturation point of water is reached more quickly at higher temperatures. As gases get less dense due to expansion on heating, so does water vapor (table). Humidity is the amount of water that air will hold at a given temperature, and the amount of vapor in the air at a given time expressed as a percentage of the total that it will hold is the relative humidity. A very small amount of water is involved in humidity. Anything used to increase room humidity, even to 100%, is futile in supplying water and preventing water loss from the lungs. Heating water with a nebulizer to produce 100% relative humidity is effective, but the temperature must be kept above body temperature until the water vapor reaches the mouth and nose. Steamers and other devices that raise the relative humidity in room air but do not put

RELATIONS DERIVED FROM STANDARD VAPOR PRESSURE, TEMPERATURE AND DENSITY AND COEFFICIENT OF EXPANSION TABLES

Temperature °C	Temperature °F	I cc water vapor & cc of water will make	II cc of water in one liter of water vapor	III Water vapor pressure	IV % of water vapor in air 100% relative humidified 760 mmHg	V cc of water per liter of air 100% relative humidified 760 mmHg
0	32	1275 cc	0.780 cc	4.6 mmHg	.61%	0.0048 cc
25	75	1382 cc	0.722 cc	23.8 mmHg	3.14%	0.023 cc
37	98.6	1400 cc	0.714 cc	47 mmHg	6.2%	0.044 cc
87	190	1681 cc	0.595 cc	468.7 mmHg	61.7%	0.367 cc
100	212	1742 cc	0.574 cc	760 mm Hg	100%	0.574 cc

(2)   J. M. A. Alabama 40:439-445, January, 1971.

enough particulate water into the nose and mouth are close to being worthless.

II. "Particulate water."—Tysinger[3] states that if the air is to put moisture into the lungs, water must be put into the air in larger than molecular size. The smallest water particles obtained from hot steam are due to the rapidly dropping dew point; their size is 2.5 μ. Larger particles form until the air is saturated with particles. The number of particles carried depends on the temperature at which air and water with particles leave the nebulizer. Hot moist air carries much less than room air or air at body temperature. Heated steam produces smaller particles than does a heated nebulizer. There are many methods of producing particles in cold solutions; all require heat and involve work. An atomizer that uses Bernoulli's principle is the most predictable nebulizer for particle size. Particle stability and "rain out" are important factors. Particles of 5 μ or less enter the lungs but must be over 1 μ to rain out effectively. The paths of particles in the lungs depend on particle size and patient position. A high water content produced by nebulization may cause denaturation of surfactant, with resultant alveolar collapse. A hypervolemic hypo-osmotic state occurs. Too much water may be as bad as, or worse than, not enough.

▶ [For those interested in humidification and the physical principles involved. It is an excellent review.—Eds.]

Carbon Dioxide Administration for Correction of Postoperative Hypoxemia. The normocapnic reduction in Pao$_2$, which most patients have after anesthesia and operation, can be attributed to ventilation-perfusion disturbance, increased venous admixture and decreased cardiac output. Tage Hald and Sophus H. Johansen[4] (Hellerup, Denmark) studied the effect of increased CO_2 concentration in the inspired air on postoperative oxygenation in 17 men and 6 women without severe cardiovascular disease. All had general anesthesia with controlled ventilation. The average patient age was 45.5 years. Humidified atmospheric air containing 2% CO_2 was given through one nostril at a rate of 30 L. per minute for 20 minutes postoperatively; the ventilatory response was recorded. Eleven other patients with an average age of 54 did not receive CO_2. The respective mean operative periods were 81.1 and 77.7 minutes. Six study patients were examined an hour after operation and the following day.

The Paco$_2$ before anesthesia and 20 minutes afterward was

(3) J. M. A. Alabama 40:503-510. February, 1971.
(4) Acta anaesth. scandinav. 14:53-59, 1970.

40.7 and 43.4 mm. Hg, respectively, in CO_2-treated patients and 41.4 and 41.9 mm. Hg, respectively, in control patients. The administration of CO_2 did not alter the $Paco_2$ significantly. Decreased oxygenation after anesthesia was most marked after abdominal operation. A distinct rise in Pao_2 was noted after 20 minutes of CO_2 inhalation. Only a few control patients showed a return of Pao_2 to normal 40 minutes after anesthesia. The average Pao_2 in 6 patients studied 20 minutes after CO_2 treatment was stopped was 3.5 mm. Hg less than the average during CO_2 administration. Three of these patients showed an increase in Pao_2 the following day as compared with immediate postoperative values, whereas 3 showed lower levels. Ventilation volumes increased an average of 43% during CO_2 administration. Patients exposed to CO_2 recovered surprisingly rapidly from anesthesia.

It is still not clear whether an increase in the inspired CO_2 level is of therapeutic value in the postoperative period, but it would seem desirable to improve ventilation as well as oxygenation postoperatively. The finding that CO_2 enhances the elimination of anesthetics supports this view.

▶ [The use of CO_2 to stimulate respiration in the recovery room is worthwhile. It not only will reverse hypoxemia, but will help to prevent atelectasis and awake the patient. However, 2% CO_2 for 20 minutes is too weak for too long.—Eds.]

Sensitivities and Response Times of Ventilatory Assistors. Most modern ventilators are said to be able to assist as well as control ventilation, but there are few reports to support this. Ralph A. Epstein[5] (Columbia Univ.) developed a method of quantifying the ability of a ventilator to assist and evaluated 6 ventilators.

METHOD.—The minimum amount of air that caused triggering when rapidly removed from the patient end of the ventilatory circuit was determined. The critical volume that caused triggering at least 90% of the time and the time from initiation of negative pressure to attainment of a positive pressure of 1 cm. water was recorded (response time).

The following ventilators were tested: 2 pneumatically powered ventilators, the Bennett PR-2 Special and the Bird Mark 8, and 4 electrically powered units, the Bennett MA-1, the Bourns model 104-150, the Dräger Spiromat 661 and the Ohio 560. All units but the Bourns were set up in a pressure-limited mode. Ten trials were made at each volume level with each ventilator; failure in more than 1 trial was considered failure to trigger.

The Bourns ventilator was triggered on withdrawal of 0.1

(5) Anesthesiology 34:321-326, April, 1971.

ml. and responded in 36 msec. The Bennett MA-1 triggered with removal of 0.5 ml. in 82 msec. The Bennett PR-2 triggered on withdrawal of 1.5 ml. and responded in 226 msec. (106 msec. on withdrawal of a larger volume). The Bird Mark 8 triggered on removal of 1.5 ml. in 157 msec. (87 msec. with withdrawal of a larger volume). The Dräger required 434 msec. to respond to withdrawal of 1 ml. and the response time remained high with a larger volume. The Ohio ventilators triggered in 123 msec. with withdrawal of 0.5 ml. and in 145 msec. with removal of a larger volume.

Peak negative pressures were reasonably constant at each level of withdrawal volume, indicating that the withdrawal technic was consistent. The Bourns ventilator was exceptionally sensitive and its response time was significantly shorter than that of the other ventilators. Reproducibility of the response times varied. The Dräger Spiromat must be considered primarily a controller, although occasional patient triggering may be allowed. The other units had response times adequate for moderate rates of assistance.

Continuous Positive-Pressure Ventilation in Acute Respiratory Failure: Effects on Hemodynamics and Lung Function. Continuous positive-pressure ventilation has been reported to improve arterial oxygenation in patients in severe acute respiratory failure by increasing the functional residual capacity secondary to prevention of terminal airspace collapse on expiration. A low end-expiratory pressure (5 cm. water) does not significantly alter cardiac output; higher pressures are needed to improve arterial oxygenation substantially.

Anil Kumar, Konrad J. Falke, Bennie Geffin, Carolyn F. Aldredge, Myron B. Laver, Edward Lowenstein and Henning Pontoppidan[6] (Harvard Med. School) studied 8 patients who had received intermittent ventilation with a constant-volume time-cycled ventilator for varying periods before continuous positive-pressure ventilation was started. The goal was a Pao_2 of 100 mm. Hg. Intermittent ventilation with an inspired oxygen level of 50% or more had not provided satisfactory oxygenation.

No patient had previously had respiratory failure. Six patients had serious cerebral, cardiorenal or hepatic complications, and none of these survived. All but 1 were in a stable circulatory state when studied. Ventilation was given with a

(6) New England J. Med. 283:1430-1436, Dec. 24, 1970.

volume-limited, sinusoid flow ventilator (Emerson). The inspired oxygen level was raised to 100% only for 30 minutes before and during study.

Continuous ventilation with use of high positive end-expiratory airway pressures significantly improved arterial oxygenation in the patients. A satisfactory Pao_2 was maintained with an inspired oxygen concentration of 50% or less. The mean intrapulmonary shunt was 19% of the cardiac output, increasing 9% with a change to intermittent ventilation. The cardiac index was normal or above in all patients but 1 during continuous ventilation and rose further on intermittent ventilation.

Six patients died after 4-16 days of continuous ventilation; the mean Pao_2 shortly before death was 356 mm. Hg. Four patients had autopsy evidence of the lung changes described in patients dying after prolonged mechanical ventilation.

This study showed significant improvement in Pao_2 in patients in severe acute respiratory failure with use of positive end-expiratory airway pressure during continuous positive-pressure ventilation. The calculated intrapulmonary shunt improved during continuous ventilation. Four patients had complications, subcutaneous emphysema in 3 of them, which did not interfere with their management. Continuous positive-pressure ventilation should be terminated gradually, with frequent analysis of arterial blood gases.

Subsequent treatment of over 100 patients by continuous positive-pressure ventilation confirmed the results of this study. However, arterial oxygenation deteriorated in 3 patients.

► [Both pulmonary edema and hypoxia can be treated with continuous positive ventilation. As long as the retard pressure is not too high, and the blood volume normal, the cardiac output should not fall, as has been shown. However, the subcutaneous emphysema is of concern.—Eds.]

Relaxed Expiratory Volume and Forced Inspiratory Volume after Bronchodilators. Response to bronchodilators is usually assessed by tests that require maximum expiratory effort, which may narrow the airways, especially in the presence of chronic airway obstruction. Changes in peripheral airways may not be detected by such tests because of masking by collapsed larger central airways. M. K. Tandon and A. H. Campbell[7] (Melbourne, Australia) compared the 1-second forced expiratory volume (FEV_1) with the relaxed expiratory volume (REV_1) and the forced inspiratory volume (FIV_1) in assessing responses to bronchodilators in patients with airway obstruction.

(7) Brit. J. Dis. Chest 64:73-77, April, 1970.

The subjects were 92 men aged 43-78 years with chronic bronchitis. All had had a productive cough for over 3 years and all but 2 reported exertional dyspnea. Some had x-ray evidence of emphysema. All measurements were recorded at spirometry. For the REV_1, the patient was asked to inhale deeply, hold his breath, put on a mask and then exhale by a deep and heavy sigh, without forcing air out. Measurements were repeated 15-30 minutes after 3 inhalations of 1% isoprenaline sulfate aerosol.

All measurements improved significantly after aerosol administration. The FIV_1 tended to respond better than the FEV_1. Forty-two patients did not show at least 10% improvement in FEV_1 after bronchodilator therapy. In these, the FEV_1 and vital capacity did not improve significantly after aerosol therapy, but the REV_1 and FIV_1 both improved highly significantly. The FIV_1 showed a significantly greater response than the FEV_1 in 2 patients with a check-valve spirogram. The 13 patients with radiologic evidence of emphysema had a relatively poor bronchodilator response as measured by the FEV_1 compared with that measured by the FIV_1 and REV_1.

The FEV_1 remains the simplest means of assessing bronchodilator responses, but it may fail to detect an actual response in some patients. The bronchodilator response in the peripheral bronchi may be partly masked during measurement of FEV_1, probably by central airways collapse.

Further Experience with Electric Stimulation of the Phrenic Nerve: Electrically Induced Fatigue. A practical method of assisted ventilation by electrophrenic respiration (EPR) has been developed but, in early studies and in a patient, diaphragmatic fatigue occurred after several hours of stimulation. Genichi Sato, William W. L. Glenn, Wade G. Holcomb and Daniel Wuench[8] (Yale Univ.) sought the site of alteration or injury in adult mongrel dogs. Bipolar stimulating electrodes were attached to the phrenic nerve trunk in the chest in ventilated, anesthetized dogs. Nerve action potentials were recorded distally from the ipsilateral phrenic nerve bundle about 4 cm. above the diaphragm. The diaphragmatic muscle action potential was measured by a pair of unipolar needle electrodes. Venous blood lactic and pyruvic acid levels were estimated. Nerve injury due to electric stimulation was assessed and end-plate potential

(8)   Surgery 68:817-826, November, 1970.

changes after stimulation were observed. Prevention of fatigue by alternating bidirectional current was assessed.

The nerve was ruled out as the site of origin of fatigue after EPR because measured nerve action potentials showed no change in strength or duration after continuous graded stimulation when no diaphragmatic contraction was observed. The diaphragm was also not the site; though muscle action potentials disappeared at the time of fatigue, the diaphragm responded to directly applied stimuli.

End-plate potential measurements showed EPR-induced fatigue to be due to interference with impulse transmission across the neuromuscular junction. Pulse parameters were significantly related to measured fatigue. With the lowest pulse frequency giving graded contraction, significantly prolonged respiration resulted without diaphragm fatigue. The pulse train duration and system tolerance time were in inverse proportion.

During repetitive stimulation, the shorter the pulse interval, the quicker the decline in muscle action potentials. The same results were obtained in studying the relationship of several pulse intervals to end-plate potentials during curarization.

Stimulation with alternating bidirectional current greatly prolonged effective diaphragmatic contractions. Avoidance of fatigue with this technic may be due to depolarization or to the lack of firing of some motor units by every anodal stimulus.

▶ [Electric stimulation of nerves sounds so simple but prolonged stimulation is exceedingly complex. Nonetheless, clinical application on an intermittent basis appears feasible.—Eds.]

Central Hypoventilation: Long-Term Ventilatory Assistance by Radiofrequency Electrophrenic Respiration. William W. L. Glenn, Wade G. Holcomb, J. Bernard L. Gee and Ranjit Rath[9] (Yale Univ.) have applied electrophrenic respiration (EPR) for 4-22 months to 4 patients with hypoventilation of central origin. All patients had an unequivocal need for chronic ventilatory assistance. Three had normal lungs and normal response of phrenic nerve and diaphragm to electric stimulation; 1 had obstructive lung disease, probably secondary to longstanding severe pulmonary hypertension and polycythemia. All 4 patients had a reduced Pao_2 and elevated $Paco_2$, especially during sleep, and reduced responsiveness of the respiratory center to 5% CO_2.

PROCEDURE.—The left phrenic nerve was isolated under local in-

(9) Ann. Surg. 172:755-773, October, 1970.

filtrative anesthesia and stimulated electrically to demonstrate its suitability for EPR. A receiver pocket was made above the costal margin in the midaxillary line. The nerve and perineural tissues were placed within an electrode cuff, which was closed with sutures and fixed to the surrounding tissue.

Chronic EPR, for 8-12 hours nightly, was usually not begun until the incisions were healed, about 10-14 days postoperatively. A pulse-width modulated radiofrequency transmitter was used in the 3 most recent patients.

Tidal volume and instantaneous flow measurements during submaximal EPR showed ventilation in excess of the resting normal state. Flow and volume tracings during EPR were similar in contour to those of spontaneous respiration; no biphasic response was apparent. Compared with normal values, radioxenon washout was faster during EPR in all parts of the lung but the right lower lobe. A rise in Pco_2 during sleep was promptly reversed by EPR. Alveolar ventilation was increased during EPR. Hypoxemia and hypercapnia were partially reversed during EPR in sleep. Alveolar-arterial oxygen gradients were not markedly affected by EPR. The contralateral diaphragm showed paradoxical motion during EPR in all patients. Decreased motion occurred after 8 hours of stimulation and progressed to 20 hours, about 24 hours being needed for full recovery. No fatigue occurred after 18 hours when a revised waveform was used. Systolic blood pressure fell by 15-20% soon after the beginning of EPR; pulmonary artery pressure changed similarly during EPR.

This treatment at present is recommended only for patients having a definite need for chronic ventilatory assistance and whose lungs are normal. This includes patients with lesions involving the respiratory center or the cervical cord above the C3 level. Other patients should be treated only if the expected improvement in lung function outweighs the risk of phrenic nerve damage.

ACUTE MEDICAL CARE

Management of Acute Respiratory Failure in a Respiratory Intensive Care Unit. Walter J. O'Donohue, Jr., James P. Baker, George M. Bell, Orhan Muren and John L. Patterson, Jr.[1] (Med. College of Virginia) report experience with patients in a respiratory intensive care unit, among whom mortality from

(1)   Chest 58:603-610, December, 1970.

acute respiratory failure has been reduced fivefold, compared with similar patients treated in the same hospital before establishment of the unit. Mortality has been reduced from over 40 to 8.6% in the first 2 years of operation of the unit. There were 269 admissions of 222 patients with acute respiratory failure during this time. Of the 130 males and 92 females admitted, 15 were under age 12 years. Average stay in the unit was 11.6 days. One third of admissions were for respiratory failure in patients with chronic obstructive pulmonary disease, who had an average stay in the unit of 15 days. In only 9 of these patients was the $Paco_2$ less than 60 mm. Hg before definitive treatment. Treatment was with low-flow oxygen and assisted ventilation by tracheostomy or tracheal intubation.

There were 22 deaths, including 7 in patients with obstructive lung disease. Mortality in patients with a $Paco_2$ of 60 mm. Hg or higher at any time during the stay was 47%. Deaths after discharge from the unit totaled 19 during the 2-year study. Low-flow oxygen therapy was adequate initially in only 11 of 56 admissions for chronic obstructive lung disease. Twelve of 21 patients with endotracheal tubes subsequently required tracheostomy. In all, 76% of patients with obstructive lung disease had tracheostomy and another 12% had tracheal intubation. Only about two thirds of the patients had pathogens in their sputum on admission. Ampicillin and tetracycline were frequently administered.

Management of acute respiratory failure has been greatly facilitated by the modern respiratory intensive care unit and by improved technics of patient care. The unit provides a center for training medical personnel in methods of respiratory care.

▶ [Concentration of patients with similar disorders will nearly always result in improved care, but at the expense of posing additional problems, e.g., expense, equipment, physical layout and highly trained personnel. Note the number of chest physicians in this article.—Eds.]

Shock Associated with Barbiturate Intoxication is discussed by Herbert Shubin and Max Harry Weil[2] (Univ. of Southern California). The patient admitted with signs of shock after barbiturate intoxication is typically in a deep coma, with a reduced rectal temperature and cool skin. Pulse rates over 130 are uncommon. The systolic blood pressure is typically below 80 mm. Hg, but intra-arterial measurements generally show pressures 10-20 mm. Hg higher than sphygmomanometer values. Rhonchi and wheezes are frequent, but moist rales are unusual. Serum

(2) J.A.M.A. 215:263-268, Jan. 11, 1971.

barbiturate levels do not necessarily reflect the severity of hypotension, respiratory depression or coma. The ECG often shows nonspecific S-T segment and T wave changes. Serum enzyme activities are increased in most cases, reflecting general tissue injury. Continuous ECG monitoring is indicated. The arterial pressure is monitored by catheter measurements, and plasma volume is studied by using central venous and arterial catheters. It is the cardiac output that is reduced, vasoconstriction compensates for this effect to keep the arterial pressure near normal levels. The central venous pressure is usually reduced, with reductions in blood and plasma volumes. The hemodynamic defect is due to an increase in vascular capacity without a concurrent increase in blood volume.

Treatment aims to maintain effective pulmonary gas exchange and effective circulating blood volume. Respiratory stimulants are contraindicated. An oropharyngeal airway is inserted, and if gastric contents are found in the aspirate, warm saline lavage is recommended. Oxygen is given if the Pao_2 is below 80 mm. Hg or the arterial oxygen saturation is less than 94%. A concentration of 40% is used initially, with 10-20% increments according to the response of the Pao_2 as measured at 2-4 hour intervals. A pressure-controlled ventilator is used for severe respiratory impairment. Antibiotics are given on the basis of staining of a tracheal aspirate, but they are not given routinely to spontaneously ventilating patients. Initially 5% normal human albumin is given; subsequently fluid therapy is with 10% dextrose in 0.9% saline. Urinary alkalinization is not uniformly effective. Dialysis is preferable to diuretic therapy when renal function is impaired or the serum long-acting barbiturate level exceeds 20 mg./100 ml. Digitalis is used only in patients who have a disproportionate rise in central venous pressure on fluid infusion in the absence of diuresis.

▶ [A good resumé of the treatment of severe barbiturate intoxication.— Eds.]

Management of Patients Unconscious from Drug Overdosage. J. W. Freeman, R. R. Beattie and C. A. Ryan[3] (Hobart, Tasmania) conducted a prospective survey of patients seen with drug overdosage in an 18-month period in 1968-69, and data on 179 of 333 patients admitted unconscious during the time were reviewed. Changes in management made during the survey period included cessation of routine forced diuresis and

(3) M. J. Australia 2:1165-1168, Dec. 19, 1970.

change in the indications for tracheal intubation. There were 73 patients asleep but rousable on admission, 70 who were comatose but reacted to painful stimuli, 14 who did not react to painful stimuli, 5 with absent reflexes and 15 with cardiorespiratory depression.

Patients were nursed semiprone. Tracheal intubation was done whenever the pharyngeal and tracheal reflexes were depressed enough for the patient to tolerate an endotracheal tube. It was done in 50 patients (28%), and 3 required tracheostomy. Endotracheal red rubber tubes were changed for Portex tubes after 24 hours. Complications were slight. Adequate humidification was vital. Pneumonia occurred in 25 patients, including 14 who had the disease on admission; it was serious in only 1. The goal in cardiovascular management was to maintain adequate tissue perfusion as judged by urine output. Usually this was possible by expanding the blood volume; vasopressors were rarely necessary. The central venous pressure was monitored in elderly patients or when larger amounts of plasma expander were used. No attempts were made to remove ingested poisons after forced diuresis was abandoned. Patients were turned every 2 hours and had chest physiotherapy and aseptic bronchial toilet. Three patients (1.7%) died, 2 with arrhythmias; 1 had ingested an organophosphate (Malathion).

The main approach to treatment in this series was conservative, attention being given to the support of cardiorespiratory function. Conservative management of patients who are unconscious after drug overdosage gives results equivalent to those obtained with more aggressive management, without the complications inherent in such management.

▶ [It is interesting that the population of all of Tasmania was 383,500 in 1968, and that 179 patients were admitted to this one hospital in 18 months.—Eds.]

Resin Hemoperfusion: A New Treatment for Acute Drug Intoxication is described by Jerry L. Rosenbaum, Mark S. Kramer, Rasib Raja and Christopher Boreyko[4] (Albert Einstein Med. Center, Philadelphia). Direct perfusion of blood through a column of activated charcoal or anion-exchange resin has toxic effects. Recently a new resin, Amberlite XAD-2, has been used in a column hemoperfusion system to remove barbiturates and glutethimide from dogs and human beings. The resin, which has a cross-linked polystyrene macroreticular structure,

(4) New England J. Med. 284:874-877, Apr. 22, 1971.

is prepared in a sterile, pyrogen-free form and has a specific adsorption attraction for high molecular weight, lipid-soluble substances.

Four patients with severe drug intoxication, in profound coma and with potentially lethal blood levels of drug, were treated using the Amberlite XAD-2 resin column hemoperfusion system (Figs. 34 and 35). The inflow catheter was inserted into the femoral vein and passed to the inferior vena cava, and the outflow catheter was inserted into a forearm vein. Patients received 4,000 units of heparin intravenously 15 minutes before the procedure was started. Blood was circulated at a rate of

Fig. 34 (top).—Diagram of the resin column hemoperfusion system.
Fig. 35 (bottom).—Photograph of a 650-G Amberlite XAD-2 resin column.
(Courtesy of Rosenbaum, J. L., et al.: New England J. Med. 284:874-877, Apr. 22, 1971.)

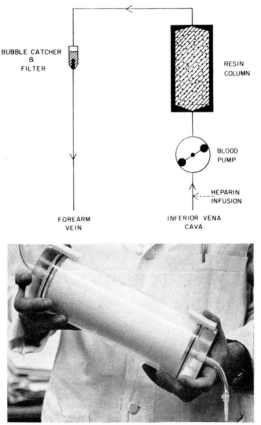

BLOOD CONCENTRATION OF DRUGS DURING HEMOPERFUSION IN 4 PATIENTS WITH DRUG INTOXICATION

CASE No.	DRUG	INFLOW BLOOD CONCENTRATION (MG/100 ML)*							OUTFLOW BLOOD CONCENTRATION (MG/100 ML)†							QUANTITY OF DRUG REMOVED (MG)
		0 TIME	AT ½ HR	AT 1 HR	AT 1½ HR	AT 2 HR	AT 2½ HR	AT 3 HR	0 TIME	AT ½ HR	AT 1 HR	AT 1½ HR	AT 2 HR	AT 2½ HR	AT 3 HR	
1	Secobarbital	9.2	8.5	7.6	7.5	6.4	6.1	5.8	1.4	2.2	2.5	2.6	2.3	3.5	3.4	2535
2	Glutethimide-butabarbital	4.3	3.9	2.6	2.5	2.2	1.8	1.5	0.8	0.8	0.6	0.5	0.7	0.7	0.8	1064
3	Ethchlorvynol	4.5	4.1	4.0	3.9	3.5	3.5	3.5	0.2	0.3	0.9	1.2	1.7	0.9	1.3	1506
	Amobarbital	5.9	4.6	4.6	4.2	4.0	4.3	3.9	0.0	0.0	0.2	0.5	0.8	0.6	0.4	1784
4	Secobarbital	13.2	9.0	7.5	7.1	6.8	6.5	6.2	0.1	0.1	0.5	1.6	1.8	2.1	2.8	3525

*Inflow blood concentration in systemic blood entering resin column.
†Outflow blood concentration in blood leaving column.

300 ml. per minute for 3 hours with a roller pump, and additional heparin was infused into the inflow line to maintain a Lee-White clotting time of 20-30 minutes.

The 3-hour perfusions through a 650-Gm. column were consistently effective in clearing drug intoxicants (table). Blood platelets decreased moderately during the procedure, but approached normal 12-24 hours after treatment. No hemorrhagic complications occurred. Leukocytes were not appreciably adsorbed in the column. Clinical improvement was not closely correlated with drug concentrations in the blood. Blood flow through the column was easily maintained at 300 ml. per minute. The pressure gradient across the column was 50-80 mm. Hg and was stable throughout all hemoperfusions.

Most sedative and tranquilizing drugs commonly responsible for acute intoxication should be within the spectrum of adsorption of Amberlite XAD-2. The only apparent side effect is a transient thrombocytopenia. Resin perfusion may provide rapid clinical improvement in acute drug intoxication. They appear to be clinically superior to hemodialysis in cases of intoxication with various barbiturates, glutethimide and ethchlorvynol, with higher clearance rates and less expense. Hemoperfusion may prove useful in less severe drug intoxication associated with coma.

▶ [It makes sense to remove excess drugs from blood using a resin with specific affinity for drugs rather than dialysis. Only 4 patients were included in this study, but the technic appears to be promising and deserves further trial. One patient died after respirator failure, re-emphasizing the need for total patient support in barbiturate poisoning.—Eds.]

Case against Use of Respiratory Stimulants is presented by Hylan A. Bickerman and E. Leslie Chusid[5] (New York). Respiratory failure is the final common path of the various physiologic defects that occur in chronic obstructive pulmonary disease. A number of reports have indicated the importance of hypercapnia with respiratory acidosis as an adaptive mechanism permitting elimination of large amounts of carbon dioxide per breath and enabling the patient to tolerate an increase in work of breathing. Correction of hypercapnia is less urgent than that of hypoxemia. Correction of acidemia is also of secondary importance, provided the pH does not fall below 7.25. Pharmacologically, there are no specific respiratory stimulants. Analeptic agents such as nikethamide and pentylene tetrazol have generally been discarded for the treatment of barbiturate poi-

(5)   Chest 58:53-56, July, 1970.

soning. Marked variations in sensitivity to the respiratory stimulants make it difficult to avoid adverse reactions.

Patients in mild to moderate respiratory failure, and some in severe failure, can be adequately treated by measures such as controlled oxygen therapy, bronchodilators and bronchial drainage. Is there a reason to use respiratory stimulants in this group? Negligible changes in oxygen tension have been found after stimulant therapy in unconscious or uncooperative patients who were becoming worse despite conservative management. The reports of the effects of stimulants on carbon dioxide tension and acidemia have been variable. A definite indication for the use of stimulants is respiratory failure precipitated or aggravated in a patient with chronic obstrucfive pulmonary disease by injudicious use of oxygen or hypnotics.

In general, "respiratory stimulants" would best be discarded as having a greater potential for harm, through inherent toxicity or delay in the use of more appropriate measures, than for benefit as documented by acceptable studies.

▶ [It is somewhat surprising to see this debate still going on. Many medical schools have dropped the analeptics from their pharmacologic curriculum.—Eds.]

Hypotension and Shock Syndrome in Myocardial Infarction are discussed by Richard S. Ross[6] (Johns Hopkins Univ.). Hypotension is a common, often benign consequence of myocardial infarction. The "shock syndrome" is less common but often fatal. Blood pressure alone is not a good index of the state of a patient with infarction. Hypotension may be related to reduced cardiac output, with normal or elevated peripheral resistance. In other cases, peripheral resistance is reduced but cardiac output is normal. The first group of patients presents with cool limbs and a small pulse volume and the second with warm extremities and a full pulse. Hypotension appears in at least 80% of patients with infarction and usually resolves with relief from pain and oxygen administration. Shock is seen in about 20% of cases and accounts for at least half the deaths that occur now that mortality from arrhythmias has been reduced. Coronary and myocardial blood flow are reduced, further impairing myocardial function and possibly increasing the size of the infarction. Arrhythmias and metabolic acidosis participate in the deterioration. Low cardiac output alone does not explain the changes noted. Total peripheral resistance is variable, but the

(6)   Ohio M. J. 66:140-141, February, 1970.

appropriate response does not occur in patients in shock, and it is inadequate to support the blood pressure at the existing level of cardiac output regardless of the extent of reduction of output.

Treatment aims to interrupt the negative feedback loop by improving cardiac function and increasing arterial pressure. A small rise in arterial pressure from vasopressor therapy may result in a sizable increase in coronary blood flow. Norepinephrine and metaraminol are the drugs of choice. Glycoside therapy will improve the function of uninfarcted myocardium and does not increase the incidence of arrhythmia or cardiac rupture. All patients in shock are given 100% oxygen continuously. Relief from pain is important, but narcotics should be used cautiously. Fluid volume replacement may be indicated, with plasma or salt-poor albumin, in patients given pressor drugs for a prolonged period if central venous pressure is low and pulmonary congestion is not evident. Vomiting or excessive sweating may also make volume replacement necessary. Many patients with the shock syndrome have severe, diffuse coronary atherosclerosis with large areas of infarcted myocardium. It is in this group that circulatory assist devices and replacement of the heart by an artificial device or a homotransplant are most useful.

▶ [We're back to morphine, digitalis, vasopressors and oxygen—just what we used 25 years ago.—Eds.]

Treatment of Shock Following Myocardial Infarction. Jay N. Cohn[7] (Georgetown Univ.) states that shock after myocardial infarction still carries a grave prognosis. Inadequate tissue perfusion impairs organ function and disrupts metabolic pathways; if it is not corrected, metabolic acidosis and progressive circulatory deterioration occur. The sooner the syndrome is recognized, the more likely treatment is to be effective. Important signs include cool, clammy skin, thready or absent pulses, confusion or somnolence, low urine output, persistent or recurrent chest pain or arrhythmia with other signs of hypotension, and a low arterial blood pH with an elevated lactate level. Blood pressure is as useful a diagnostic guide as the peripheral pulses, although an absent auscultatory pressure usually indicates inadequate blood flow and a need for treatment. These signs, in a patient with infarction, are presumptive evidence of shock. It is important to determine the adequacy of the blood volume; central venous pressure should be monitored in all patients with

---

(7)   Ohio M. J. 66:137-139, February, 1970.

shock. A low pressure is an indication for a trial of volume expansion; if this does not correct shock, significant left ventricular failure can be assumed to be present. Indicator dilution cardiac output data are helpful in evaluating myocardial function in selected cases.

Therapy in shock aims to restore adequate organ perfusion. Isoproterenol is probably the drug of choice when cardiac output is severely reduced, especially when reflex vasoconstriction is present. A concentration as great as 2 mg./100 ml. is sometimes needed for a satisfactory response. Lidocaine may help control ventricular irritability during isoproterenol infusion. Levarterenol or metaraminol is used only when isoproterenol is ineffective and in the smallest amount necessary. Digitalis may be given orally. Atropine may be helpful if sinus bradycardia occurs. Furosemide can help establish urine output in the oliguric patient. Bicarbonate is given if the arterial pH is below 7.35. Catheter electrode pacing may be helpful if shock and marked bradycardia coexist. Use of sympathetic blocking drugs and other inotropic agents such as dopamine and glucagon is still experimental. Cardiovascular function must be monitored continuously. Adrenergic drugs are stopped as soon as possible. Mechanical circulatory support may be indicated when medical management is ineffective.

Arrhythmias in Acute Myocardial Infarction: Assessment of Incidence among 250 Patients Treated in a Coronary Care Unit. Eugene Mascarenhas and Henry A. Zimmerman[8] (St. Vincent's Charity Hosp., Cleveland) reviewed data on 250 consecutive patients with acute myocardial infarction admitted to a coronary care unit in 1965-68. A light diet was given, with access to a bedside commode. Oxygen was given by nasal mask or cannula. Sedation was with oral barbiturates or chlordiazepoxide. Anticoagulants were given 86% of the patients. Heart failure was managed with digitalis and diuretics and shock with metaraminol, isoproterenol, norepinephrine or steroids. Supraventricular arrhythmias with a rapid rate were treated with intravenous lanatoside-C or digoxin and, if necessary, with synchronized countershock. Frequent ventricular ectopic beats were treated with procainamide or, more recently, lidocaine. Ventricular tachycardia was managed with procainamide and if sustained, with d-c countershock. Sinus bradycardia or A-V block with a slow ventricular rate was treated with atropine or iso-

(8)   Ohio M. J. 66:565-575, June, 1970.

proterenol. Steroids were used in incomplete and complete heart block. Cardiac arrest was managed by external heart massage and ventricular fibrillation by d-c countershock followed by intramuscular procainamide or intravenous lidocaine.

Mortality was 17.2%. It increased with advancing age, with severity of infarction, with pre-existing heart disease and with multiple arrhythmias. The 1st day of hospitalization was most critical. Mortality was 22% for the 43% of patients admitted within 4 hours of onset of symptoms. Arrhythmias occurred in 86% of patients; fewer than a third had only one arrhythmia. The mortality with multiple arrhythmias was 46%. A combination of supraventricular and infranodal arrhythmias was particularly lethal. Ventricular fibrillation was fatal in all 6 patients with pre-existing atrial fibrillation. The mortality of bundle-branch block was 13% with supraventricular arrhythmia and 53% with associated infranodal arrhythmia. Arrhythmias of pump failure increased with advancing age, but mortality in this group did not depend on age. Women had more arrhythmias of pump failure. The response of ventricular fibrillation was greatly influenced by the severity of infarction. The prognosis of arrhythmias of potential electric instability was also related to the severity of infarction. Six of 8 patients with complete heart block responded to treatment. Ventricular ectopic beats and ventricular tachycardia were generally relatively transient and benign in patients with mild infarction.

Central Venous Pressure in Acute Myocardial Infarction. Central venous pressure measurement is the simplest and safest invasive technic available to indicate cardiac performance. J. V. Collins, T. J. H. Clark, T. R. Evans and M. A. Riaz[9] (Guy's Hosp., London) evaluated the technic as part of the management of patients with acute myocardial infarction in an intensive care unit. Study was made of 20 males and 5 females with acute infarction. A central venous pressure line was introduced aseptically, percutaneously or by cutdown, using a 60-cm. opaque Intracath, and measurements were made on a saline manometer with the patient supine. Dynamic and mean pressures were measured in 14 patients; mean values were closely correlated with simultaneous manometer readings. No patient had a systolic blood pressure below 80 mm. Hg.

The mean central venous pressure in the first 6-hour monitoring period was 7.9 cm. water. There was no clear relation be-

(9) Lancet 1:373-375, Feb. 20, 1971.

tween admission pressure and radiographic evidence of left ventricular failure. Two patients with evidence of severe ventricular failure had pressures of 7 and 9 cm. water, respectively, and neither ever had a rise above 9 cm. Two patients with pressures of 20 cm. or higher had mild evidence of left ventricular failure; both died within 2 weeks of admission. Mean pulse and mean blood pressure were not correlated with clinical or x-ray evidence of left ventricular failure or with the mean central venous pressure. Of the 25 patients studied, 21 had a mean 6-hour central venous pressure above the normal range within 36 hours after infarction.

The central venous pressure is elevated in patients with severe acute myocardial infarction, especially of the inferior type. An elevated pressure is commonly associated with x-ray evidence of left ventricular failure and cardiac dysrhythmias. A pressure of 20 cm. water or higher seems to be associated with death. This measurement is of some value in the management of acute infarction. It is useful when infusions are given to increase circulatory volume, when α-adrenergic blocking drugs are given and to monitor the effects of cardiac glycosides and diuretics. Measurement of pulmonary artery end-diastolic pressure may be the best indirect index of left ventricular performance in the presence of normal pulmonary vascular resistance.

Effect of Glucagon Infusion on Cardiovascular Function in the Critically Ill. John H. Siegel, Michael J. Levine, Rita McConn and Louis R. M. Del Guercio[1] (Albert Einstein College of Medicine) examined the cardiovascular effects of glucagon in surgical patients with venous critical illnesses due to sepsis, shock and/or hyperdynamic state. Hemodynamics and oxygen consumption were studied in 20 patients, in 1 of them on 3 occasions 2 days apart, and in 10 control patients, 1 of them twice. Control patients were of about the same age as the study patients but were not critically ill and had a stable cardiovascular state.

Eight study patients were in septic shock; 5 had severe sepsis but were not hypotensive, 3 had a hyperdynamic state secondary to hepatic cirrhosis with portal hypertension, 2 of them being postoperative after portal decompression and 1 in frank hepatic failure; and 4 were neither septic nor cirrhotic. Many patients had been fully digitalized and some were on isoproterenol infusion when glucagon was given. An intravenous dose

(1) Surg., Gynec. & Obst. 131:505-515, September, 1970.

of 4 mg. glucagon was followed by infusion of 3.3 mg. per hour for as long as the response was favorable.

Cardiac output was increased in 14 of the 22 studies on critically ill patients. In septic patients, cardiac output increased in 8 instances and decreased in 7. The greatest decreases occurred in patients who were the most markedly hyperdynamic. No patient had arrhythmia during glucagon infusion. Vascular tone increased in 8 of the 10 control patients; it increased in only 9 of 22 studies on critically ill patients and in 8 instances decreased. Ventricular function increased in 15 of the 22 studies on critically ill patients, sometimes profoundly. Oxygen consumption increased in 14 instances, sometimes markedly; the most marked increases occurred in the most hyperdynamic patients. The integrated index of cardiovascular function increased in 16 of 22 instances in critically ill patients, but generally decreased in control patients. A serial study in 1 septic patient showed an additive effect of glucagon and a β-adrenergic catecholamine effect on myocardial function.

These results suggest that glucagon is an effective cardiodynamic agent that can be used safely in critically ill surgical patients, either alone or with digitalis and catecholamine inotropic agents. In patients with sepsis or cirrhotic disease, glucagon can often reduce the abnormalities in oxygen consumption that characterize the hyperdynamic state.

Hospital-Acquired Infections are discussed by David S. Feingold[2] (Harvard Med. School). The major infectious disease problems in most hospitals today are the so-called nosocomial infections, found in 3.5 to 15.5% of various hospital populations. The epidemic is worldwide in institutions that care for the sick. The hospitalized patient is often an "altered host" with enhanced susceptibility to infection because of either disease or treatment. Some conditions that compromise defenses against infection in hospital patients are shown in the table. Procedures done to treat underlying diseases create many situations that predispose to infection. Recognition of all the factors involved precludes optimism about effecting a major decrease in the prevalence of nosocomial infections.

The difficult problem at present is the treatment of infections due to antibiotic-resistant gram-negative organisms. Gentamicin and carbenicillin have somewhat improved the ability to

(2)   New England J. Med. 283:1384-1391, Dec. 17, 1970.

SOME CONDITIONS THAT COMPROMISE DEFENSE MECHANISMS
AGAINST INFECTION

CONDITIONS CAUSING IMPAIRED HUMORAL OR CELLULAR PHAGOCYTIC FUNCTION

Decreased numbers of polymorphonuclear leukocytes
   Drug-induced granulocytopenia including antitumor therapy
   Myelophthisic processes
Defective function of polymorphonuclear leukocytes
   Chronic granulomatous disease
   Diabetic acidosis or acidosis in general
   Corticosteroid therapy
Defective cellular immunity
   Hodgkin's disease
   Swiss-type agammaglobulinemia
   Sarcoid
Defective humoral systems (immunoglobulins)
   Sex-linked agammaglobulinemia
   Immunosuppressive therapy
   Cancers involving lymphatic system

CONDITIONS COMPROMISING MECHANICAL BARRIERS AGAINST INFECTION

Urinary bladder instrumentation
Indwelling venous catheterization
Surgical procedures
Burns
Tracheostomy

treat pseudomonas infections, but resistant strains already have been observed in several institutions.

Generally a particular preventive technic only reduces the number of organisms in some part of the environment of the patient. Several epidemiologic aspects change in different wards and different patients. The risk of infection must be weighed before cytotoxic or immunosuppressive drugs or corticosteroids are administered. There is little to offer the patient with profoundly depressed cellular or humoral defenses.

Most procedures aimed at preventing infections are designed to block colonization. Isolation of patients with infected lesions is useful if thoughtfully applied. Contact spread is much more important than airborne spread of virulent organisms. In a few situations, simple measures can effectively minimize the risk of infection associated with certain procedures, such as bladder catheterization and indwelling venous catheterization. Nosocomial infections must be surveyed in individual institutions.

There is a real risk of further increases in nosocomial infections. It is unlikely that immunization can effectively stimulate the immune bactericidal reaction against virulent gram-negative bacilli. Generally, prophylactic antimicrobial drug therapy is ineffective and should be condemned. A unique class of anti-microbials against gram-negative organisms may exist which inhibits the synthesis of the somatic antigen of the cell wall complex. Manipulation of the "normal flora" is also being attempted.

▶ [To the list of conditions we must add anesthesia, since there are data to indicate a depression of neutrophil mobilization, phagocytosis and the immune response. Anesthesia for a patient already receiving immunosuppressive drugs or cancer chemotherapy represents a major challenge to our ability to avoid infection.—Eds.]

Glucagon in Resistant Heart Failure and Cardiogenic Shock. D. E. L. Wilcken and R. Lvoff[3] (Sydney) administered glucagon intravenously in hourly doses of 2.5-7.5 mg. for 24-72 hours to 6 patients in gross heart failure unresponsive to conventional therapy, including 5 in cardiogenic shock, and to 1 patient with cardiomegaly and controlled heart failure. The 7 patients received lyophilized porcine glucagon in 5% aqueous dextrose solution, given by continuous infusion at an initial rate of 5 mg. per hour.

There was marked improvement in 5 of the 6 with gross heart failure. The likeliest cause of the diuresis that occurred in these patients is a positive inotropic effect of glucagon on the myo-cardium, with an increase in cardiac output and renal blood flow. Improved myocardial contraction was observed directly at thoracotomy in 1 case. Frequent arrhythmias were abolished by treatment with glucagon in another case. Left bundle-branch block was converted to normal intraventricular conduction in 2 cases. Even virtually moribund patients showed good evidence of an additional inotropic effect above that obtained by full digitalization. Two patients failed to respond; 1 was the only patient in whom congestive cardiac failure had been controlled by conventional therapy. Three patients had nausea, requiring a reduction in dose in 1. Only 1 patient, who had a large diuresis, had a reduction in serum potassium.

Glucagon has a definite place in the management of resistant heart failure, even in the presence of gross myocardial disease and cardiogenic shock. It may be particularly important as an adjunct to the treatment of patients in cardiogenic shock after myocardial infarction or heart surgery. Glucagon therapy should

(3)   Lancet 1:1315-1318, June 20, 1970.

be considered in such cases before deciding that medical treatment has nothing further to offer.

► [It seems strange, somehow, that a pancreatic protein that raises blood sugar by promoting hepatic glycogenolysis would be useful in treating cardiogenic shock.—Eds.]

Bronchopulmonary Lavage: A "New" Approach to Old Problems is discussed by Robert M. Rogers and Kermit R. Tantum[4] (Univ. of Pennsylvania). In disease states, mechanisms for clearing the tracheobronchial tree are often impaired or the quantity of secretions makes them less effective. Ramirez-R. developed a method of "pulmonary segmental flooding" to treat pulmonary alveolar proteinosis. The method was later modified so that an entire lung could be lavaged while the other was ventilated.

METHOD.—All lavages are performed under general anesthesia with topical laryngotracheal anesthesia, permitting an inspired oxygen level of 95-98%. A Carlen catheter is placed to isolate the two lungs, and bronchospirometric measurements are made, after which respiration is controlled to maintain a normal $Paco_2$.

With the patient in lateral decubitus position (Fig. 36), a volume

Fig. 36.—Diagram of patient during bronchopulmonary lavage. (Courtesy of Rogers, R. M., and Tantum, K. R.: M. Clin. North America 54:755-771, May, 1970.)

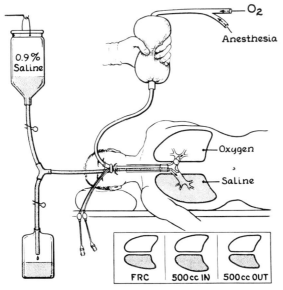

(4) M. Clin. North America 54:755-771, May, 1970.

of saline equal to the measured oxygen consumption of the lung to be treated is flowed in. When the volume in the lung is equal to the functional residual capacity (FRC), volumes of 300-500 ml. are allowed to flow rapidly into the lung and a similar volume is drained into a bottle. Total fluid volumes have ranged from 5 to 25 L.

After the procedure, as much fluid as possible is drained from the lung, using endotracheal suctioning and the Trendelenburg position. Oxygen is continued for 24 hours or longer. Mechanical ventilation is continued if the patient was in respiratory failure before lavage.

Lavage depends on mechanical debridement; therefore no significant amount of fluid should be absorbed during the procedure. Actually, insignificant absorption of saline occurs. Pulmonary blood flow to the treated lung decreases during lavage. Hypoxemia has not been a problem in 15 lavages, but hypercarbia develops readily if the lung not being lavaged is not hyperventilated. The total amount of surfactant removed is small. Most patients require only supplemental oxygen after lavage, although 1-2 L. of saline remain in the lung.

Indications for lavage include alveolar proteinosis, status asthmaticus and cystic fibrosis in older children. Other likely candidates are aspiration pneumonia, Pneumocystis carinii infestation and microlithiasis. This procedure can achieve in one sitting what may be attempted by many medications and maneuvers and does so dramatically. It is especially useful when the other measures prove ineffective.

▶ [This seems rather heroic but it is probably worthwhile in the unusual case refractory to less dramatic therapy. Good chest physical therapy still remains the best way to treat most of these patients.—Eds.]

Psychoreactive Problems of Intensive Therapy are discussed by H. G. Schroeder[5] (Univ. of Sheffield). Intensive therapy units are becoming an accepted part of the hospital scene, but they present psychoreactive problems for patients, relatives and staff. Any illness requiring admission to such a unit causes the patient and his relatives acute anxiety and apprehension. The patient is affected by placement in a world of machines and mechanized confusion. Reassurance and simple explanations are important at this time and may preclude the need for sedation. Confused, hypoxic patients do require sedation initially. The relatives must also be reassured. Exhaustion, disorientation and confusion must be considered in patients staying on an intensive care unit. An active effort must be made to reduce the impact of sensory and sleep deprivation. Constant verbal reassurance, newspapers and television are important. Relatives

(5)   Anaesthesia 26:28-35, January, 1971.

should be encouraged to go home and sleep. Exhaustion is also a problem for the nursing staff, as is overinvolvement with patients. Communication problems must be considered for patients with tracheostomies or indwelling tracheal tubes.

Review was made of data on 332 patients admitted to an intensive therapy unit in 1 year, 263 of whom were discharged alive. Most accepted the stress of intensive therapy without untoward effects. They provided much guidance for improving the management of psychoemotional distress in such patients. No attempted suicides occurred, excluding patients admitted as a result of such attempts, but there were depressive episodes triggered by associated domestic and personal concerns. Patients were more accepting of procedures done on themselves with accompanying explanations than of those done on other patients that were not necessarily explained. This effect could be minimized by placing beds so that patients could not observe one another. The procedures performed on intensive therapy units, rather than the environment of the unit itself, are what contribute most markedly to the psychoreactive disturbances of patients, relatives and staff.

▶ [The author's concerns are justified. In Utopia, the inhabitants of an intensive care unit would be discharged alive, well and psychologically normal. In reality, we hope they at least are alive, thankful and understanding.—Eds.]

Accidental Hypothermia. Keith G. Tolman and Arthur Cohen[6] (Baylor Univ.) report 11 cases of accidental hypothermia, 5 of them fatal. All patients were admitted on an emergency basis during the winter of 1967-68. Hypothermia was defined as a rectal temperature below 95 F. Patients with recognized causes of hypothermia were not included. The average age of the 10 males and 1 female was 60 years. The patients were comatose or semicomatose, found in unheated rooms or outdoors where the temperature was 27-48 F. All were adequately clothed. Four patients had an alcoholic breath. The average rectal temperature on admission was 76 F. (range, 69-86). All patients had acrocyanosis and most had generalized muscular rigidity. Six had athetoid-like movements intermittently and 5 had proximal muscle fasciculations. Nine were hypotensive and 7 had bradycardia. The 4 with the lowest temperatures had slow, shallow respirations. Hypothermia lasted an average of 22 hours. Five patients had anemia and 7 had leukocytosis. Four of 7 patients with a platelet count below 150,000/cu. mm.

(6) Canad. M. A. J. 103: 1357-1361, Dec. 19, 1970.

died with thrombotic complications. Hyperglycemia was present in 7 patients, including 6 with diabetes. Arterial blood pH averaged 7.32. Serum 17-hydroxycorticosteroids were elevated in all 5 patients in whom they were studied. Seven patients had J waves on ECG study. Five patients were known alcoholics.

Infection occurred in 4 patients and intravascular thrombosis in 4. All patients who died had one of these complications and 3 had both. Nine patients had mechanical respiratory assistance. Initially 5% dextrose in 0.9% saline was infused. Dextran was given 6 patients. No patient was actively rewarmed. Antibiotics were used only for overt infection. The last 6 patients did not receive steroids, and only 2 of them died. The 6 patients who survived had an average admission rectal temperature of 77 F. and an average duration of hypothermia of 18½ hours, not significantly different from nonsurvivors. A low platelet count or serum fibrinogen level was a poor prognostic sign.

Accidental hypothermia is not confined to extremes of environmental exposure. Absence of infection and intravascular thrombosis was the most important factor in survival in this series. Not all patients should be given antibiotics and steroids. Patients should not be actively rewarmed. Theoretically at least, the method of choice for rewarming hypothermic patients is probably dialysis.

▶ [One wonders if improved survival might have occurred with active but gentle rewarming and guarding against metabolic acidosis.—Eds.]

Massive Steroid Therapy in Severe Fat Embolism. In 1965, Josef E. Fischer, Roderick H. Turner, James H. Herndon and E. J. Riseborough[7] (Massachusetts Gen'l Hosp.) administered large doses of steroids to a patient with multiple injuries and a downhill course with fat embolism despite standard treatment and observed reversal of the hypoxic course. They now report experience with 17 patients seen during the past 5 years who had a definitive diagnosis of clinically severe fat embolism, evidenced by presence of petechiae in the axilla and upper part of the neck. There were 13 male and 4 female patients; the mean age was 29 years.

All patients but 1 had fractures of the long bones and many also had extensive contusion of soft tissue. One patient had undergone total hip replacement. All patients had fever, tachycardia and tachypnea and all manifested at least mild confusion; 5 were comatose. Petechiae, often transient, were noted in 11

(7)   Surg., Gynec. & Obst. 132:667-672, April, 1971.

patients. A drop in hematocrit was noted in 12 patients. Chest x-rays showed changes in all 15 patients examined. All patients evaluated had arterial hypoxemia, often severe.

Various types of supportive therapy were given. At present, such therapy is limited to oxygen given by mask with humidity, rapid-acting diuretics on occasion and steroids. For specific therapy, 5 patients received intravenous alcohol and 6, low doses of heparin. The 13 most severely affected patients received steroids in doses similar to those used in gram-negative sepsis; administration was stopped abruptly, with no tapering of dosage. Some patients appeared to be dying from hypoxia when steroids were begun. The pulse rate generally responded within 12-24 hours; the Po_2 was the first parameter to respond. Chest x-rays showed improvement at 24-48 hours. Pulmonary compliance measured in 4 patients did not improve until 60-72 hours after the start of steroid therapy. The neurologic status was often the slowest factor to clear.

Large doses of steroids appear to be beneficial in severe fat embolism. Steroids may improve the ventilation-perfusion ratio and response of the pulmonary arterial tree to some substances released by platelets or by an injured lung. Steroids are also believed to exert a general effect in stabilizing membranes that may contribute lipids to serum lipids and thereby to embolization.

▶ [Sounds interesting, but to quote the authors, ". . . this is not a controlled study and . . . we are basing our suggestion . . . on our clinical impression." More data, particularly describing the patient's condition, would be desirable.—Eds.]

Reserpine in Thyrotoxic Crisis. Although rare, thyrotoxic crisis remains an emergency requiring prompt recognition and energetic management. Using only reserpine, Pauline T. Dillon, John Babe, C. R. Meloni and John J. Canary[8] (Georgetown Univ.) have successfully treated eight episodes of thyroid crisis in 7 women, aged 32-78, all with established thyrotoxicosis.

Four patients had an infection, 2 had subtotal thyroidectomy, 1 had radioiodine therapy and 1 had an extrathyroidal operation. Rectal temperatures were 101 F. or higher, with an average pulse of 138 and an average 24-hour radioiodine uptake of 63%. One patient had a substantial rise in the blood urea nitrogen concentration. Initially the patients received 1-5 mg. reserpine intramuscularly, with a total dose of 3-15 mg. in the first 24 hours (0.07-0.3 mg./kg.).

---

(8)   New England J. Med. 283:1020-1023, Nov. 5, 1970.

All the patients survived and had improvement within 8-24 hours of the start of treatment. The average dose given in the first 24 hours was 7.5 mg. and the total dose averaged 16.1 mg. Treatment lasted from 15 to 120 hours. Body temperature was 99.8 F. or less at 48 hours in all patients. Tachypnea resolved in 8-10 hours and the pulse rate declined promptly. Atrial fibrillation was not converted in any of 3 patients but the ventricular rate was reduced after reserpine therapy. No hypotensive phenomena were noted. Congestive heart failure, present in 3 patients, improved during treatment. Psychomotor activity slowed markedly in the 1st day of treatment. Two patients had diarrhea and 1 had a transient cutaneous blush. None had depressive reactions or gastrointestinal bleeding.

The basic cause of thyroid crisis remains unknown but the sympathetic system has been implicated. Reserpine is a safe and effective form of treatment for the manifestations of thyroid crisis. Administration of large doses had few side effects in the present patients.

Drugs that alter the availability or actions of the chemical intermediates of the adrenergic system should be a part of the therapy of thyrotoxic crisis.

▶ [It appears that we now have a choice between reserpine and β-blockers for this syndrome. Perhaps reserpine is the choice because of its longer action.—Eds.]

TRACHEOSTOMY AND COMPLICATIONS

Incidence and Pathogenesis of Tracheal Injury Following Cuffed-Tube Tracheostomy with Assisted Ventilation: Analysis of a Two-Year Prospective Study. Awareness is increasing that tracheal stenosis may result from use of cuffed tracheostomy tubes with assisted ventilation. M. J. Andrews and F. G. Pearson[9] (Univ. of Toronto) reviewed data from 220 patients who had cuffed-tube tracheostomy with assisted ventilation in a respiratory failure unit in 1967-68. There were 103 evaluable survivors, including 34 with chest trauma, 31 with postoperative respiratory insufficiency, 20 with acute and chronic lung disease, 3 with drug overdosage and 15 with other conditions. Mortality in patients requiring assisted ventilation was 42%. Ventilation with a cuffed tube was not maintained for over 72 hours; tracheostomy was generally done using general anes-

(9) Ann. Surg. 173:249-263, February, 1971.

thesia. Both incisional and excisional technics have been used. A gamma-irradiated PVC tube was usually employed. Well-humidified gas was given at all times, with aspiration of the tracheobronchial tree every 30 minutes. The tube cuff was deflated every 2 hours for 30 seconds and reinflated with the minimal amount of air needed to prevent leakage around the cuff as determined by auscultation. Dressings were changed every 2 hours and the tube was changed weekly. Patients were examined 3 weeks and 3 months after extubation.

Almost all patients had some loss of airway size at the stomal level on soft-tissue radiographs. Twelve patients had 25-50% reductions in airway diameter without clinical disability. Eighteen symptomatic tracheal strictures developed in 17 patients (17.5%). Twelve strictures occurred at the tracheostomy level and 6 at the level of the cuff. Ten resulted in life-threatening disability. Two patients died of airway obstruction due to severe stomal stenosis before treatment was given. Two patients in whom tracheoesophageal fistulas developed are living. Significant stenosis was less frequent after a pliable rubber connector

INCIDENCE OF TRACHEAL STENOSIS AFTER TRACHEOSTOMY WITH ASSISTED VENTILATION

Author	No. of Patients with Tracheostomy	No. of Patients Surviving for Analysis (Studied)	No. of Patients with Tracheal Stenosis	"Apparent" Incidence of Tracheal Stenosis	True Incidence of Tracheal Stenosis
Falbe-Hansen 1955	270	116	6	2.2%	5.2%
Aboulker 1960	600	Not given	22	3.7%	—
Paloschi 1965	76	Not given	2	2.6%	—
Johnston et al. 1967	325	Not given	4	1.2%	—
Deverall 1967	104	Not given	6	5.8%	—
Gibson 1967	154	116	4	2.6%	3.5%
Kucher et al. 1967	223	57 Studied	5 Severe	2.2%	8.8%
Stoeckel 1967	358	63 Studied	6 Severe	1.6%	9.5%
Andrews and Pearson	220	103 Studied	18 10 Severe	8.2% 5.5%	17.5% 9.7%

was introduced between the tube attachment and the Y connector on the respirator to permit freer head and neck movement and reduce traction on the tube. Only 2 of 10 patients with significant stomal stenosis had unusually large stomas at extubation. Three of 4 with significant cuff level strictures had circumferential ulceration at that level.

The incidence of symptomatic tracheal stenosis in this series was much higher than that reported in others (table). Circumferential mucosal ulceration at the cuff level was always a prelude to symptomatic stenosis. Tracheostomy tubes of large diameter predispose to stricture formation at both stomal and cuff levels. Steroids also predispose to stomal stenosis, and hypotension and airway infection are probable predisposing factors. Improved technics of tracheostomy management are required, as is routine follow-up examination to evaluate tracheal injury.

▶ [A good analysis of the dangers of a life-saving therapy.—Eds.]

THE TRAUMATIZED PATIENT

Analysis of Pulmonary Function Following Nonthoracic Trauma, with Recommendations for Therapy. H. J. Proctor, T. V. N. Ballantine and N. D. Broussard[1] undertook to determine what changes, if any, occur in the pulmonary function of massively injured combat casualties without primary thoracic injury, who have been resuscitated from hemorrhagic and traumatic shock. Study was made of 33 massively injured patients with a systolic pressure of 80 mm. Hg or less and no primary thoracic or intracranial injury (group I); 15 bed rest control patients who sustained minor injuries (group II); and 4 patients with congestive atelectasis or "shock lung" (group III) with a Pao_2 below 60 mm. Hg while breathing room air and typical chest x-ray changes and clinical signs of respiratory insufficiency. Group I patients received lactated Ringer's solution and whole blood.

The chest x-rays of group I patients remained clear to death or for the 120 hours of study. The 3 deaths were not due to pulmonary causes. Only 1 group III patient survived the 120-hour study period. Group I patients had a reduced tidal volume and an increased respiratory rate, with little change in minute volume. Pulmonary compliance was only slightly reduced, and

(1) Ann. Surg. 172:180-189, August, 1970.

there was little change in total work per breath, although resistive work per breath was increased. There was a large increase in pulmonary arteriovenous shunting in this group. These changes were significant. Bed rest alone did not cause significant changes in group II patients, except for a decrease in tidal volume and an increase in resistive work per breath. Differences between groups I and II were quantitative only. Resistive work returned toward normal in the 1 group III survivor.

Altered mechanical properties, a need for increased alveolar ventilation, or both, resulted in increased work of breathing in massively injured patients in this study. Endotracheal suction and intermittent deep breathing are recommended in such patients. Supplemental oxygen is not needed by young patients unless the Pao_2 drops below 65 mm. Hg. Ventilation should instead be increased and controlled by a respirator. Sepsis should be controlled and fluids restricted once resuscitation is achieved. Use of diuretics should be considered.

▶ [The best guide to the need for supplemental oxygen remains the arterial Po_2.—Eds.]

Hypoxemia during First 12 Hours after Battle Injury. Arterial hypoxemia occurring soon after injury indicates pulmonary insufficiency and may be a premonitory sign of lethal respiratory failure. Roger V. Moseley and Donald B. Doty[2] (Walter Reed Army Med. Center, Washington, D. C.) studied 58 patients in whom hypoxemia developed within 12 hours after combat injury, with a Pao_2 below 80 mm. Hg.

Penetrating chest injury was present in 26 cases and nonpenetrating chest injury in 3. These patients had physiologic intrapulmonary shunting of blood, often exceeding 30% of cardiac output and related to the extent of pulmonary contusion. The most effective treatment was tracheostomy and assisted ventilation. The principal chest injuries in this group were hemopneumothorax and pulmonary contusion. Six patients had hypoxemia attributable to pulmonary fat embolism. An increasing intrapulmonary shunt was evident in all 3 with definite fat embolism, which paralleled increasing hypoxemia and a deteriorating clinical state. The shunt decreased slowly in the single survivor. Chest x-rays were normal when hypoxemia was present in these cases. Fourteen patients had aspiration of foreign substances accounting for hypoxemia. Seven aspirated gas-

---

(2) Surgery 67:765-772, May, 1970.

tric contents and 7, blood. All 7 who aspirated gastric contents were critically ill, with severe respiratory distress making tracheostomy and assisted respiration necessary. Abnormalities disappeared in a week in the 5 who survived. The average intrapulmonary shunt in the 7 patients with maxillofacial wounds who aspirated blood was 25% of cardiac output. None had symptomatic respiratory insufficiency. Overtransfusion occurred in 1 patient without and in 3 with spinal cord injury. The intrapulmonary shunt increased as pulmonary edema developed. The response to phlebotomy and controlled ventilation was good. Five hypoxemic patients had severe brain injuries and died within a few hours of admission. Physiologic shunts ranged from 26 to 50% of cardiac output in this group.

Functional deficits appeared to be similar in the various groups of hypoxemic injured patients in this series. This uniformity of response, regardless of underlying cause, may be the reason why the term "traumatic wet lung" persists. Mechanical ventilation is often required to obtain normal arterial oxygenation in such patients. The absence of "shock lung" is probably due to rapid aeromedical evacuation, eliminating prolonged episodes of hypotension.

▶ [Early attention to blood gas values and adequacy of ventilation may save the life of a severely wounded patient, whether injured on the battlefield or behind the wheel of an automobile. As seen in this study, a normal chest x-ray is no guarantee of normal pulmonary function.—Eds.]

Mechanism of Hepatic Dysfunction Following Shock and Trauma. Geoffrey Nunes, F. William Blaisdell and William Margaretten[3] (Univ. of California) studied 12 cases of postoperative jaundice seen among about 500 patients admitted to the hospital in 1965-69 with major life-threatening injuries. Jaundice was clinically apparent in these cases; the peak total serum bilirubin was 3 mg./100 cc. or above. Patients with cirrhosis, hepatic abscesses or major liver injuries were excluded from the study. Trauma resulted from automobile accidents in 8 cases. Ten patients had major fractures; 3 had flail chest. Nine were hypotensive on admission. Twenty-five inhalation anesthetics were given to the 12 patients. Five patients received halothane, 4 of them twice.

The mean peak serum bilirubin level in these cases was 19.4 mg./100 cc.; the direct fraction constituted 57-90% of the total bilirubin. The SGOT and alkaline phosphatase values were variable. Jaundice appeared 1-12 days after injury. Five pa-

(3)   Arch. Surg. 100: 546-556, May, 1970.

tients had an initial marked elevation of SGOT when the bilirubin and alkaline phosphatase levels were only slightly elevated. Five had a second rise in bilirubin, usually to a higher level, sometimes in relation to surgery or renal failure. Four patients had marked elevations of SGOT and alkaline phosphatase after jaundice had subsided. Two of 4 patients with generalized bleeding had good evidence of disseminated intravascular coagulation. An average of 31 units of blood was administered. Infection was present in all cases. Six of the 8 patients who did not survive had progressive respiratory insufficiency with decreasing lung compliance and hypoxia. Three patients developed acute renal failure. Histologic findings included centrilobular congestion, centrilobular intracellular bile accumulation and in 2 cases, true centrilobular necrosis. None of the 4 survivors has had recurrent jaundice; the 3 retested after discharge had normal liver function values.

The primary mechanism of jaundice in these cases appears to be a hepatic cellular excretory defect resembling intrahepatic cholestasis, probably due to hepatic anoxia. The increased bilirubin load from extravasated and transfused blood results in more marked jaundice in patients with livers damaged from anoxia. Jaundice is a grave prognostic sign in the patient recovering from shock, since the ultimate outcome in severe shock is profoundly affected by impairment of hepatic function.

▶ [These were severe cases of trauma, in which the liver surely was not being supplied adequately with well-oxygenated blood. It is well to remember that hepatic failure may develop in such cases, no matter what anesthetic management is chosen.—Eds.]

Intracranial Pressure Changes Following Head Injury. I. H. Johnston, J. A. Johnston and Bryan Jennett[4] (Univ. of Glasgow) attempted to find differences between patients who develop a significantly elevated intracranial pressure after head injury and those who do not, to correlate alterations in perfusion pressure with changes in the cerebral circulation and to seek a better understanding of the relative efficacy of the methods for controlling raised intracranial pressure. Study was made of 32 patients aged 1-68 years with severe head injury, seen in an 18-month period. A catheter was placed in the right lateral ventricle via a frontal burr hole. Recording was usually continued for 4-5 days, starting as soon as possible after injury.

Some patients had wide variations in pressure over the recording period. Five of 9 with normal pressures below 20 mm.

(4) Lancet 2:433-436, Aug. 29, 1970.

Hg died. All had been rendered unconscious when injured and showed signs of primary brain stem injury. Eleven patients with pressures of 20-40 mm. Hg showed a variety of clinical pictures; 6 of them died. Only 1 of 12 patients with a mean maximal ventricular fluid pressure exceeding 40 mm. Hg recovered satisfactorily; 3 remain in coma, and the rest have died. Six patients in this group talked at some time after their injury. There was an apparently high incidence of cerebral infarction in this group. The ventricular fluid and systemic arterial pressures were very inconstantly related to one another. No single method of controlling the intracranial pressure was uniformly effective. Mannitol was very effective in some cases but not with prolonged and pronounced elevations of ventricular fluid pressure. Repeated doses of mannitol tended to be progressively less effective. Withdrawal of ventricular fluid and hyperventilation were both very effective in reducing elevated intracranial pressure. The effect of bony decompression was sometimes short-lived, and the pressure could return to very high levels despite removal of a large bone flap.

Some patients without a space-occupying hematoma develop a progressive rise in intracranial pressure after severe head injury, and most of these die within a few days after injury. The perfusion pressure is probably more significant than the intracranial pressure alone in such cases. Whether a given level of intracranial pressure will threaten the cerebral circulation depends on the systemic arterial pressure at the time. The best guide to the effectiveness of treatment is continuous monitoring of both the ventricular fluid and systemic arterial pressures. Such monitoring, with the combined use of controlled hyperventilation, mannitol and ventricular drainage, may reduce the mortality and morbidity of head injury in patients who have a progressive rise in intracranial pressure in the absence of any surgically correctable expanding lesion. The value of spinal fluid aspiration in an acutely developing pressure situation argues for a monitoring method that involves ventricular catheterization rather than the placement of sensors on the brain surface.

▶ [No mention of dexamethasone, now used so commonly to combat cerebral edema.—Eds.]

Application of the "G-Suit" to Control of Hemorrhage in Massive Trauma was evaluated by Bruce S. Cutler and Willard M. Daggett[5] (Massachusetts Gen'l Hosp.) because of a recent resurgence of interest in use of external counterpressure to control intra-abdominal hemorrhage. The technic was assessed in 8 massively injured patients at a forward clearing company in a combat zone in Vietnam that was distant from definitive surgical facilities. Mine and booby trap injuries incurred in Vietnam lead to extensive damage to the lower limbs, perineum and pelvis, which has been uniformly fatal despite vigorous resuscitation including massive transfusion. The patients were males aged 18-24 years. None had injuries above the diaphragm. All had a poor prognosis. Abdominal hemorrhage was controlled by implantation of commercial G-suits inflated to 30-40 cm. water during helicopter evacuation of the patient to a surgical hospital.

Seven of the 8 patients on whom the G-suit was used were successfully evacuated, and 4 of them survived. Experience showed the best approach to be immediate application of the G-suit and simultaneous administration of whole blood through upper limb or subclavian veins. The suit increases arterial resistance and causes venous blood to be translocated centrally, permitting more adequate perfusion of the head and heart. Generally, there was a rise in blood pressure of the same order of magnitude as the compressive force applied, but in some cases it was substantially greater.

External counterpressure can help support the circulation and improve the chance for survival while blood is replaced in patients with extensive injuries of the lower part of the body. This approach has potential civilian applications. In smaller hospitals with limited personnel and blood reserves, use of the G-suit may help resuscitate severely injured patients during their transportation to larger medical facilities where definitive surgical care is available.

▶ [A temporary but apparently worthwhile measure deserving more of a trial. As the authors point out, there are data indicating prolonged application of the G-suit can decrease survival.—Eds.]

Acute Laryngeal Trauma. The commonest cause of laryngeal injury is a traffic accident. A. G. D. Maran and P. M. Stell[6] reviewed 9 such injuries seen in the past 3 years. The larynx may be injured in automobile accidents if lap-type belts are worn and the face fails to hit the dashboard, the larynx being

(5) Ann. Surg. 173:511-514, April, 1971.
(6) Lancet 2:1107-1110, Nov. 28, 1970.

driven against the cervical spine. Similar injury may occur in sports such as karate and basketball. A fall onto a sharp object may also injure the laryngeal cartilage. The injury depends in part on how much the thyroid cartilage is calcified. An uncalcified cartilage forced against the cervical spine will expand and flatten and fracture down its prominence anteriorly. Any compression will tend to shatter a calcified thyroid cartilage. Symptoms may not be present initially, and laryngeal fracture is easily missed if unsuspected. A laryngoscope or endotracheal tube may pass a detached epiglottis, with dyspnea occurring on its removal. If the mucosa is torn, air will pass into the soft tissues of the neck when the patient coughs, resulting in subcutaneous emphysema. Pain may occur on coughing or swallowing. Dyspnea may not be present for some hours. Hemorrhage is unusual. Mirror examination is always worth attempting. Laryngography is the definitive diagnostic measure. Direct laryngoscopy should be done in all cases.

No treatment is required for a mild injury except to insure that laryngeal edema does not occur. If respiratory distress appears, steroids and oxygen may be tried, but tracheostomy and open exploration should not be delayed. Tracheostomy is mandatory in severe cases. Repair must be done to prevent laryngotracheal stenosis. Only wiring may be needed if there is no soft-tissue injury. Otherwise the larynx is opened through the fracture line, the vocal cords are stitched in position and the arytenoids are replaced. If the thyroid cartilage is shattered, a stent of Verone may be placed in the laryngeal lumen and held in place by wire sutures for at least 2 months, after which it is removed with use of a laryngoscope.

Factors Affecting Prognosis in Patients with Flail Chest. Most who have used early tracheostomy and mechanical ventilation to treat flail chest have noted benefit, but many large series show a higher mortality for patients treated in this way. S. Sankaran and Robert F. Wilson[7] (Wayne State Univ.) analyzed factors that influence prognosis in 100 patients with flail chest seen in 1962-69. About two thirds of the injuries were due to automobile accidents. There were 24 deaths in the series. Most occurred in patients with shock, three or more associated injuries, head injury or over seven fractured ribs. Fourteen of 23 patients with a systolic pressure below 80 mm. Hg on admission died, as did 10 of the 77 other patients, a highly significant

(7) J. Thoracic & Cardiovas. Surg. 60:402-410, September, 1970.

difference. Eleven of 19 patients with three or more associated injuries, 13 of 33 with head injury and 16 of 49 with seven or more fractured ribs died. None of 9 patients aged 30 or under died, although 5 were in shock when admitted. The mortality of 16 patients aged 61 or over was 38%.

Ten patients had no initial treatment for flail chest. Nine each had external traction only and tracheostomy only, 25 had tracheostomy with external traction and 47 had tracheostomy with respirator assistance. Five of the 10 untreated patients died, with relatively uncomplicated injuries. Eight of the 25 having tracheostomy and traction died, not significantly different from the mortality among those having respirator assistance. All 10 patients with the most numerous and severe associated injuries had early tracheostomy and traction or respirator assistance, but 9 died. Initial treatment was important only in patients with injuries of intermediate severity. Only 1 of 15 such patients having tracheostomy and respirator assistance died, as did 5 of 10 having tracheostomy and external traction, a significant difference. The difference was even more striking if patients aged 30 or under were excluded from consideration.

Early tracheostomy and respirator assistance are extremely important in patients with flail chest and injury of intermediate severity.

▶ [We doubt if anyone could argue with these general conclusions.—Eds.]

DIAGNOSIS, EFFECTS AND TREATMENT OF SHOCK

Shock after Acute Myocardial Infarction: Clinical and Hemodynamic Profile. Current treatment for cardiogenic shock is unsatisfactory. Stephen Scheidt, Robert Ascheim and Thomas Killip III[8] (Cornell Univ.) reviewed data on 547 patients seen in 1965-69 with acute myocardial infarction, including 19 with shock in whom hemodynamic studies were carried out. Cardiogenic shock developed in 73 patients in all (15%), as defined by a systolic pressure of 90 mm. Hg or lower and signs of poor peripheral circulation. The hospital mortality was 86% for patients in shock and 15% for the others.

The physical findings in patients in shock are shown in the table. These patients tended to be older, and shock developed

(8)   Am. J. Cardiol. 26:556-564, December, 1970.

PHYSICAL FINDINGS IN 73 PATIENTS

Physical Findings	Percent of Patients
Skin	
Cool and moist	87
Warm and dry	13
Brain	
Mental status normal	46
Depressed brain function, confusion, lethargy, agitation	37
Frank coma	17
Urine output	
Oliguria (<20 ml/hour)	71
Normal (>20 ml/hour)	16
Anuria (no urine for at least 1 hour)	13
Pulmonary edema	
None	54
Overt (rales covering more than 50% of both lung fields)	46

more often in women. The interval between infarction and onset of shock varied. Serious arrhythmias rarely preceded onset of shock, and drugs and infections could not be implicated. Shock was usually rapidly fatal. Neither vasopressor nor vasodilator therapy influenced survival. Survivors were somewhat younger than those who died, were admitted sooner and had shock sooner after infarction. All survivors showed improved peripheral perfusion within 1 or 2 hours after the start of drug therapy. Cardiac index and stroke volume were reduced in all cases. Peripheral resistance was generally increased in patients with shock. Large infarcts predominated at autopsy in patients with and without shock.

Clinical observations fail to predict which patients with acute myocardial infarction will have cardiogenic shock. The frequency of a delayed onset of shock suggests that progressive cardiac damage may follow initial acute infarction. Any treatment for cardiogenic shock should provide circulatory support, reduce myocardial work and improve coronary flow and oxygen delivery. For temporary mechanical support to be effective, there must be significant improvement in intrinsic cardiac function after a "rest" period.

Practical Considerations in Management of Shock Complicating Acute Myocardial Infarction: Summary of Current Prac-

tice is presented by Herbert Shubin and Max Harry Weil[9] (Univ. of Southern California). The systolic pressure is usually below 90 mm. Hg in shock after myocardial infarction in 12% of such patients, and signs of impaired peripheral perfusion are present. Only a few patients have overt congestive failure. Urine output is reduced. Central venous and arterial catheters and ECG monitoring facilitate assessment of the hemodynamic state of patients in shock and their response to treatment. Arterial blood gases should also be monitored.

Treatment is outlined in the table. Morphine is usually effective in relieving pain. Dramamine reduces the risk of vomiting, and diazepam may be given to allay anxiety. Administration of 100% oxygen by mask or nasal catheter at a rate of 6-8 L. per minute is advisable. Ventilatory support may be required for respiratory failure. Volume deficits are corrected with equal amounts of half-normal saline in glucose or 5% albumin solution. The volume given should be reduced if central venous pressure increases progressively, and phlebotomy may prevent pulmonary edema if the pressure rises more than 5 cm. during a fluid challenge period. Metaraminol may be given by infusion as 100-200 mg./L. of 5% glucose in water. Levarterenol is given as 8-16 mg./L. of 5% aqueous glucose. Glucagon and dopamine have been advocated as vasoactive agents, but no definite ad-

TREATMENT OF SHOCK DUE TO MYOCARDIAL INFARCTION

Condition	Treatment*	Guide
Pain	Morphine sulfate 5 to 10 mg i.v.	Symptomatic relief
Nausea	Dimenhydrinate (Dramamine®) 50 mg i.v.	Symptomatic relief
Hypoxia	Oxygen 100 percent by nasal catheter, flow 6 to 8 liters/min; ventilatory support with intermittent positive pressure or volume respirator	Arterial O_2 saturation, pO_2, pCO_2, pH
Hypotension	Fluid challenge (see text); metaraminol (Aramine®) 0.3 to 1.0 mg/min in 5 percent G/W i.v. or levarterenol (Levophed®) 3 to 30 μg/min to maintain systolic pressure 30 mm Hg below "normal" level	Central venous pressure; arterial pressure; peripheral pulses; skin temperature; urine flow
Congestive failure	Digoxin (Lanoxin®) 0.75 mg i.v. followed by 1 to 3 subsequent injections of 0.25 mg at ½ to 3 hour interval6; or lanatoside C (Cediland®) 0.8 mg i.v. followed by 1 to 3 subsequent injections of 0.4 mg at 1 to 3 hour intervals	Central venous pressure; circulation time; cardiac output
Atrial tachycardia, flutter, fibrillation	Electrical cardioversion; or digoxin (see text); or methoxamine (Vasoxyl®) 3 to 5 mg i.v.; or phenylephrine (Neo-Synephrine®) 0.5 to 2 mg i.v.	Electrocardiogram
Sinus bradycardia	Atropine sulfate 1 mg i.v.	Electrocardiogram
Atrioventricular block	Electrical pacing; in interim isoproterenol (Isuprel®) 5 mg/liter of 5 percent G/W i.v., infusion rate to increase ventricular rate to between 60 and 80 beats/min	Electrocardiogram
Ventricular tachycardia	Lidocaine (Xylocaine®) (see text); or procainamide (Pronestyl®) 50 to 100 mg/min i.v. until arrhythmia terminated, up to a maximum of 3 g	Electrocardiogram
Ventricular fibrillation	Resuscitation; d-c countershock	Electrocardiogram
Thromboembolism	Heparin, 50-150 units/kg body weight i.v. every 4 hours	Coagulation time

*G/W: glucose in water; i.v.: intravenously.

(9) Am. J. Cardiol. 26:603-608, December, 1970.

vantage over metaraminol and levarterenol has been demonstrated.

Rapid digitalization is indicated for acute congestive heart failure in previously undigitalized patients. Cardioversion with d-c current is often effective in controlling tachyarrhythmias that are immediately life threatening. Mechanical assistance must be considered experimental, as must cardiac transplantation. Surgery has proved clinically feasible, however, for management of such complications as myocardial aneurysm and perforation of the ventricular septum.

▶ [This article and the preceding one stress the need for vigilance in following patients with acute myocardial infarction and the need for a definitive plan of therapy for them. The results of treatment of cardiogenic shock are disappointing and may simply indicate a degree of cardiac pathology that will, in most cases, make any therapy fruitless.—Eds.]

Clinical Management of Shock is discussed by Robert M. Hardaway, III[1] (US Army Gen'l Hosp., Frankfurt, Germany). The dramatic improvement in saving lives in Vietnam has been largely due to the more prompt and efficient treatment of hemorrhagic and traumatic shock. The most important factor is the speed with which the patient can be treated. Critically wounded patients with rapid blood loss, who formerly would have been "killed in action," are now delivered to a hospital shortly after being injured. They may have unobtainable blood pressure and high lactate levels, with severe alkalosis or acidosis. Massive bicarbonate administration may lead to cardiac arrest.

Upon admission to the hospital central venous and urethral catheters are placed, the ECG is monitored, fluids are given until the arterial pressure is normal and oxygen is given if the Pao_2 is below normal. Tracheal intubation or tracheotomy is indicated if nasal oxygen by catheter is inadequate. Normal blood pH is maintained. The best treatment of metabolic acidosis is restoration of capillary perfusion with adequate intravenous fluids. Phenoxybenzamine is given in a dose of 1 mg./kg. if the central venous pressure reaches 15 cm. water when the arterial pressure is still inadequate. Isoproterenol may be given as a vasodilator but not if the pulse is over 120. A cyanoacrylate adhesive Freon spray has been developed to control hemorrhage from visceral wounds and has proved to be quite effective and safe. Central venous pressure measurements are the best way of determining volume requirements in shock. Urine output and systemic pressure are also helpful. Lactate levels are a good

(1) Cincinnati J. Med. 52:43-53, February, 1971.

index of tissue perfusion. Blood volume measurements are not useful for determining volume requirements in acute shock, but red blood cell mass is the best index of red blood cell requirements. The kind of fluid given is initially less important than the amount; a combination of fluids is generally used. Vasodilators are limited to refractory shock in the presence of a high central venous pressure. The usefulness of steroids in shock is unproved.

Corticosteroids as Effective Vasodilators in the Treatment of Low-Output Syndrome. Vasopressors and volume replacement have not effectively altered the mortality due to low-output syndrome after cardiac surgery. Ronald H. Dietzman, Aldo R. Castaneda, C. Walton Lillehei, Robert A. Ersek, George J. Motsay and Richard C. Lillehei[2] (Univ. of Minnesota) found methylprednisolone to be an effective vasodilator for use in this syndrome. Low-output syndrome was induced in 98 adult dogs by embolizing plastic microspheres into the coronary arteries. Methylprednisolone was given in a dose of 15 mg./ kg. to 17 dogs and in a dose of 30 mg./kg. to 23, 5 minutes after infarction. Cardiac index was markedly reduced after infarction and then stabilized at about half the preinfarct level 1-4 hours after injury. Changes in stroke index paralleled those in cardiac index. Mean blood pressure was about 85% of control level. A sustained increase in total peripheral resistance occurred. Tissue perfusion was reduced. Only 22% of 58 control dogs survived over 72 hours. The lower dose of steroid had a positive inotropic effect, but vasoconstriction persisted, and only 35% of the dogs survived. Tissue perfusion improved after the larger dose of steroid, and 65% of these dogs survived, representing significant improvement.

Nineteen patients, including 12 survivors, were studied after heart valve replacement. They received 30 mg. methylprednisolone per kg. intravenously after treatment with isoproterenol and volume replacement. Steroid therapy increased the cardiac and stroke indexes within an hour in surviving patients. Total peripheral resistance decreased significantly. Urine output increased after steroid therapy, and the limbs became better perfused. Lactic acid levels returned to normal within 24-48 hours. Three of the 7 nonsurvivors were treated in the first 12 hours of low-output syndrome, as were all the survivors. All 3 had autopsy evidence of mechanical obstruction in the aortic area.

(2)   Chest 57:440-453, May, 1970.

Steroid did not increase the cardiac index markedly in patients who did not survive. Peripheral resistance decreased but then increased. Oxygen consumption rose but less markedly than in the surviving patients.

The findings indicate the effectiveness of methylprednisolone, combined with isoproterenol and adequate volume replacement, in patients with low-output syndrome after cardiac surgery.

▶ [The authors may have proved to themselves the effectiveness of the steroid in treating low-output syndrome, but they have not done so to the editors.—Eds.]

Dilemma of Vasopressors and Vasodilators in Therapy of Shock. Experiments have suggested that blood flow, rather than pressure, is the key to maintenance of circulatory integrity. The immediate goal of vasodilator therapy is improvement of blood flow in shock. It is based on the assumptions that flow is reduced by vasoconstriction, and that α-adrenergic blocking agents increase flow by reducing peripheral resistance. William C. Shoemaker and Robert S. Brown[3] (Mt. Sinai School of Medicine) compared the hemodynamic effects of sympathomimetic agents, blocking agents and hydrocortisone in various types of clinical shock. Responses to sympathomimetic amines were compared in 17 patients in shock, 9 with a mean arterial pressure of 50 mm. Hg or below at some point. Shock was primarily due to trauma and hemorrhage in 15 patients, but 9 had sepsis. The patients received 0.4-0.5 μg. norepinephrine per kg. per minute, 9-13 μg. metaraminol per kg. per minute, 9-13 μg. methoxamine per kg. per minute or 0.03-0.15 μg. isoproterenol per kg. per minute. Hydrocortisone was given intravenously in doses of 5-50 mg./kg. to 12 patients in shock, with a mean lowest arterial pressure of 51 mm. Hg. Vasodilators, given in 42 instances to 34 patients, included 25 mg. phentolamine, 15-40 mg. chlorpromazine and about 1 mg. phenoxybenzamine per kg. Cardiac output was measured by the indicator dilution technic.

Responses to the agents are shown in Figure 37. Isoproterenol produced the greatest rise in cardiac output, but only about 80% of patients had an increase greater than 0.5 L./minute/sq. m. Steroid therapy did not lead to significant hemodynamic changes. Responses to the three blocking drugs were similar. The mean increase in cardiac index was 0.4 L./minute/sq. m., not a significant change, but in 15 instances an increase of over 0.5 L. occurred. Generally, significant increases in cardi-

(3)   Surg., Gynec. & Obst. 132:51-57, January, 1971.

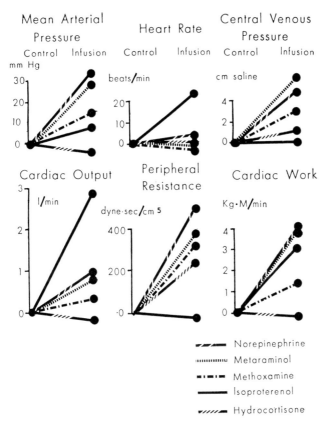

Fig. 37.—Incremental changes in arterial pressure, heart rate, central venous pressure, cardiac output, peripheral resistance and cardiac work after administration of norepinephrine, metaraminol, methoxamine, isoproterenol and hydrocortisone. (Courtesy of Shoemaker, W. C., and Brown, R. S.: Surg., Gynec. & Obst. 132:51-57, January, 1971.)

ac index occurred in the middle stage of shock. About half the responses occurred in postoperative patients. Peripheral resistance fell significantly after administration of blocking agents.

The findings do not support the assumptions that underlie the treatment of shock with either vasopressors or vasodilators. Shock therapy cannot be simplified to the point of considering only maintenance of arterial pressure or blood flow. Changes in volume and oxygen transport and pressure-flow relations must also be considered. The greatest usefulness of vasodilators is primarily to permit volume loading without producing excessively high venous pressures. In such instances a mild, short-acting agent such as phentolamine can be given, provided great care is taken to prevent or minimize hypotension.

▶ [It is interesting that these authors found steroids did not lend to significant hemodynamic changes whereas in the preceding article steroids are described as being very effective (although combined with isoproterenol).—Eds.]

Hemodynamic Changes, Treatment and Prognosis in Clinical Shock. Robert F. Wilson, Edward J. Sarver and Joseph Rizzo[4] (Wayne State Univ.) reviewed the records of 151 patients studied in a shock unit in 1963-68. The criteria for shock, three of them required for the diagnosis, included a systolic blood pressure below 80 mm. Hg; cold, clammy skin or a cardiac index below 2.5 L./minute/sq. m.; arterial standard bicarbonate below 20 mEq./L.; urine output below 25 ml. per hour; and a need for vasopressors or vasodilators to maintain adequate cerebral, cardiac or renal function. Liver disease was present in 41 patients who had abnormal function tests with a history of previous liver disease or heavy alcoholism. It was confirmed at biopsy or autopsy in all but 4.

There were 81 deaths in the shock unit and 41 later deaths; 19% of the patients went home alive. Thirteen patients with liver disease improved, but none left the hospital alive, compared with 26% of the patients without liver disease. Among 49 patients without sepsis or liver disease, hemodynamics were similar in those who died or survived. Nine of 12 patients with a cardiac index below 2 that could not be raised died in the shock unit, compared with only 4 of 15 in whom the index could be elevated. Vasopressors were detrimental in patients with a low cardiac index. Peripheral resistance also did not distinguish patients who died from survivors. The same was true for the 61 patients with sepsis but no liver disease. Vasodilators led to increased mortality in this group, especially in moderately to severely dilated patients as judged from the peripheral resistance. Cardiac indexes were higher in patients who died in the shock unit than in those who improved among the 41 with liver disease, especially in those without sepsis. Nonseptic patients who died in the shock unit tended to have a lower peripheral resistance than those who improved.

Patients with low cardiac output should not be given vasoconstrictors. It is not clear why septic, vasodilated patients did poorly with vasodilator therapy.

(4)   Arch. Surg. 102:21-24, January, 1971.

▶ [It is increasingly apparent that vasodilator therapy is of benefit in vasoconstrictive shock states and is of little value or contraindicated in shock accompanied by vasodilation per se.—Eds.]

Skeletal Muscle Hydrogen Ion Activity in Endotoxin Shock. The surface pH of skeletal muscle has been shown to be a sensitive indirect indicator of peripheral blood flow, in accord with the concept that increased hydrogen ion activity is a result of anaerobic glycolysis and lactic acid production, which in turn resulted from reduced tissue perfusion. Jan R. Dmochowski and Nathan P. Cough[5] (Boston) measured muscle pH in endotoxin shock in mongrel dogs, and the effects of volume infusion, sodium bicarbonate and vasodilators. A pH electrode was placed on the surface of the sortorius muscle and connected to an electrometer. Two dogs were used for controls and were

Fig. 38.—Endotoxin shock-treated dogs. Mean arterial blood pressure, skeletal muscle surface pH, arterial blood pH, hematocrit values and lactate concentration are shown for 1 of the 2 dogs given Dibenzyline as well as Ringer's solution and sodium bicarbonate; the dog weighed 20 kg. (Courtesy of Dmochowski, J. R., and Couch, N. P.: Surg., Gynec. & Obst. 131:669-674, October, 1970.)

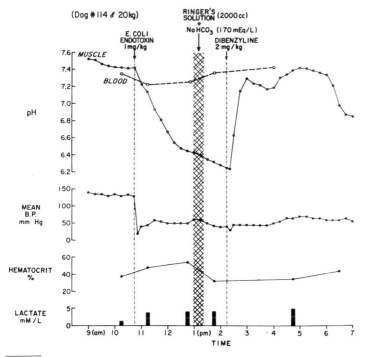

(5)   Surg., Gynec. & Obst. 131:669-674, October, 1970.

subjected to all surgical and testing procedures but were not given endotoxin or any form of treatment. Thirteen dogs received Escherichia coli endotoxin, 1 mg./kg., intravenously. Two shocked dogs received Ringer's solution, 79 ml./kg., and sodium bicarbonates, 4 mEq./kg., after 2 hours. Four others received similar treatment as well as phentolamine, 203 mg./kg., intravenously, within 10 minutes of fluid administration. Two dogs received phenoxybenzamine, 1 mg./kg., intravenously as well as Ringer's solution and sodium bicarbonate.

Blood pressure and muscle pH dropped steeply in endotoxin shock. Blood pH fell more gradually and lactate increased, with no change in blood Po_2 or Pco_2. Untreated animals had progressive muscle acidosis, acidemia and hemoconcentration and died within 12 hours. Infusion of Ringer's solution and bicarbonate had a beneficial but transient influence, without changing the muscle pH; the dogs died within 24 hours. Phentolamine increased muscle pH and reduced blood pressure without altering the elevated lactate level. In the 2 dogs receiving phenoxybenzamine there was a greater and more prolonged effect (Fig. 38). Blood pressure was lowered, while muscle pH returned to normal for about 3 hours. These dogs, however, died at 36 and 72 hours, respectively.

Muscle acidosis occurs throughout endotoxin shock and if the current theory is correct is due initially to reduced flow secondary to low cardiac output and later to reduced flow from vasoconstriction and arteriovenous shunting evoked by catecholamine release. The method may be useful in monitoring a variety of low-flow states both in animals and in patients.

► [It is of interest that the muscle pH increased dramatically after phenoxybenzamine, suggesting marked improvement of muscle blood flow. —Eds.]

Epidural Blockade in Treatment of Septic Shock. M. J. Silverstein (Boston, Mass., City Hosp.), I. O. Mehrez (Tufts Univ.) and A. E. Ogden[6] (Mt. Auburn Hosp., Cambridge, Mass.) recently evaluated preganglionic splanchnic blockade via fractional epidural lidocaine injection as an adjunct to the standard treatment of septic shock in 2 severe cases.

Man, 66, was admitted with right lower lobe atelectasis and a temperature of 101 F. The fever resolved, but epigastric and right upper quadrant discomfort developed, and an oral cholecystogram showed nonfilling. Fever of 103 F. and profuse sweating ensued, and ampicillin was given intravenously. Shaking chills and more profound pyrexia followed, with disorientation and recurrent chills. The

(6)   J. Cardiovas. Surg. 11:122-128, Mar.-Apr., 1970.

serum bilirubin rose to 4.1 mg./100 ml. Kanamycin and penicillin were substituted for ampicillin, and a hypothermia blanket was utilized. Cholecystostomy was performed with removal of a single large stone. Drainage stopped after 24 hours, with a temperature spike to 105 F. and hypotension as well as a fall in urine output. The patient was cold and clammy. Ringer's lactate was infused with THAM-E, and isoproterenol was given, with a rapid rise in the central venous pressure without improvement in blood pressure. Limb temperatures were 85 F. An epidural catheter was placed at T12, and 2% lidocaine with 1:200,000 epinephrine was given. Blood pressure, urine output and leg temperature soon increased. Injections of 8-10 ml. lidocaine solution were given every 2-4 hours for 24 hours. Bile and blood cultures yielded group C Aerobacter; cultures were sterile after 2 weeks, when the serum bilirubin was 1.5 mg./100 ml. Cholangiography showed a common duct stone, which was removed, along with the gallbladder. The patient was discharged after removal of the T-tube.

A woman aged 53, with a pelvic abscess, was treated similarly after conventional treatment was ineffective. The response to epidural blockade was dramatic. Central venous and pulmonary congestion was relieved by diverting blood to the splanchnic areas and the periphery, with a fall in central venous pressure and a rise in both arterial pressure and urine output resulting. Monitoring of skin temperatures was important in these cases. Epidural blockade appears to have a potentially major role in current shock therapy.

▶ [There are more ways than one of blocking the autonomic nervous system.—Eds.]

Depletion of Alveolar Surface-Active Material by Transbronchial Plasma Irrigation of the Lung. The terms "shock lung" and "wet lung" have been applied to a condition of deteriorating lung compliance and inadequate blood oxygenation with pink frothy tracheobronchial fluid in severely injured subjects in shock. Sidney Levitsky, Charles A. Annable, Benjamin S. Park, Allen L. Davis and Paul A. Thomas[7] (Valley Forge Gen'l Hosp., Phoenixville, Pa.) examined 5 lung specimens taken at autopsy from Vietnam casualties. Surface activity of tracheobronchial fluids and lung extracts was measured in dogs with acute pulmonary edema. Measurements were repeated after in vitro transbronchial irrigation with 0.9% saline, canine plasma or 4% human albumin. Measurements were made of lung extracts 24 hours after in vivo transbronchial irrigations with saline or canine plasma and after in vivo transbronchial irrigations in dogs kept on positive-pressure ventilation with

(7) Ann. Surg. 173:107-115, January, 1971.

or without oxygen enrichment for 12 hours. Pulmonary edema was induced by infusing 6% low molecular weight dextran in saline.

Examination of the lungs of battle casualties showed edema and hyaline membrane formation, with a reduced surface tension stability index. Experimentally produced pulmonary edema in dogs resulted in surfactant appearing in edema fluid, but without evidence of alveolar depletion. The surface tension stability index decreased in plasma-irrigated lung lobes but not markedly in saline-filled lobes. Findings were analogous with in vivo irrigations. Addition of a highly concentrated oxygen atmosphere for 12 hours of assisted ventilation did not result in discernible surfactant changes besides those found after plasma irrigation.

The findings support the hypothesis that a plasma factor, introduced into the alveoli, contributes to the removal of surface-active material and may explain the apparent irreversibility of the "shock lung" syndrome. Surfactant is depleted by mechanical removal, probably aided by an affinity for protein carried in the plasma. Agitation of free surfactant-bearing fluid by assisted ventilation further depletes surface-active substance. Resurfacing of the alveoli and establishment of an air-liquid interface is prevented by metabolic depression of alveolar cells that produce surfactant, and this may result in an irreversible terminal state.

Adult Acute Respiratory Insufficiency Syndrome Following Nonthoracic Trauma: The Lung in Shock. Edward H. Bergofsky[8] (New York Univ.) observes that the syndrome of acute pulmonary insufficiency after shock or trauma has become increasingly well defined. Generally tachypnea, dyspnea, cyanosis, respiratory alkalosis and diffuse pneumonic or interstitial infiltration appear after a latent period of several hours, and pure oxygen inhalation does not relieve the cyanosis. Respiratory acidosis develops and tracheostomy is often required. The predominant pathologic changes are hyperemia and capillary or interstitial edema with diffuse microatelectasis with or without bacterial pneumonia. Hyaline-like membranes are present in some instances. Inflatability of the lungs at autopsy is reduced or absent.

Compliance is reduced in this state, but it is unclear whether this is due to the anatomic changes or to a loss of surfactant

(8)   Am. J. Cardiol. 26:619-621, December, 1970.

with consequent exaggeration of surface tension at the alevolar air-liquid interface. There is considerable disagreement as to the type of pulmonary vessel that is most damaged. The author's data favor direct capillary damage. Animal studies suggest a loss of pulmonary surfactant and increased surface tension in the lung in experimental shock. The end result in either instance is widespread alveolar microatelectasis with or without alveolar fluid, stiff lungs and ventilation-perfusion imbalance with venous admixture predominating.

Stiff, atelectatic lungs can be inflated with brief periods of high pressure, and once inflated, they become less stiff and are far more easily ventilated. The most important measure is maintenance of continuous positive pressure throughout the respiratory cycle. Endotracheal pressures at the end of expiration are set at about 6 cm. water. The importance of overinfusing noncolloidal fluid in aggravating pulmonary transudation during shock is unclear, nor is it clear to what degree oxygen concentrations over 60% superimpose toxic effects on pre-existing respiratory insufficiency. Present knowledge of lung mechanics permits a hopeful treatment approach to the stiff, collapsed lung, even though the initiating factors and detailed mechanisms of the syndrome have not been definitely determined.

▶ [Chest physical therapy and postural drainage, insofar as can be done in these patients, are also important therapeutic measures.—Eds.]

Lung Pathology in Respiratory Distress Following Shock in the Adult. Parallel with the rapid development of intensive care, severe lung lesions have been noted with increasing frequency in patients dying in shock of varying etiology. S. R. Orell[9] (Danderyd, Sweden) reviewed the autopsy findings in 20 patients with progressive respiratory distress and shock seen since 1964 (group 1). All these patients had had ventilation with an Engström respirator, with a high oxygen concentration. The findings in 12 patients who died after a period of mechanical ventilation not associated with progressive respiratory distress (group 2) were also reviewed.

Nine group 1 patients had postoperative complications. All 20 patients had circulatory failure and signs of respiratory insufficiency requiring tracheotomy and artificial ventilation. Generally the circulation was restored, but respiratory distress developed after a few days and, with other complications, re-

---

(9)   Acta path. et microbiol. scandinav. 79-A:65-76, 1971.

sulted in death. During progression of respiratory distress, oxygen concentration, ventilatory volume per minute and inspiratory pressure had to be progressively increased to maintain an acceptable arterial oxygen tension. Thrombocytopenia was a common finding. Chest x-rays showed widespread flecks and blurred shadows, with later massive consolidation. Complex treatment was given to these patients.

Group 2 patients were ventilated for 1-34 days. Respiratory function was fairly stable. Shock treatment was given in 8 cases. X-rays showed no characteristic lesions.

All group 1 patients had advanced pulmonary changes; group 2 patients had similar but more variable changes. The central, dorsal and basal parts of the lungs were most consolidated. The earliest lesions were alveolar and interstitial edema and alveolar wall thickening. Alveolar hemorrhage and, in all cases but 1, hyaline membranes were also present. The membranes were first noted on the tips of the alveolar walls along the ducts. In patients with longer survival, fibroblastic proliferation was seen in the membranes (Fig. 39). In 1 case, new cellular fibrous

Fig. 39 (left).—Transversely cut alveolar duct lined by dissolving membrane infiltrated by inflammatory and fibroblastic cells. Case 11. Ladewig; reduced from ×150.
Fig. 40 (right).—Respiratory bronchiole and alveolar ducts filled by young cellular fibrous tissue. Case 18. Van Gieson; reduced from ×135.
(Courtesy of Orell, S. R.: Acta path. et microbiol. scandinav. 79-A:65-76, 1971.)

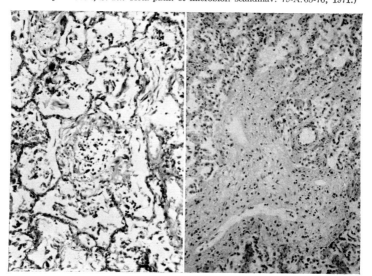

tissue filled many bronchioles and alveolar ducts (Fig. 40). Inflammatory lesions were present in most cases. Microscopic thrombi in the small muscular pulmonary arteries and arterioles were present in 16 group 1 and 8 group 2 patients.

Severe lung lesions were associated with large ventilatory volumes and high oxygen concentrations. Development of hyaline membranes was not definitely related to a high oxygen concentration or to duration of mechanical ventilation. Organization of the membranes in group 1 cases was related to the period of survival after onset of progressive respiratory distress. Extensive bronchopneumonia was more frequent with longer periods of treatment.

Lung lesions in progressive respiratory distress are precipitated by inadequate tissue perfusion and possibly also by intravascular coagulation during shock, leading to endothelial damage and reduced alveolor surfactant. "Respiratory distress lung" as an appropriate term for this type of lung lesion, which may also be precipitated by viral pneumonia and uremia and greatly resembles hyaline membrane disease in the newborn.

▶ [Many factors have been incriminated as *the factor* in causation of "respirator lung"—high oxygen tension, high airway pressure, loss of surfactant, etc. Orell adds hypoperfusion of the lung and intravascular coagulation leading to endothelial damage and reduced surfactant. It is extremely difficult to sort out the etiology in complex situations such as these.—Eds.]

Central Nervous System in Experimental Hemorrhagic Shock: Cerebrospinal Fluid Pressure. F. A. Simeone and M. Witoszka[1] (Brown Univ.) studied the effect of experimental hemorrhage and blood "reinfusion" on cerebrospinal fluid pressure in 25 rabbits and 7 dogs.

Experiments were done in heparinized animals anesthetized with pentobarbital. Animals had tracheal intubation but breathed spontaneously. Access to the subarachnoid space was by a stainless steel, conical, threaded tube, which tightened its grip into the inner and outer tables of the skull as it was screwed into place through a drill hole in the parietal bone. The inner margin barely touched the dura mater. Adapters could be fitted to the tube lumen. Cerebrospinal fluid pressures were recorded across the intact dura, or the dura was opened and pressures were measured directly. Measurements were made with a manometer primed with isotonic saline or through Statham strain gauges connected to a direct-writing Grass Polygraph. Animals

(1)   Am. J. Surg. 119:427-432, April, 1970.

were bled rapidly into a Lamson bottle to induce and maintain oligemic hypotension at 30-35 mm. Hg. Rabbits were reinfused after 1 hour and dogs after 2 hours. Cerebrospinal fluid pressures were measured during a 2-hour control period, during oligemic hypotension and after reinfusion (for about 1 hour in rabbits and 2½-4 hours in dogs). Animals were killed at the end of the studies, and skulls and their contents were prepared for histologic examination.

During the control period under anesthesia, mean cerebrospinal fluid pressure was 7.4 mm. Hg in the rabbits and 10 mm. Hg in the dogs. With bleeding, mean aortic pressure in rabbits dropped 68% and mean cerebrospinal fluid pressure, 77% from the control value (table). In 6 of 7 dogs, cerebrospinal fluid pressures were negative during oligemia-hypotension. When blood from the reservoir was reinfused, aortic blood pressure rose but did not equal the control value in either dogs or rabbits. The course of aortic blood pressure after infusion suggested that no rabbit but all dogs would have survived. In both species, cerebrospinal fluid pressure rose sharply after infusion, and in 5 rabbits, it was 5 or 6 times the control pressure. In some rabbits the brain herniated into the implanted tube and blocked the pressure-recording system. After the acute rise of cerebrospinal fluid, pressure that followed infusion, the pressure fell rapidly to a sustained level distinctly higher than the control value. Whereas ratios of mean cerebrospinal fluid to mean aortic pressure in rabbits were 13.9 (control), 19 (oligemia-hypotension) and 4.7 (postinfusion), ratios of mean cerebrospinal fluid to mean central venous pressure were 1, 0.4 and 1.8, respectively. Histologic examinations of brains and meninges showed congestion of pial vessels, hemorrhage into the brain and cerebrospinal fluid and areas of focal necrosis.

Irreversibility of prolonged shock has been attributed to

CEREBROSPINAL FLUID PRESSURE IN EXPERIMENTAL HEMORRHAGIC SHOCK
(MEAN PRESSURE IN MILLIMETERS OF MERCURY; 25 RABBITS)

	Control	Oligemia and Hypotension	Infusion of Reservoir Blood
Aortic blood pressure	103.8	32.6	72.6
Central venous pressure	7.4	4.5	8.8
Cerebrospinal fluid pressure	7.4	1.7	15.5

breakdown in the delicately interrelated mechanisms that comprise the organization for circulatory homeostasis. The present studies suggest that in the dog and rabbit, some of the disorganization occurs in the central nervous system.

▶ [If any of this applies to man, we should think of elevated intracranial pressure in patients deteriorating after massive transfusion and be prepared to attempt lowering it when indicated.—Eds.]

Effect of Adrenalectomy and Complete Blockade of Adrenergic Function on Mortality from Histamine, Endotoxin, Formalin and Tourniquet Stress in Rats was investigated by J. J. Krawczak and B. B. Brodie[2] (Nat'l Inst. of Health).

METHOD.—Experiments were made on adrenalectomized and adrenal demedullated adult male rats. Until used in experiments, the former were given free access to drinking water containing 1% saline-glucose; the latter received 1% saline-5% glucose for 7 days and then free access to drinking water. Sympathetic function was blocked in adrenal demedullated animals by intraperitoneal injection of BW392C60 (20 mg./kg.), a potent bretylium-like drug, or chlorisondamine (10 mg./kg.), a ganglionic blocking agent. Cortisone and epinephrine were given subcutaneously 10 minutes before the experiments. Shock was produced with histamine, Escherichia coli endotoxin, neutral formalin and tourniquet trauma applied after local anesthesia to the thighs.

Adrenalectomy greatly reduced the lethal dose of histamine. Although histamine shock appeared in adrenalectomized animals pretreated with cortisone, partial protection was evident, 50% of the animals surviving at 24 hours. Animals pretreated with both cortisone and epinephrine showed few signs of toxicity and none died. Sympathetic blockade also greatly increased the toxicity of histamine. Epinephrine pretreatment ameliorated the effects of histamine toxicity, nearly 90% of the animals surviving.

Endotoxin toxicity was greatly increased by both adrenalectomy and sympathetic blockade. Epinephrine alone was protective after sympathetic blockade, but cortisone was also required after adrenalectomy. Adrenalectomy but not sympathetic blockade decreased the lethal dose of formalin. Pretreatment with cortisone alone greatly ameliorated the effects of formalin and provided almost complete protection from the lethal effects of tourniquet application in adrenalectomized rats. Reduction of sympathetic tone did not increase the mortality rate from formalin, nor did it increase the effects of tourniquet shock; if anything, it decreased the lethal effects of occlusion of the blood supply.

(2) Pharmacology 3:65-75, 1970.

Formalin and tourniquet shock is initiated by a mechanism different from that elicited by histamine and endotoxin, and protection against such shock does not primarily involve the sympathetic nervous system. The increased toxicity of endotoxin and histamine after adrenalectomy is due largely to impaired sympathetic responses.

Redistribution of Cardiac Output during Hemorrhage in the Unanesthetized Monkey. Ralph P. Forsyth, Barry I. Hoffbrand and Kenneth L. Melmon[3] (Univ. of California) used a microsphere technic to study the effects of different levels of bleeding in the unanesthetized monkey free from the influences of recent operations. Circulating blood volume was measured in 12 supine male rhesus monkeys about a week after placement of catheters. Cardiac output and arterial and central venous pressures were measured before and after bleeding. Microspheres were injected after removal of a 10% increment of blood volume and after removal of two 20% increments from 5 monkeys. Similar measurements were made on 7 controls. Measurements of regional blood flow were made with 40-70-μ microspheres labeled with ^{125}I, ^{46}Sc, ^{85}Sr or ^{51}Cr injected into the left ventricle.

Arterial and central venous pressures, cardiac output and stroke volume were significantly reduced after 30% bleeding. Hematocrit and plasma bradykininogen also fell significantly. Two monkeys were moribund after 50% bleeding. The other 3 had a significantly higher peripheral resistance and heart rate than controls. The fraction of cardiac output to brain, heart, adrenal gland and hepatic artery was increased progressively at the expense of skin, spleen and pancreas. The largest change in fraction of cardiac output in controls, among organs receiving more than 1% of the output, was 14% in bone at the third injection of microspheres. After 10% bleeding, the heart received 146% of baseline output and the skin, 67%. Blood flow fell significantly after 30% bleeding in the kidneys, skeletal muscle, small and large intestines, spine, mesentery and diaphragm. After 50% bleeding, most organs showed significant changes in fraction of the cardiac output they received (Fig. 41). No remarkable gross pathologic findings were evident at autopsy. The monkeys did not become comatose until about 40-50% bleeding, but they did not struggle or show other signs of discomfort.

A different pattern of regional flow changes has been found

(3) Circulation Res. 27:311-320, September, 1970.

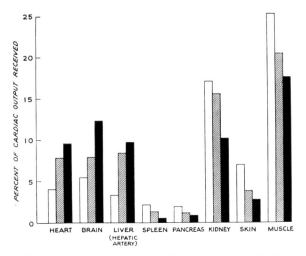

Fig. 41.—Mean per cent of cardiac output delivered to 8 organs of 5 bled monkeys before (*open bars*) and after 30 (*hatched bars*) and 50% (*solid bars*) of blood volume had been removed. Mean cardiac outputs at baseline, 30 and 50% bleeding were 1.22, 0.66 and 0.28 L. per minute, respectively. (Courtesy of Forsyth, R. P., *et al.*: Circulation Res. 27: 311-320, September, 1970.)

in acute endotoxin shock in monkeys, with a similar fall in systemic arterial pressure due to decreased peripheral resistance. A lack of bradykinin production, the integrity of cardioregulatory mechanisms and the fall of hematocrit found in hemorrhage may help account for some of the hemodynamic differences between the two types of shock.

Renal Effects of Hemorrhage in Normal Man. Alex M. Stone and William M. Stahl[4] (New York Univ.) assessed the importance of various factors on renal function after arterial hemorrhage in normal man. Eighteen studies were done on 14 subjects aged 25-40. Supine patients were loaded with 0.45% saline, 10-20 ml./kg., and infused with inulin and para-amino-hippurates. In 14 studies, 5% mannitol was also infused. Rapid hemorrhage was done in amounts of 11.2-16.6 ml./kg. at a rate of 55 ml. per minute; a total of 900-1,190 ml. was bled. Measurements were repeated at 30 minutes, and shed blood then was reinfused rapidly with anticoagulant. Four 30-minute post-reinfusion clearance periods were then obtained.

The results are given in the table. The mean arterial blood pressure fell from 80 to 62 mm. Hg with hemorrhage and re-

(4)   Ann. Surg. 172: 825-836, November, 1970.

RENAL EFFECTS OF HEMORRHAGE AND REINFUSION IN 14 NORMAL SUBJECTS

		Hemorrhage		Reinfusion			
	Control	30′	60′	30′	60′	90′	120′
Urine sodium excretion (μEq./min.)							
No mannitol	166	51	43	115	157	163	208
Mannitol	190	102	74	148	176	215	238
Urine potassium excretion (μEq./min.)							
No mannitol	71	41	55	78	74	64	78
Mannitol	78	48	46	77	64	56	66
Urine Na/K ratio							
No mannitol	2.33	1.26	0.77	1.49	2.13	2.55	2.66
Mannitol	2.44	2.13	1.61	1.92	2.75	3.48	3.61
Osmolar clearance (ml./min.)							
No mannitol	2.8	1.1	1.3	2.4	2.6	3.4	3.2
Mannitol	3.8	2.4	2.7	3.1	3.0	3.5	3.6
Urine volume (ml./min.)							
No mannitol	2.5	0.5	0.6	1.1	2.9	6.2	5.8
Mannitol	2.7	1.0	1.1	1.8	3.1	2.8	3.2

covered to 67 mm. Hg an hour after bleeding. Reinfusion restored the pressure to normal over 1 hour. Individual variations in blood pressure response were unrelated to the volume of bleeding or to mannitol infusion. With hemorrhage, cardiac output fell from 6.2 to 3.8 L. per minute and recovered to 4.5 L. at 1 hour. Central venous pressure fell to 2.8 mm. Hg after hemorrhage. Peripheral vascular resistance was markedly reduced after reinfusion. It was essentially normal an hour after reinfusion.

Effective renal blood flow fell from 1,040 to 784 ml. per minute after hemorrhage and rose above the control level with reinfusion. The portion of total cardiac output perfusing the kidneys rose from 16.8 to 20.6% immediately after hemorrhage. Renal vascular resistance changed little with acute hemorrhage. Wedged renal vein pressure fell from 29.3 to 19.4 mm. Hg immediately after hemorrhage and returned to normal after reinfusion of shed blood. The glomerular filtration rate fell with hemorrhage and returned to normal on reinfusion of shed blood. The filtration fraction fell markedly in the first 30 minutes after reinfusion. Urine volume was higher after hemorrhage in patients given mannitol. Osmolar clearance was also higher in those given mannitol. The urine sodium-potassium ratio fell 40% in the mannitol group and 67.5% in the other patients

during hemorrhage. Free water resorption occurred in all periods in the mannitol group.

Subjects vary considerably in their response to acute arterial
hemorrhage. It is not clear whether excretion of a water load in
subjects not receiving mannitol is a normal response, which is
blocked by mannitol infusion, or whether it is a pathologic response to hemorrhage, masked or protected by mannitol. The
routine infusion of mannitol may lead to erroneous results in
clearance studies.

► [Since mannitol is alleged to have a specific tubular effect, it would in-
deed be unwise to give this agent when doing clearance studies.—Eds.]

CARDIOPULMONARY RESUSCITATION

**Serial Blood Gas Studies during Cardiopulmonary Resusci-
tation** were evaluated by Sidney J. Fillmore, Mario Shapiro
and Thomas Killip[5] (Cornell Univ.) in 10 men and 4 women,
aged 34-84 years, in whom 15 episodes of cardiac arrest complicated ischemic heart disease. All received prolonged closed
chest cardiac massage for circulatory support. Treatment consisted of mouth-to-mouth ventilation, external cardiac compression, sodium bicarbonate, d-c countershock, isoproterenol, norepinephrine, epinephrine and atropine as prescribed for individual situations. A nurse-technician kept a prospective record of
treatment. Arterial blood specimens were taken about every 5
minutes. Blood gas analyses were done with a Radiometer pH
meter 27 with gas monitor. Arterial oxyhemoglobin saturation
was calculated from oxygen tension and pH. Lactates were determined by enzymatic technic.

In 9 arrests in 9 patients (group I), resuscitation failed to restore an effective circulation; 6 patients had blood samples
taken before and after intubation. In 5 arrests in 4 patients
(group II), resuscitation restored blood pressure and spontaneous ventilation, but all 4 eventually died in cardiogenic
shock. None had preintubation blood samples. Patients in the
two groups did not differ in age, clinical severity of disease before arrest or promptness of initial treatment (except for
tracheal intubation). The fourteenth patient was discharged
from the hospital and was well 1 year later. The table gives

----

(5)   Ann. Int. Med. 72:465-469, April, 1970.

ARTERIAL P_{CO_2}, OXYHEMOGLOBIN SATURATION, pH AND LACTATE
DURING TREATMENT OF CARDIAC ARREST

| | Group I | | | | Group II | |
| | Preintubation | | Postintubation | | Postintubation | |
	Mean	Range	Mean	Range	Mean	Range
Minutes between arrest and intubation	14	3–30	—	—	5	1–10
Arterial P_{CO_2}, *mm Hg*	66	31–120	41	19–59	46	31–94
Oxyhemoglobin saturation, %	79	41–98	82	39–98	90	72–99
pH, *units*	7.31	7.06–7.32	7.39	7.03–7.57	7.37*	7.15–7.68
Lactate, *mg/deciliter*	122	87–155	152	9–254	74	16–211

*Excludes 1 patient with hydrothorax.

mean and range values for time between cardiac arrest and tracheal intubation, arterial P_{CO_2}, oxyhemoglobin saturation, pH and blood lactate concentration for the two groups. Figure 42 shows the effect of tracheal intubation on arterial P_{CO_2} in 6 group I patients. Differences in postintubation P_{CO_2} values in groups I and II were not significant. All 9 group I patients re-

Fig. 42.—Serial Pa_{CO_2} after cardiopulmonary arrest in 6 patients. Circles enclosing *A* indicate time of arrest, solid lines indicate serial carbon dioxide measurements and arrows indicate time of successful endotracheal intubation. (Courtesy of Fillmore, S. J., *et al.*: Ann. Int. Med. 72:465-469, April, 1970.)

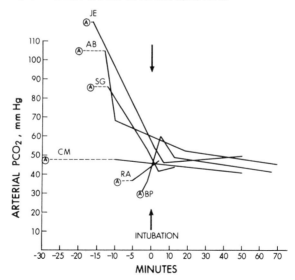

ceived comparable amounts of bicarbonate (mean, 400 mEq.) in the 1st hour. In 5 whose mean pH was 7.45, mean Pco_2 was 37 mm. Hg, and in 4 whose mean pH was 7.24, Pco_2 was 52 mm. Hg. The more promptly intubated group II patients required less bicarbonate (mean, 100 mEq. per hour) to prevent acidemia. In group II, the rise in blood lactate concentration was significantly slower than in group I and then declined when adequate ventilation was provided and circulation resumed. Oxyhemoglobin saturation was maintained at significantly higher levels in group II. Of 6 group I patients on whom autopsy was performed, those with the highest oxyhemoglobin saturation and lowest arterial Pco_2 had the lightest lungs, with 1 exception. Lungs of the latter, who had nearly normal gas values after over 1 hour of attempted resuscitation, weighed 850 Gm./sq. m. body surface area and had areas of consolidated infarction; noninfarcted parenchyma was not edematous. Time between study and death in group II patients precluded meaningful correlation of blood gas and lung findings. Temporary support of the arrested circulation is more likely to be effective if prompt ventilation and tracheal intubation are performed.

▶ [The conclusion is right, but don't delay ventilation to do tracheal intubation unless the equipment is immediately at hand and prepared for use (which is unlikely).—Eds.]

Experimental Comparison in Dogs of Expired Air and Oxygen Ventilation during External Cardiac Massage. Cardiopulmonary function deteriorates steadily during external cardiac massage even when 100% oxygen is administered, and question arises as to the effects of expired-air ventilation used as a first aid measure outside the hospital. W. R. Lee, H. D. Baillie, A. D. Clarke, L. S. Levy, S. Zoledziowski and A. A. E. Massoud[6] studied survival in dogs with electrically induced ventricular fibrillation, which had external cardiac massage and expired-air ventilation. Oxygen was used for artificial respiration in 20 dogs and a gas mixture equivalent to expired air in 18, consisting of 16% oxygen, 4% carbon dioxide and nitrogen. Anesthesia was induced with thiopentone before positive-pressure ventilation was begun at a minute ventilation of 250 ml./ kg. Ventricular fibrillation was induced by an a-c shock after the endotracheal tube was disconnected from the ventilator, and manual external heart massage was performed as the dog was ventilated by hand with oxygen or expired air. Massage was

(6) Brit. J. Anaesth. 43:38-50, January, 1971.

done at 80-100 compressions per minute to maintain an aortic pressure of 40-60 mm. Hg. The lungs were inflated after each fourth sternal compression, at a gas flow of 12-15 L. per minute. Metabolic acidosis was corrected with bicarbonate shortly before cardiac arrest was ended with a defibrillator.

Sixteen dogs recovered consciousness, with evidence of full cerebral recovery, including 6 in the oxygen group and 10 in the expired-air group. Four dogs in each group survived after 40 minutes of heart massage; 1 and 2, respectively, after 50 minutes; and 1 and 4, respectively, after 60 minutes of heart massage. Systolic blood pressures remained nearly constant during heart massage in both groups of dogs. The $Paco_2$ was better maintained in the expired-air group. The Pao_2 fell in the oxygen group but remained fairly constant in the expired-air group after initially decreasing. The mean pH fell to 7.09 in the oxygen group and to 6.85 in the expired-air group. Pulmonary complications occurred in about half the dogs in the oxygen group and in 9 in the expired-air group. None of 17 dogs examined at necropsy showed evidence of mechanical damage to the heart or hemothorax.

Expired-air resuscitation with external heart massage is as likely to provide satisfactory oxygenation as is ventilation with oxygen in previously fit human patients. Determined efforts should not be abandoned because oxygen is unavailable.

▶ [It would never have occurred to the editors to give up a resuscitative effort because 100% oxygen was not available. On the other hand, judgment when to attempt resuscitation is a less difficult decision than when not to attempt resuscitation.—Eds.]

HYPERBARIC OXYGENATION AND OXYGEN TOXICITY

Mechanism of Pulmonary Injury after Oxygen Therapy was investigated by Arthur N. Thomas and Albert D. Hall[7] (Univ. of California). Lung function deteriorates with prolonged oxygen therapy. Pulmonary oxygen toxicity is probably related to poisoning of cell enzyme systems and membrane integrity. Both intermittent oxygen therapy and arterial hypoxemia have been suggested as means of increasing lung tolerance for oxygen.

Eight rabbits (group 1) received a single 2-hour exposure to

(7) Am. J. Surg. 120:255-263, August, 1970.

humidified 98% oxygen at 3 atmospheres; in group 2, 12 had six 1-hour sessions at 3 atmospheres pressure absolute (ATA) alternated with 3 hours of air at 1 ATA; 12 in group 3 had a 20-day regimen of six 1-hour exposures every 24 hours at 2 ATA alternated with 3-hour periods of air at 1 ATA; and in group 4, 20 were exposed at 2 ATA with six 1-hour treatments alternated with 1 hour of air at 1 ATA, followed by 12 hours of air at 1 ATA, for 20 days.

All in the first group died of acute pulmonary edema, congestion and atelectasis during oxygen exposure. Surviving animals in the second group had proliferative alveolar changes and hyaline membrane deposition in the lungs. Animals in the third group all survived, with proliferative lung changes. All animals in the fourth group survived. Alveolar cellularity and patchy atelectasis were less marked in this group; at 10 days, residual proliferative changes were minimal.

Constant tidal volume ventilation was compared with intermittent hyperinflation with oxygen in 13 mongrel dogs ventilated with pure oxygen. The Po_2 rose transiently to extremely high levels on compression to 2 ATA but then declined. Periodic hyperinflation raised the Pao_2 to 1300-1700 mm. Hg. The alveolar-arterial oxygen gradient remained relatively constant for 4-7 hours with arterial hypoxemia maintained.

In other dogs, different blood oxygen tensions were provided to perfuse each lung by intrapericardial right pulmonary artery ligation or by left pulmonary-left atrial anastomosis followed by right middle lobe pulmonary artery ligation. The most severe lung changes after exposure to hyperbaric oxygen occurred in the lungs with the ligated artery.

Hypoxic patients tolerate prolonged oxygen therapy better than other patients. The inspiratory Po_2 should not exceed the measured need of the patient and should be raised to a level that relieves hypoxia whenever possible. The need for a high inspiratory Po_2 must be minimized where possible. Oxygen requirements increase with infection, hyperthermia and the work of breathing.

▶ [As the authors say in closing the discussion of their article, ". . . we have stressed the importance of tailoring the concentration of administered oxygen to the patient's therapeutic response." They have!—Eds.]

Response of the Lung to 6-12 Hours of 100% Oxygen Inhalation in Normal Man was studied by Joseph M. Van De Water, Karen S. Kagey, Ian T. Miller, David A. Parker, Nicholas E.

O'Connor, Jaen-Min Sheh, John D. MacArthur, Robert M. Zollinger, Jr., and Francis D. Moore[8] (Harvard Med. School). High oxygen concentration is often necessary for prolonged periods for seriously ill patients, and some such patients are found at autopsy to have lung changes associated with oxygen toxicity, although the changes are nonspecific. The toxic effect of oxygen on the animal lung has been well established.

In the present study, 9 healthy males, aged 21-26, were exposed to 100% oxygen at ambient pressure and 2 others to compressed air. Gas was administered with a face mask at a rate of 45 L. per minute, a rate adequate for deep inspirations. A slightly positive mask pressure was maintained throughout the respiratory cycle. All subjects were told that 100% oxygen was to be given. Exposure was for periods of 6-12 hours.

Four subjects exposed to oxygen had a burning sensation in the eyes and conjunctival injection, which responded to a brief reduction in flow rate. Heart rate, systemic pressure and central venous pressure remained constant during the study. Total body water values were normal. Respiratory rate did not change. The $Paco_2$ declined from 38.4 to 34.7 mm. Hg on pure oxygen inhalation. The Pao_2 on 100% oxygen was 485-562 mm.

Fig. 43.—Effects of 100% oxygen on A-aDo2 showing no significant change from the control period. (Courtesy of Van De Water, J. M., *et al.*: New England J. Med. 283:621-626, Sept. 17, 1970.)

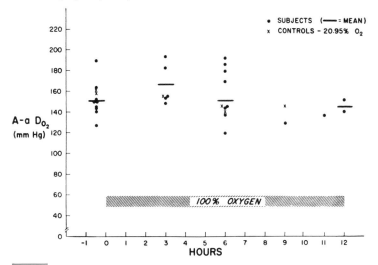

Hg, with an alveolar-arterial oxygen gradient (A-aDo$_2$) of 193-89 mm. Hg, with no significant change during the study period (Fig. 43). Physiologic pulmonary shunt did not change significantly during the study. The mean pulmonary artery pressure did not change significantly. Total pulmonary resistance rose insignificantly during the study period. Pulmonary extravascular water volume also failed to change significantly during the study. Chest x-rays taken at the end of exposure showed no changes.

This study failed to show significant pulmonary changes during oxygen inhalation in healthy young men. Trauma, anesthesia, shock and resuscitation, however, all involve components of lung injury that could make the lungs more vulnerable to the effects of oxygen inhalation than the normal lungs of healthy subjects.

▶ [This study shows that only minimal physiologic change occurs when fit young men breathe 100% oxygen at ambient pressure for 12 hours. Because patients who are found to have "respirator lung" at autopsy have often been ventilated with intermittent positive pressure, it would be of interest to know whether oxygen or air at elevated pressures might be responsible. As the authors point out, many factors are at play in the very ill patient who requires long-term oxygen therapy. It is interesting that there were only 2 more subjects in this study than there were investigators. —Eds.]

Oxygen Toxicity in Man: Prospective Study in Patients after Open Heart Surgery. It would be advantageous in some clinical circumstances to administer oxygen in concentrations higher than those needed to maintain a normal Pao$_2$. If such exposure can cause lung lesions in man, it is important to know the critical duration of exposure and oxygen concentration with which damage might be expected. Morley M. Singer, Frederick Wright, Loren K. Stanley, Benson B. Roe and William K. Hamilton[9] (Univ. of California) carried out a prospective study of the pulmonary effects of oxygen in adult postoperative patients requiring artificial ventilation. Study was made of 40 patients having cardiac surgical procedures, usually valve replacement, under cardiopulmonary bypass. Alternate patients were ventilated with pure oxygen or a sufficient inspired oxygen concentration to maintain a Pao$_2$ of 80-120 mm. Hg. The respective mean durations of bypass were 98 and 120 minutes. After stabilization for 1-3 hours after operation, compliance and intrapulmonary shunting were determined after 20 minutes' inhalation of 100% oxygen. Most patients had isoproterenol in-

(9)   New England J. Med. 283:1473-1478, Dec. 31, 1970.

fusion at some time, and all received morphine for analgesia. None received phenothiazines during the study. Both groups had periodic tracheal suction, frequent position changes and chest physiotherapy.

The mean inspired oxygen concentration for the limited-oxygen group was 32% and the mean duration of exposure, 21 hours. The mean exposure for 18 patients given pure oxygen was 24 hours; 2 patients were exposed for 5 and 7 days, respectively. Initial right-to-left shunts were similar in the two groups. No differences were found after oxygen exposure in intrapulmonary shunting, effective compliance, ratio of dead space to tidal volume or clinical course. One patient given oxygen for a prolonged period died of massive pulmonary hemorrhage related to a clotting deficit. The other recovered.

Further studies are needed to determine the dose and duration of oxygen exposure that may cause lung damage in man, especially in the specific environment of intermittent positive-pressure ventilation. Ventilation with oxygen had no apparent adverse effect in these patients with intrapulmonary shunting after heart operations. Fear of pulmonary oxygen toxicity should not prevent use of elevated inspired oxygen concentrations in critically ill patients requiring artificial ventilation.

Oxygen Toxicity in Man: Prospective Study in Patients with Irreversible Brain Damage. Studies of pulmonary oxygen toxicity in patients have been retrospective and the interpretations have been complicated by the presence of cardiopulmonary disease. Prospective studies have been done on healthy subjects. Richard E. Barber, Joseph Lee and William K. Hamilton[1] (Univ. of California) examined patients who sustained massive cerebral trauma and who had irreversible, ultimately fatal brain damage. They had no evidence of pre-existing cardiopulmonary disease or metabolic disease that might modify oxygen toxicity. Ten patients aged 15-45 years were examined. Five were ventilated with air and 5 with oxygen. The interval between admission and onset of artificial ventilation ranged from 30 minutes to 49 hours. All patients received dexamethasone. Studies were continued until terminal cardiovascular deterioration occurred or a kidney was removed for donation. Four patients in each group had transient hypotensive episodes, treated with increased fluids and isoproterenol.

The initial Pao_2 during oxygen inhalation was about 500 torr

(1) New England J. Med. 283:1478-1484, Dec. 31, 1970.

in both groups. The value remained well above 300 torr in the air group but dropped precipitously after pure oxygen inhalation for about 40 hours. Right-to-left shunting was significantly greater in the oxygen group at 41-50 hours. The $Paco_2$ was near normal in both groups throughout the study. The ratio of dead space to tidal volume was greater in the oxygen group from 30 hours of ventilation. Compliance values and mean cardiac indexes were similar in the two groups. Lobar consolidation developed in 2 patients in the air group. All those in the oxygen group had definite radiologic changes in time, and all but 1 had multiple lobar involvement. Lung sections were similar in the two groups, showing bronchopneumonia, congestion, edema, atelectasis, hemorrhage and, in 8 of 9 cases, intravascular coagulation. Hyaline membranes were not noted in either group.

Prolonged artificial ventilation with oxygen adversely affects pulmonary function in patients with cerebral trauma but with normal lungs. The most sensitive index of involvement is a decreasing Pao_2. Hyaline membranes may not be present at a time when pulmonary oxygen toxicity is demonstrable by other means.

▶ [This article and the preceding one document the philosophy that if oxygen is needed, use it liberally. If not needed, and often the patient does well with an F_{IO_2} of 30%, excessive oxygen is hazardous.—Eds.]

Pulmonary Oxygen Toxicity in Experimental Hemorrhagic Shock. Clinical use of 100% oxygen in shock is based on the tissue oxygen deficit known to occur in low flow states, but prolonged ventilation with high oxygen concentrations apparently can produce progressive pulmonary insufficiency. Lazar J. Greenfield, William C. McCurdy, III, and Jacqueline J. Coalson[2] (Oklahoma City, Okla.), with the technical assistance of Dennice Noel, examined the vulnerability of the canine lung to 100% oxygen in the presence of hypovolemic shock.

Warmed, humidified oxygen was supplied at ambient pressure to ventilated adult mongrel dogs anesthetized with pentobarbital. A rebreathing circuit was used. Animals were bled to a mean femoral artery pressure of 50 mm. Hg. Oxygen, started with the onset of shock, was given for 4 hours to 39 dogs (group I). Sixteen (group II) received air for 2 hours of shock and then 100% oxygen for 2 hours. Seven dogs (group III) were subjected to shock alone for 4 hours, and 6 (group IV) were given oxygen alone for 3-4 hours.

(2)   Surgery 68:662-675, October, 1970.

Group III dogs, bled an average of 34.6% of their blood volume, had a sustained fall in arterial pH to 7.22. Hypocapnia persisted during the shock period; the Pao_2 increased slightly for the first 3 hours of shock. Pulmonary vascular resistance rose markedly but dropped after 2 hours of shock. Group IV animals did not show a significant change in pulmonary vascular resistance. The arterial pH fell to 7.31 in the last hour of shock. Group I animals had a sustained elevation of Pao_2 above 300 mm. Hg and little change in $Paco_2$. Arterial pH fell to 7.29. Cardiac output decreased in the 1st hour of shock but then rose gradually, as pulmonary vascular resistance returned to moderately elevated levels after an early sharp rise. Group II animals had elevations of Pao_2 to less than 250 mm. Hg when oxygen was begun. The arterial pH fell continuously and was 7.22 after 4 hours of shock. Cardiac output remained low, and pulmonary resistance remained elevated.

Studies of excised lungs suggested premature closure of alveolar spaces; this was less marked in the lungs from group I dogs than in those from group II and III dogs. Pulmonary surfactant remained within normal limits in all groups. Group IV animals acquired diffuse congestive atelectasis with pulmonary edema and intra-alveolar hemorrhage. Moderate to severe changes occurred in group III animals. Changes in group I dogs were focal and less marked than after shock alone. The changes in group II dogs resembled more closely those after pure oxygen alone. At electron microscopy, endothelial damage was more marked after oxygen alone.

Ventilation with high concentrations of oxygen after more than 2 hours of shock in the dog appears to be more detrimental than beneficial.

▶ [It is unfortunate that another group of dogs wasn't studied—one in which the arterial Po_2 was maintained between 90-100 mm. Hg.—Eds.]

Protective Effects of Acetazolamide and Hyperbaric Oxygenation on Experimentally Induced Syncope. Acetazolamide is a potent cerebral vasodilator, and recent studies indicate that a combination of acetazolamine and hyperbaric oxygenation may be of value in patients with cerebral ischemia. Yihong Kong, Steven Lunzer, Albert Heyman and Herbert A. Saltzman[3] (Duke Univ.) evaluated this possibility in normal young subjects in whom transient cerebral ischemia was induced by brief periods of hypocapnia and hypotension, produced by

---

(3)   Stroke 1:69-76, Mar.-Apr., 1970.

vigorous hyperventilation and the Valsalva maneuver. Seven healthy males, aged 18-25 years, were studied on a tilt table in a hyperbaric chamber. Room air or 9 or 100% oxygen was administered. Syncope was induced by hyperventilation for 1 minute in a 40-degree head-up tilt position, followed by a vigorous 10-second Valsalva maneuver. The maneuvers were repeated 15 minutes after 10 ml. saline was given intravenously during room air breathing; after saline injection during 100% oxygen inhalation at 2.36 atmospheres absolute; during 9% oxygen-91% nitrogen inhalation at 2.36 atmospheres; and after injection of 500 mg. acetazolamide during inhalation of 100% oxygen at 2.36 atmospheres.

With comparable changes in $Paco_2$ and blood pressure during hyperventilation and the Valsalva maneuver, syncope occurred in 91% of maneuvers done at ambient pressure, in 86% done with 9% oxygen inhalation at high pressure, in 67% done with 100% oxygen inhalation at high pressure and in 33% done with acetazolamide injection with hyperbaric oxygenation. Syncope was completely prevented by hyperbaric oxygenation in 1 subject and by the combination of acetazolamide and hyperbaric oxygen in 4 subjects. In an ambient environment, syncope almost always occurred when the $Paco_2$ fell below 26 mm. Hg and the mean blood pressure below 90 mm. Hg. Increased pressure and hyperbaric oxygenation alone did not significantly reduce these critical levels, but with acetazolamide and hyperbaric oxygen, syncope did not occur until mean arterial pressure fell below 64 mm. Hg and the $Paco_2$ below 26 mm. Hg.

The exact mechanism by which acetazolamide increases cerebral blood flow is unclear. A combination of high arterial oxygen tension from hyperbaric oxygenation and increased cerebral perfusion may increase oxygen delivery to the brain enough to preserve cerebral function despite the hypocapnia and hypotension produced by the hyperventilation-Valsalva maneuver. The potential benefits of acetazolamide with hyperbaric oxygenation in patients with acute cerebrovascular insufficiency and those having cerebrovascular surgery are yet to be determined.

▶ [Although interesting physiologically and pharmacologically, as the authors point out the potential benefits of using such therapy are unknown.— Eds.]

THE INFORMED ANESTHESIOLOGIST

The Anterior Spinal Artery Syndrome, a Complication of Abdominal Aortic Surgery: Report of Five Cases and Review of the Literature are presented by William F. Zuber, Max R. Gaspar and Philip D. Rothschild[4] (Univ. of Southern California). In 5 new cases and 8 previously reported, a syndrome of paraplegia or paraparesis, usually with dissociated sensory loss and loss of rectal and urinary sphincter tone, followed abdominal aortic surgery. This is termed the anterior spinal artery syndrome.

The anterior median spinal artery extends the length of the cord, varying markedly in diameter (Fig. 44). The anterior spinal arteries supply the anterior horns, central gray matter, lateral horns, Clarke's columns and anterior and lateral tracts of the cord. A review of 25 unselected aortograms done for aor-

Fig. 44.—Diagram of a common pattern of formation of anterior spinal artery by intercostal and lumbar arteries. Inset shows how anterior spinal artery may become almost nonexistent before being joined by the major anterior radicular artery. (Courtesy of Zuber, W. F., *et al.*: Ann. Surg. 172:909-915, November, 1970.)

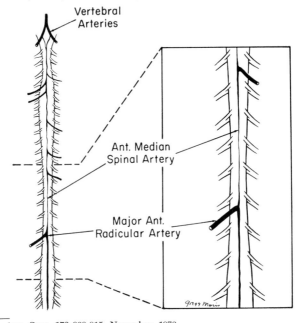

(4) Ann. Surg. 172:909-915, November, 1970.

toiliac occlusive disease showed frequent hypertrophy of L4 arteries, but no consistent pattern to the lumbar collaterals. Only the large lumbar vessels in 1 of the present cases apparently functioned as vessels supplying the major anterior radicular artery to the cord. All efforts must be made to preserve large lumbar arteries and to insure that they are not occluded by thrombus at operation.

Two of the 5 patients seen had suprarenal aortic occlusion coincident with hypotension, and 1 had proved thrombosis of extremely large collateral lumbar arteries at the L4 level. Two others had prolonged hypotension. All had reduced or absent flow through all lumbar arteries.

It is possible in any case for the major anterior radicular artery to be damaged as it can arise anywhere from the T10 to the L4 level. The cord thus could be injured by simple infrarenal aneurysmal resection. Also, arteriosclerotic disease might narrow the lumbar vessel supplying the major anterior radicular artery at the usual supradiaphragmatic level, stimulating a lower lumbar collateral to acquire the function of the latter vessel; injury to this second collateral would then produce paraplegia. The collaterals can be occluded by an organized clot being forced into them when a partially occluding clamp is placed on the aorta, as occurred in 1 case. Where the major anterior radicular artery or its collateral counterpart arises below the renal arteries, routine infrarenal clamping for over 20 minutes theoretically could cause permanent paraplegia.

Of the total of 13 cases, 8 occurred with resection of ruptured aneurysms and 3 with elective aneurysmal resections. Two occurred at bypass grafting for arteriosclerotic occlusive disease. Major anterior radicular arterial blood flow should be maintained at all times.

Neurologic Complications of Prevertebral Surgery under Regional Anesthesia. Jose E. Usubiaga, Jose Kolodny and Lilia E. Usubiaga[5] (Univ. of Miami) report 2 grave neurologic syndromes that followed excision of the terminal aorta and the lumbar sympathetic chain, respectively. The sequelae appeared to be due to section of the nutrient arteries to nerve plexuses and the spinal cord in both cases.

CASE 1.—Man, 75, had a 2-year history of abdominal aortic aneurysm, with a recent increase in size, and abdominal pain. Bronchitis and anemia were present. An aneurysm extending from 2 cm. below

(5) Surgery 68:304-309, August, 1970.

the renal arteries, including both iliac branches, was resected, and an aortobifemoral Y graft was inserted under epidural anesthesia. The aorta was cross clamped for 45 minutes during the operation. Bicarbonate was given to correct metabolic acidosis. Motor and sensory losses were apparent in the left lower limb immediately after operation. Tendon reflexes were absent and all muscle groups distal to the knee were completely plegic. The patient died with pneumonia after several days. Autopsy showed lower intestinal infarction. The left psoas muscle was totally liquefied, and infarction of the lumbosacral plexus and sciatic nerve was evident.

CASE 2.—Man, 49, with thrombotic disease of the left leg, underwent left lumbar sympathectomy under epidural anesthesia. Loss of power in the legs and numbness were reported just after operation, and urinary retention was present. Examination showed flaccid paralysis of both lower limbs and hypesthesia up to T10, with preservation of deep sensation. The epidural catheter was withdrawn intact. Decubitus ulcers developed, and the patient died with respiratory tract infection without recovering from the cord lesion. Autopsy showed atrophic kidneys and necrosis over the anterior two thirds of the spinal cord below T7. The ventral roots showed wallerian degeneration.

Surgery in the abdominal prevertebral area may cause serious neurologic sequelae. Damage was ischemic in both these cases. Arterial anastomoses within the spinal cord are rare, and occlusion of an important tributary may lead to ischemic necrosis of the cord. Presence of the greater anterior radicular artery in 80% of subjects explains the low incidence of paraplegia after prevertebral surgery. A normal arterial pressure must be maintained during operation.

▶ [The anesthesiologists would do well to read this article and the preceding one, both about the arterial blood supply to the lower spinal cord. The information might come in handy.—Eds.]

Direct Revascularization with Coronary Gas Endarterectomy is discussed by Philip N. Sawyer[6] (State Univ. of New York Downstate Med. Center). About 100 coronary gas endarterectomies have been done, most in the right coronary artery. About half the vessels treated were patent after 18 months. The technic had been used in peripheral vessels. All side branches became patent when coronary gas endarterectomy was applied at autopsy in a patient who had died in cardiogenic shock. Studies also were done in dogs. Lactate metabolism reverted to normal in the first patient treated, a premenopausal woman, aged 50, who is still alive.

The right coronary is dissected out and gassed. The artery is incised, and a gas endarterectomy spatula is inserted. The

(6)   New York J. Med. 70: 1995-2002, Aug. 1, 1970.

vessel core is extracted and, if dissection must be extended distally, a more distal incision is made. The most distal dissection is in a small intramuscular branch with considerable outflow through opened side branches and distal run-off. Distal gassing is done largely to separate all of the distal core. A Christmas tree trunk is then pulled out proximally with all its branches. In many cases, combined technics were used, including gas endarterectomy in the right coronary artery with venous bypass into the arteriotomy used to carry out the endarterectomy from the aortic route. Right gas endarterectomy has also been combined with left anterior descending venous bypass, with single or double Vineberg implants into the left ventricular wall.

Five of 28 patients died, 4 after attempted right and left or left total coronary reconstruction. The 23 survivors had 16 early patent vessels. Patency could often be predicted at operation. All the operations were done on totally occluded coronary arteries; most had little wisps of retrograde back-filling. Reocclusion occurred almost immediately if good backflow and, thus, good run-off were not obtained at operation. Arteries with good backflow tended to remain open.

Diagnosis of Hyperthyroidism and Hypothyroidism by Laboratory Methods. Colum A. Gorman and William M. McConahey[7] believe that a small number of carefully chosen, properly used thyroid function tests will provide a correct diagnosis of thyroid overactivity or underactivity in almost all instances. In primary hypothyroidism the thyroid cannot respond even to the large amount of thyroid-stimulating hormone (TSH) released by the pituitary, nor does it respond to injected TSH. In secondary hypothyroidism the pituitary cannot release enough TSH even to maintain normal thyroid function, but the response to injected TSH is normal. Nearly all of the thyroid hormone carried in the blood is bound to serum proteins, and binding anomalies can cause the total serum thyroxine (T_4) to vary widely without corresponding changes in metabolic status. Free thyroxine determination is helpful in these circumstances.

Recent drug use and contrast medium administration should be inquired about. Protein-bound iodine (PBI) and ^{131}I uptake should not be determined when iodide contamination is likely. Protein-bound iodine and total circulating hormone should not be measured when binding is affected, as by oral contraceptives or estrogens; instead, free T_4 should be determined. A single

(7)   M. Clin. North America 54:1037-1047. July, 1970.

CHOICE OF THYROID FUNCTION TESTS IN SPECIAL CLINICAL SITUATIONS

TESTS FOR DIAGNOSIS OF THYROID DISEASE

PROBLEM	Suitable	Not Suitable
Graves' disease	BMR,* PBI, BEI,† total and free T_4, ^{131}I uptake, T_3 test, T_3 suppression test	TSH stimulation test, TSH immunoassay, Achilles tendon reflex (our opinion, because of considerable overlap of values from normal and hyperthyroid subjects)
Toxic nodular goiter	BMR, PBI, BEI, total and free T_4, radioiodine thyroid scan	Routine ^{131}I uptake without thyroid scan. (In many cases of this disease, over-all uptake of ^{131}I is normal, but *distribution within gland* is abnormal, and only scan can show it.)
Primary hypothyroidism	PBI, BEI, total and free T_4, BMR, TSH stimulation test, TSH immunoassay, Achilles tendon reflex	Thyroid scan. (Even standard ^{131}I tracer may be misleading, since some hypothyroid subjects, especially with Hashimoto's thyroiditis, may have ^{131}I uptake in normal range.)
Secondary hypothyroidism	PBI, BEI, total and free T_4, TSH stimulation test, head x-ray, visual-field examination, measurement of other pituitary hormones	Thyroid scan, TSH immunoassay. (Assay system is still not sensitive enough to distinguish between normal and subnormal values, but once hypothyroidism is diagnosed by other means, TSH assay will distinguish primary from secondary form.)
Hyperthyroidism in pregnancy	Free T_4, T_3 test. (T_3 test ordinarily gives low values in pregnancy. High-normal or above-normal values suggest hyperthyroidism.)	BMR, PBI, total T_4, ^{131}I uptake. (Values from all are increased during normal pregnancy.)
Hypothyroidism in pregnancy	Achilles tendon reflex, free T_4, TSH immunoassay	BMR, PBI, total T_4, ^{131}I uptake. (Values from these may be normal when patient is truly hypothyroid. If low, they are diagnostic of hypothyroidism.)

Thyroid dysfunction; recent gallbladder x-ray	BMR, total‡ and free T_4, red blood cell or resin T_3, Achilles tendon reflex (for hypothyroid patients)	PBI, BEI, ^{131}I uptake, T_4 by column, thyroid scan
Hyper- or hypothyroidism; patient taking estrogens, androgens, diphenylhydantoin or salicylates	BMR, ^{131}I uptake, free T_4, Achilles tendon reflex	PBI, BEI, total T_4
Euthyroid on thyroid hormone. Receiving thyroid hormone unnecessarily?	Stop medication, recheck thyroid function in 8-10 weeks, TSH stimulation test	(Any other tests performed during replacement therapy merely reflect combined effects of patient's own thyroid plus drug.)
Patient receiving Lugol's solution for control of Graves' disease. Is therapy adequate?	BMR, serum total and free T_4	PBI, BEI, ^{131}I uptake

*BMR, basal metabolic rate.
‡BEI, serum butanol-extractable iodine.
‡Murphy Pattee method or resin-sponge method.

test should not be relied on for definitive diagnosis. When feasible it is often wise to determine the thyroidal ^{131}I accumulation, the circulating thyroid hormone level and the impact of thyroid hormone on the organism. Tests such as the immunoassay measurement of TSH and the Achilles tendon reflex are more effective in diagnosing hypothyroidism than hyperthyroidism. The TSH stimulation test and the triiodothyronine (T_3) suppression test may be used to confirm the diagnosis. Even the best tests are only indirect measures of thyroid function. The results should be interpreted in the light of clinical evidence, and the tests should be repeated if results seem inconsistent. If results are still inconsistent, another parameter of iodide metabolism or thyroid function should be measured. Tests to be used in special clinical situations are indicated in the table.

► [Those interested in this area should read the article in its entirety, as the newer tests are explained quite clearly. We must understand the significance of these tests if we are to avoid the pitfalls well-known to exist in anesthetizing patients with abnormal thyroid function.—Eds.]

Hemodynamic Response to Chronic Renal Failure as Studied in the Azotemic State. J. W. Mostert, J. L. Evers, G. H. Hobika, R. H. Moore, G. M. Kenny and G. P. Murphy[8] (Roswell Park Mem'l Inst., Buffalo) report 59 hemodynamic studies in 9 men and 12 women patients, aged 19-61, who had chronic renal failure and were maintained on periodic hemodialysis during 1969; the patients were studied when blood urea nitrogen was between 75 and 125 mg./100 ml.

METHOD.—Radiopaque polyethylene tubing, 1.65 mm. in external diameter and 90 cm. long, was passed percutaneously via subclavian or right internal jugular vein into the right ventricle and sometimes into the pulmonary artery under continuous ECG and pressure monitoring. Care was taken not to "float" the catheter more than about 1 cm. distal to the tricuspid valve to avoid catheter coiling in a dilated cardiac chamber or its tributaries (Fig. 45). Blood was sampled from a cannulated brachial artery. Blood volume was measured by the Volemetron computer with radioiodinated serum albumin-^{125}I as indicator. Cardiac output was measured by a dye dilution technic in which 3.75 mg. indocyanine green was rapidly flushed into the cavity of the right ventricle. Blood gas analysis was done within 20 minutes of sampling with the use of Radiometer equipment. An arterial gauge was used to measure airway pressure during the Valsalva maneuver in which the patient tried to blow a column of mercury under direct vision to 40 mm. Hg for 10 seconds. For comparison, the Valsalva maneuver was similarly used in 7 patients with lung cancer but without diseased kidneys.

―――――――
(8) Brit. J. Anaesth. 42:397-411, May, 1970.

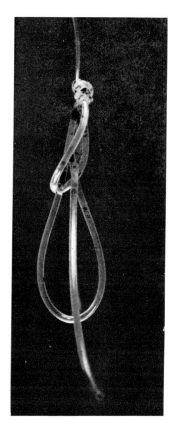

Fig. 45.—Multiple knots in miniature cardiac catheter after it was allowed to curl in cavity of right atrium, where movement of heart spontaneously initiated formation of knots. Attenuated part just proximal to knots shows the force that had to be overcome to pull knots free from the vascular system. (Courtesy of Mostert, J. W., *et al.*: Brit. J. Anaesth. 42:397-411, May, 1970.)

Of 21 patients, 15 had radiologic evidence of pulmonary edema during at least 1 of the studies. Hemodynamic measurements showed that mean cardiac output and right heart and arterial pressures were high but that total peripheral resistance was only slightly increased; heart rates were normal. Metabolic acidosis with respiratory alkalosis was common. Studies also showed increased arteriovenous oxygen content difference and zero or negative base excess in every case. Average travel time of indocyanine green from right ventricle to the densitometer was 7.7 seconds. The 32 studies in 20 patients showed that blocked arterial response to the Valsalva maneuver was the rule and pulse pressure was abnormally maintained during strain. Pulse pressure widened significantly during phases 2

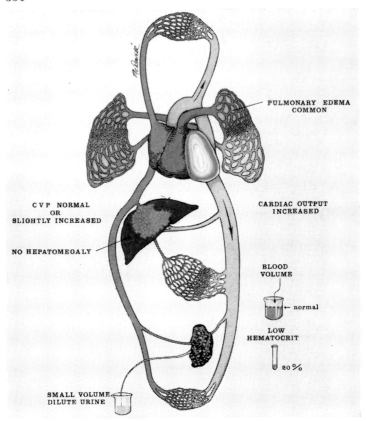

MEAN ARTERIAL HYPERTENSION

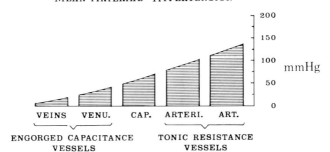

Fig. 46.—Circulation in patients with chronic renal failure. Severe anemia and elevated cardiac output is usually accompanied by hypertension and pulmonary edema. There is absence of an expanded blood volume and normal or only slightly increased central venous pressure. (Courtesy of Mostert, J. W., *et al.*: Brit. J. Anaesth. 42:397-411, May, 1970.)

and 3 of the maneuver. Although the 7 patients with lung cancer also responded abnormally to the Valsalva maneuver, reduced pulse pressure constriction of uremic patients showed significantly more cardiac failure (Cudkowicz, 1968). On the basis of ideal predicted blood volumes (Nadler et al., 1962), measured blood volumes were not expanded, although the mean increase was some 200 ml. When the catheter was floated into the right ventricle, no untoward effects were noted, except occasional, transient, premature ventricular contractions; the catheter was advanced beyond the pulmonary valve in 32 studies. At 6 studies, 4 patients showed a square-wave arterial response indicating heart failure; in each case, this response was associated with x-ray evidence of acute pulmonary edema and expanded blood volume. Of 3 chronically uremic patients in whom acute interstitial pulmonary edema was diagnosed on the basis of dyspnea, orthopnea and mental distress and x-ray patterns of perihilar and interstitial edema, all had normal right atrial pressure; 2 of the 3 patients had pulmonary arterial hypertension and 2, significantly expanded blood volume. Figure 46 shows the outstanding features of circulation in patients with chronic renal failure as ascertained in the present study.

Brain Metabolism in Experimental Uremia. Abnormally high nucleotide and sugar phosphate levels have been reported in the red blood cells of uremic patients; incubation of erythrocytes with adenine increases total adenine nucleotide levels. Stanley van den Noort, Robert E. Eckel, Katherine L. Brine and Jeffry Hrdlicka[9] (Case Western Reserve Univ.) studied changes in rat brain and blood nucleotide levels after the infusion of adenosine or adenosine monophosphate (AMP).

Intact and nephrectomized rats received 0.5 mM. adenosine or AMP intraperitoneally in 6 hours. Six rats had 75% nephrectomy and were followed for 3 months.

Spontaneous behavior was reduced and responses to noise were excessive 48 hours after nephrectomy. The blood urea nitrogen level rose from 18 to 240 mg./100 ml. and the blood pH value fell to 7.16. Subtotally operated animals had no symptoms and an average blood urea nitrogen level of only 40 mg./100 ml. Rats given adenosine or AMP were unusually tame and had an average blood urea nitrogen level of 53 mg./100 ml.

Blood nucleotide concentrations were not significantly altered in uremic rats. Both types of infusion increased total

(9) Arch. Int. Med. 126:831-834, November, 1970.

adenine nucleotide levels. Acutely uremic and infused animals had a significant increase in brain adenosine triphosphate (ATP) concentrations but also a significant reduction in adenosine diphosphate (ADP) and AMP levels. Total adenine nucleotides were unchanged.

The brain creatine phosphate level was elevated. The brain lactate level was low and the glucose concentration was high in uremic and infused animals. Utilization of ATP was markedly deficient in acutely uremic rats; glucose utilization was enhanced. The adenylate kinase ratio was unaffected by uremia and fell with ischemic anoxia. The whole brain Na-K-ATPase value was normal in uremic rats. The brain metabolic rate was reduced in uremic rats.

Uremia, like anesthesia, depresses brain utilization of ATP without apparent inhibition of the capacity to produce ATP. Adenosine infusion, like sleep, permits normal utilization of ATP but enhances the potential for ATP synthesis.

Diagnosis and Treatment of β-Adrenergic Receptor Hyperresponsiveness: Critical Appraisal is presented by Henry R. Bourne, Pate D. Thomson and Kenneth L. Melmon[1] (Univ. of California). Patients with irritable or "hyperkinetic" hearts often have labile tachycardia, palpitations, chest discomfort and varying degrees of exercise intolerance. Frohlich *et al.* (1969) suggested that at least some of these patients have hyperresponsive cardiac β-adrenergic receptors. Isoproterenol increased the heart rate of such patients threefold more than in normal control subjects. Other workers found a much greater cardioacceleration during isoproterenol infusion. Several factors in the studies might account for this difference, including variable dose calculations. Frohlich treated normal subjects with a body surface area 11% greater than that of the patients, and the drug apparently was not given on a weight basis. Studies with atropine indicate that "hypersensitive" patients have normal vagal tone. Controversy on the role of the sympathetic nervous system in thyrotoxicosis provides a parallel situation. The evidence for β-adrenergic supersensitivity is far from conclusive. The isoproterenol infusion test must be standardized, and effects of variations in vagal tone should be ruled out in further experiments.

No treatment may be necessary to improve longevity and productivity in these patients. A double-blind therapeutic trial might establish whether a "pure" β-antagonist could effectively

(1) Arch. Int. Med. 125: 1063-1066, June, 1970.

abolish the syndrome. The finding that specific β-blockade was superior to sedation and placebo in these patients would strengthen the view that their β-receptors are abnormal. Even if pure β-blockade abolished the syndrome, abnormal β-receptors might not be the primary cause. No controlled trial has been reported showing propranolol to be more effective than any other therapy, including placebo, in patients with a hyperkinetic circulatory state. At present, sources of anxiety should be sought, and psychotherapy or sedative-tranquilizing agents tried. Pharmacologic β-adrenergic blockade should be kept as a last resort for patients whose activities are severely limited by their symptoms.

Involvement of Peripheral Nerves in Radical Neck Dissection. Thomas R. Swift[2] (Cornell Univ.) assessed incidence and distribution of peripheral nerve involvement after radical neck dissection in 24 patients in whom 15 unilateral and 9 bilateral dissections were done by standard technic (Martin *et al.*, 1951)

Fig. 47.—Nerve structures that might be involved by radical neck dissection. (Courtesy of Swift, T. R.: Am. J. Surg. 119:694-698, June, 1970.)

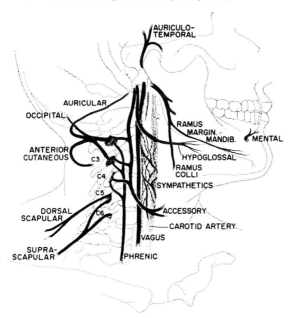

(2)   Am. J. Surg. 119:694-698, June, 1970.

during 1951-67. Patients had epidermoid carcinoma of the tongue (2), nasopharynx (1), tonsil (3), floor of the mouth (2) and larynx (1); adenocarcinoma of the thyroid (2); squamous carcinoma of the palate (2), tongue (5) and larynx (4); and papillary carcinoma of the thyroid (2). Follow-up was 2 months to 16 years. Routine maneuvers were used in testing for muscle weakness; strength was graded on a 5-point scale. Sensory loss was identified and mapped by testing with a pin. Phrenic nerve paralysis was judged by comparing pre- and postoperative chest x-rays. Operative summaries and pathology reports were reviewed. Four patients had electromyography to confirm evidence of denervation in muscles believed to be clinically involved and to see if there was evidence of denervation in muscles believed to be normal. Figure 47 shows the area exposed by radical neck dissection and the neural structures which might be damaged.

The table lists the peripheral nerves involved in the 33 radi-

INVOLVEMENT OF PERIPHERAL NERVES IN 33 RADICAL
NECK DISSECTIONS

	Nerve	Involved in Radical Neck Dissection	Noted to be Excised in Operative Report	Percentage Involved
I.	Facial (excluding branches of platysma) Ramus marginalis			
	mandibularis	22	3	67
	Other	0	0	0
II.	Glossopharyngeal	3	2	10
III.	Vagus	5	4	15
IV.	Accessory	33	33	100
V.	Hypoglossal	13	7	39
VI.	Dorsal scapular (rhomboids)	2	0	6
VII.	Medial and lateral thoracic nerves (pectoralis)	2	0	6
VIII.	Sympathetic	11	0	33
IX.	Cervical plexus and supraclavicular nerves	33	0	100
X.	Suprascapular	2	0	6
XI.	Phrenic	3	0	10

cal neck dissections. Muscle power and sensation subserved by the 7th, 9th, 10th, 11th and 12th cranial nerves and the 2d through 5th cervical roots (and possibly lower) were involved. Weakness of the orbicularis oris and depressor anguli oris after 21 dissections produced only slight corner-of-the-mouth drooping. The 3 patients with glossopharyngeal involvement did not complain of loss of taste or sensation in the pharynx. All 5 patients with vagus nerve involvement complained of persistent hoarseness but not of dysphagia. Most acknowledged shoulder weakness, but all had shoulder drooping and slight scapular winging. All 13 with tongue involvement acknowledged disability, but none volunteered this as a complaint. Only 1 patient complained of sensory loss despite the large hypoesthetic area. His sensory loss extended anteriorly to just above the nipple line, laterally to below the deltoid insertion (overlapping the area supplied by the upper lateral cutaneous nerve of the arm) sparing the axilla skin, posteriorly across the scapular spine, superiorly to the occiput and including almost the entire ear. The 3 with phrenic nerve involvement had no complaints or clinical signs referable to this. Although Horner's syndrome occurred after 11 operations, the only alteration was miosis, often with slight ptosis. An electromyograph could not be obtained from 2 patients with rhomboid weakness and 2 with pectoralis muscle weakness. One patient showed massive hypertrophy of the levator scapulae, and denervation was also found on electromyography.

Except for the high incidence of postoperative Horner's syndrome, the frequency of unsuspected phrenic nerve involvement and the large hypoesthetic skin areas, neurologic complications of radical neck dissection in this series conform to what might be predicted from knowing the nervous structures at risk. Any patient with neurologic disability going beyond this characteristic clinical picture should be suspected of having recurrent cancer.

Implantable Nuclear-Powered Cardiac Pacemakers are discussed by John C. Norman, Glenn W. Sandberg, Jr., and Fred N. Huffman.[3] The possibility of using isotopic energy to provide long-lived implantable electric power sources for cardiac pacemakers is receiving international attention. The units, comparable in size to conventional pacers, last 10-20 years and are reliable. The primary components are an isotopic fuel capsule;

(3) New England J. Med. 283:1203-1206, Nov. 26, 1970.

a direct thermodynamic converter, either thermoelectric or thermionic; thermal insulation; and an optional power conditioner to convert the low-voltage output to the higher voltage required by conventional pacemaker circuitry. Most groups have used ^{238}Pu as the fuel; it has a long half-life, reasonable power density, low radiation output and relatively reasonable cost. Usually a thermopile of thermocouples connected in series is used to convert heat to electricity. Vacuum foil insulators are now available.

So far the effects of prolonged intracorporeal irradiation from ^{238}Pu sources more than 2 orders of magnitude larger than pacemaker fuel capsules have been benign in dogs, except for minor pathologic changes and subtle chromosome alterations not unlike those reported after diagnostic irradiation. Exposure of other persons by the bearer of an isotopic pacer will probably be inconsequential. Patients will have to be clearly identified if such devices come into widespread use. Accurate cost analyses are not now available, but fuel loadings indicate a ^{238}Pu cost of from $150 to $400 for each unit. The cost, although high initially, is not prohibitive. These pacemakers may require licensing to assure quality control. The primary problem is continued maintenance of fuel capsule integrity under all conditions. Restricted clinical application may be expected in the near future.

▶ [This seems an excellent use for nuclear power and will spare the patient the problems and cost of repeated battery implantation. The isotope has a very long half-life and emits the high-energy alpha particle along with low-energy gammas, both of which are readily contained. There would be a distinct hazard if the fuel capsule were broken, as might occur, for instance, in an automobile accident.—Eds.]

Electric Hazards in the Operating Room, with Special Reference to Electrosurgery are discussed by K. W. Taylor and J. Desmond[4] (Univ. of Toronto). The hazard of explosion and fire in the operating room has been much reduced by replacement of cyclopropane and ether by noncombustible anesthetic agents, but adherence to safety codes has been relaxed. Materials used for cleaning and sterilizing may be flammable and demand the same care as anesthetics. Electrosurgery should not be used in the presence of explosive anesthetics, especially cyclopropane.

About twenty electrocutions occur in Ontario annually, about half of them due to high voltages. However, electrocution is

(4) Canad. J. Surg. 13:362-374, October, 1970.

TABLE 1.—PHYSIOLOGIC EFFECTS OF ELECTRIC CURRENTS

FREQUENCY	CURRENT	EFFECT	RESULT
60 cps	About 100 μa.	Possible fibrillation when passing directly through heart wall via catheter	Fibrillation and possible death
		Local nerve stimulation when passed through skin via small contact close to nerve ending	Nerve pain like pin prick
	About 1 ma.	Some stimulation of sensory nerves in the hand	Tingling feeling
	About 10 ma.	Continuous stimulation of sensory and motor nerves and muscles	Pain and muscle contraction. Electric shock Unable to release grip
	About 100 ma.	Continuous massive stimulation of muscles and nerves. Fibrillation Local heating of tissues	Death from fibrillation, burns
Direct current	100 μa. to 100 ma.	Increasing severity as for 60 cps but only single stimulation of nerves and muscles on first contact	Shock on contact. Able to release grip. Death less likely but burns just as likely
Above 100,000 cps	1 amp.	No nerve or muscle stimulation. Intense tissue heating	Burns
Single pulsed discharges	10 ma. to 10 amp.	Increasing severity of single nerve and muscle stimulation	Shock. Cardiac arrest. Burn

TABLE 2.—SITUATIONS IN WHICH ELECTROSURGERY MAY CAUSE ACCIDENTAL BURNS

SITUATION	EFFECT	REMEDY
Ground plate correctly sited but:		
1. Drying saline pad or towels	Painful skin burn at plate varying in size and severity Surgeon asks for more power	Use only for short operations and minimal use of electrosurgery
2. Drying electrode jelly	As in 1	Use correct electrode jelly for long operations and extensive use of electrosurgery
3. Patient contact with grounded table, clamps, conductive mattress, arm rests direct or through saline-soaked drapes	Burns as in 1 at contact areas. Usually small	Keep such contact away from operative site and ground plate Avoid soaking drapes in saline if possible. Insulate with oiled silk where position creates hazard
4. ECG electrodes	Deep local burn possibly requiring plastic surgery	Keep electrodes away from site of operation and ground plate. Use ECG monitor with high impedance to high frequencies
5. Broken ground lead	Severe burns at any grounded contact possibly needing plastic surgery	Careful inspection and maintenance Use machines with ground alarm
6. Power accidentally applied to active electrode which is resting on drapes	Deep local burn possibly needing plastic surgery	Do not rest electrode on bare tissue Avoid saline-soaked drapes. Use sound alarm to warn of activation of machine

Ground plate poorly sited:

7. Thin bony patient	Skin burn, deep burn Cooking effect with tissue swelling and rigidity	Apply ground plate where patient contact will be greater
8. Plate far from site of operation	Use of more power; greater danger of burns and other tissue heating	Site plate as close as possible to area of operation; otherwise see 9
9. Plate far from site of operation, contact with grounded table, etc. as in 3 between sites of plate and operation	As in 8	Avoid soaking drapes in saline. If not possible insulate all ground contacts with oiled silk

Contact of operating room (OR) personnel with high voltage:

10. Through capacitive leakage to OR table and other metal objects	Small skin burns	Avoid contact when electrosurgery is in use
11. By spark breakdown of gloves	Small skin burns, side effects from unexpected mechanical reaction	Use thick gloves or avoid contact with bare metal to which active electrode is applied. Use forceps with insulated handles

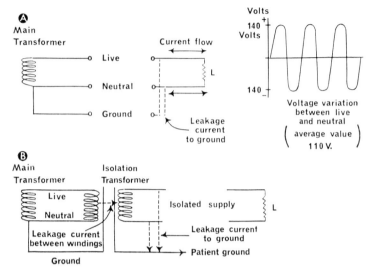

Fig. 48.—Grounded (A) and isolated (B) power supplies. (Courtesy of Taylor, K. W., and Desmond, J.: Canad. J. Surg. 13:362-374, October, 1970.)

rare in Ontario hospitals. When it occurs, it is usually due to poor maintenance of electric equipment or power supply or to inferior equipment design. The patient should be isolated from ground, but this is often not possible with present equipment. Electric shock is a warning of danger; methods of prevention are the same as for electrocution. Leaking current or static electricity from intracardiac catheters may cause fibrillation or arrest. Simple limeters are available to reduce the current that can flow along a cardiac catheter. Deep electrosurgical burns are relatively frequent and are commonly due to multiple grounding of the patient and the operator's ignorance or carelessness. Defibrillation burns are now uncommon. Operating room personnel must be instructed in the hazards of using electric equipment.

The physiologic effects of electric currents depend on strength of current frequency of alternation and site of entry into the body (Table 1). A 60-cycle current of sufficient strength continuously stimulates nerves and muscles. A current of 100 μa. can cause sharp pain and withdrawal reactions. Operating room personnel should be familiar with the characteristic situations in which electrosurgical burns may occur (Table 2). Both the site of the ground plate and its manner of application are important. The electrode contact should be checked if the effectiveness of electrosurgery decreases at a given power setting. Complete isolation is impossible at electrosurgical frequencies because of capacitive leakage of current. ECG electrodes should still be placed away from the operative area and the ground plate. Grounded and isolated power supplies are illustrated in Figure 48. Equipment must be well maintained if it is to function properly and safely.

▶ [A detailed report by a director of medical engineering (K. W. Taylor). How often have you seen the circulating nurse increase the cautery current because it wasn't working well—usually due to poor ground rather than inadequate amount of power?—Eds.]

Professional Liability of Anesthesiologist is discussed by Frank A. Manthey and William R. Murphy[5] (New Haven, Conn.). Anesthesiology is highly exposed to medical malpractice claims. In a study of 700 liability claims in California in 1957, anesthesiologists ranked second to surgeons in total claims. Generally, a plaintiff must establish that the physician failed to exercise the degree of skill or diligence ordinarily exercised by physicians engaged in the same type of practice in the same general area. Anesthesiologists cannot guarantee a favorable result nor are they liable for bona fide errors in judgment when the requisite care and skill are exercised. Application of this doctrine to particular cases is difficult. The locality has been eroded in certain jurisdictions and, in some, a general practitioner is not required to use the care commensurate with that exercised by experts in a given specialty.

Certain national standards of care have been established in the practice of anesthesiology, departure from which is likely to render an anesthesiologist liable in a malpractice suit if injury results. Examples of substandard practices are the sterilization of spinal anesthesia ampules in alcohol and the performance of general anesthesia without suctioning equipment reasonably available. True standards of care must be distinguished from mere differences in technic. Where differences in technic are involved, the development at trial of a factual record showing that the technic at issue is accepted by numerous specialists throughout the country will help protect an anesthesiologist against an unwarranted finding of malpractice.

An express written consent for anesthesia given by an adult in the presence of an independent witness is desirable wherever

---

(5) Connecticut Med. 34:714-718, October, 1970.

possible, but it is not absolutely necessary that the consent be written, or even expressed. There are few cases in which claims based on informed consent have been made against anesthesiologists. When advising a patient of risks would be detrimental, it is best to advise a relative of such risks.

It is important to make adequate records of pertinent discussions, observations, treatments and medications in all aspects of medical practice. Such records are helpful in protecting the physician against unmeritorious malpractice claims.

▶ [We would all do well when criticizing a colleague to recall that standards of care must be dissociated from mere differences in technic.—Eds.]

PAIN PROBLEMS

On the Language of Pain. R. Melzack and W. S. Torgerson[6] point out that although the description of pain is of daily concern to physicians, few studies have attempted to specify the dimensions of pain experience. The emphasis on measuring over-all pain intensity has led to neglect of the qualities of pain, reflecting the wide acceptance of Frey's concept of pain as a specific modality of cutaneous sensation. There is evidence that a multitude of nerve impulse patterns is transmitted centrally from the skin by various stimuli. "Pain" must refer to an endless variety of qualities categorized under a single linguistic label. An attempt has now been made to specify the qualities of pain. Dallenbach collected 44 words describing pain qualities and classed them into groups characterizing the temporal course of the experience, its spatial distribution, its fusion or integration with pressure, its affective coloring and purely qualitative attributes. Other words were added to provide a total of 102, classed in three major groups and 13 subgroups. The classes were words describing sensory qualities, those describing affective qualities and evaluative words describing the subjective over-all intensity of the total pain experience.

Words were presented to 20 educated subjects of both sexes, with a mean age of 29.9 years, for evaluation as to correctness of classification in a forced-choice format. Significant agreement was found for only one word, "itchy," placed in the brightness subclass. A significant pattern nevertheless emerged (table). Groups of students, physicians and patients were then

---

(6)   Anesthesiology 34:50-59, January, 1971.

CLASSES AND SUBCLASSES OF PAIN DESCRIPTORS* AS RATED BY
DOCTORS, PATIENTS AND STUDENTS

		Doctors			Patients			Students	Scale Value	Dis-criminal Dis-persion Value
		Mean	SD		Mean	SD				
SENSORY										
Temporal										
	FLICKERING	1.40	.50	FLICKERING	1.89	.94	FLICKERING		−1.57	.94
	QUIVERING	1.60	.75	QUIVERING	2.50	.83	QUIVERING		−.74	.81
	PULSING	2.30	1.03	PULSING	2.56	.92	Thumping		−.52	.78
	THROBBING	2.55	.94	Thumping	2.68	.67	PULSING		−.27	.84
	Thumping	2.55	.94	THROBBING	2.68	1.00	THROBBING		.09	.94
	BEATING	2.75	.97	BEATING	2.70	.98	BEATING		.19	.83
	POUNDING	3.10	.97	POUNDING	2.85	1.14	POUNDING		.21	.91
Spatial										
	Spreading	1.80	.77	JUMPING	2.60	.75	JUMPING		−1.05	.93
	JUMPING	2.10	.79	FLASHING	2.75	.97	Radiating		−.68	1.13
	Radiating	2.30	.80	Spreading	3.30	.98	Darting		−.58	.76
	FLASHING	2.55	1.05	Radiating	3.38	1.15	Spreading		−.34	.95
	SHOOTING	3.15	.74	SHOOTING	3.42	.90	FLASHING		−.17	1.11
							SHOOTING		.44	.92
Punctate pressure										
	PRICKING	1.60	.68	PRICKING	1.94	1.11	PRICKING		−1.04	.99
	BORING	2.75	1.02	BORING	2.05	.83	BORING		−.34	1.18
	DRILLING	2.75	.79	DRILLING	2.75	1.37	Digging		.05	.90
	Penetrating	2.90	.64	STABBING	3.45	.89	Penetrating		.11	.92
	Piercing	3.30	.66	LANCINATING	3.50	.98	Piercing		.76	.86
	STABBING	3.40	.75	Penetrating	3.72	.89	STABBING		.95	.97
	LANCINATING	3.65	.67	Piercing	3.78	.58				
Incisive pressure										
	SHARP	2.70	.73	SHARP	2.95	.94	SHARP		.32	.90
	CUTTING	3.10	.55	CUTTING	3.20	.95	CUTTING		.35	.97
	LACERATING	3.50	1.02	LACERATING	3.64	1.16	LACERATING		.93	1.05
Constrictive pressure										
	PINCHING	1.55	.51	PINCHING	1.95	.82	Nipping		−1.10	.96
	Nipping	1.70	.66	Nipping	2.00	.94	Tight		−.73	.69
	Tight	1.70	.73	Tight	2.25	.91	PINCHING		−.70	.94
	PRESSING	1.80	.62	Squeezing	2.35	.81	PRESSING		−.65	.69
	GNAWING	2.05	.69	PRESSING	2.42	.90	Gripping		−.15	.81
	Binding	2.20	.77	Binding	2.50	.86	Biting		−.05	.73
	Gripping	2.25	.91	GNAWING	2.53	.77	GNAWING		.01	.82
	Biting	2.30	.57	Biting	2.70	1.08	CRAMPING		.36	1.01
	Squeezing	2.30	.80	CRAMPING	2.75	.79	CRUSHING		1.20	.83
	CRAMPING	2.50	.83	Gripping	3.10	.74				
	CRUSHING	3.20	1.40	CRUSHING	3.58	1.02				
Traction pressure										
	TUGGING	1.70	.66	TUGGING	2.16	.60	TUGGING		−.84	.72
	PULLING	1.85	.74	PULLING	2.35	.59	PULLING		−.66	.80
	WRENCHING	2.70	.92	WRENCHING	3.47	.90	WRENCHING		.69	.71
Thermal										
	HOT	2.30	.99	HOT	2.47	.85	HOT		−.26	.92
	BURNING	2.95	.76	BURNING	2.95	.85	BURNING		.89	1.02
	SCALDING	3.65	.67	SCALDING	3.50	.98	SEARING		1.40	1.00
	SEARING	3.95	.89	SEARING	3.88	.89				
Brightness										
	Tickling	1.10	.31	Tickling	1.55	.60	TINGLING		−1.79	.87
	TINGLING	1.20	.41	TINGLING	1.60	.68	Tickling		−1.71	.97
	ITCHY	1.35	.74	ITCHY	1.70	.80	ITCHING		−1.25	.71
	SMARTING	1.85	.59	SMARTING	2.00	.82	SMARTING		−.62	.91
	STINGING	2.05	.82	STINGING	2.25	.85	STINGING		−.35	.83
Dullness										
	DULL	1.55	.60	DULL	1.60	.68	DULL		−.97	1.04
	Blurred	1.67	.91	SORE	1.90	.64	SORE		−.86	.88
	SORE	1.80	.69	Numbing	2.10	.88	Drawing		−.71	1.15
	Drawing	2.10	.79	HURTING	2.45	1.14	Steady		−.56	1.05
	Numbing	2.15	.81	ACHING	2.50	1.28	HURTING		−.39	.71
	HURTING	2.20	.62	Drawing	2.53	.84	ACHING		−.34	.81
	ACHING	2.20	.89	Blurred	2.59	1.12	HEAVY		−.33	1.03
	HEAVY	2.40	.75	Steady	2.65	1.22	Numbing		−.26	1.09
	Steady	2.40	.60	HEAVY	2.95	.94	Blurred		1.12	.98

*In each category, capitalized words have same rank order in all three groups of
subjects. Absence of one or more words in several subclasses reflects minor variations in lists during course of study.

(*cont.*)

(*cont.*) CLASSES AND SUBCLASSES OF PAIN DESCRIPTORS* AS RATED BY
DOCTORS, PATIENTS AND STUDENTS

		Doctors			Patients			Students	
		Mean	SD		Mean	SD		Scale Value	Dis-criminal Dis-persion Value
Sensory: miscellaneous									
	TENDER	1.80	.69	TENDER	1.35	.59	TENDER	−1.49	.96
	TAUT	1.85	.81	TAUT	2.36	1.01	TAUT	−.46	.92
	RASPING	2.50	.83	RASPING	2.61	.92	RASPING	−.06	.83
	Tearing	3.25	.79	SPLITTING	3.10	1.21	SPLITTING	.83	.82
	SPLITTING	3.30	.66	Tearing	3.68	.93			
AFFECTIVE Tension									
	Nagging	1.95	.51	Nagging	2.25	.79	TIRING	−1.26	.66
	Dragging	2.16	.83	Fatiguing	2.35	.61	Fatiguing	−.99	.76
	TIRING	2.20	.62	TIRING	2.42	.69	EXHAUSTING	−.63	.76
	Fatiguing	2.40	.68	EXHAUSTING	2.63	.96	Nagging	−.50	.69
	EXHAUSTING	3.20	.77	Dragging	2.95	.78			
Autonomic									
	Nauseating	3.10	1.07	Nauseating	2.74	.93	SICKENING	.24	1.00
	Choking	3.30	.73	SICKENING	2.75	.79	Nauseating	.42	1.15
	SICKENING	3.37	.68	SUFFOCATING	3.45	1.14	Choking	.65	.71
	SUFFOCATING	3.75	.85	Choking	3.55	1.10	SUFFOCATING	1.03	.87
Fear									
	FEARFUL	3.45	.89	FEARFUL	3.30	.92	FEARFUL	−.16	.69
	Dreadful	3.72	.85	FRIGHTFUL	3.53	.77	FRIGHTFUL	−.06	.70
	FRIGHTFUL	3.80	.70	TERRIFYING	3.95	1.08	Dreadful	.03	.65
	TERRIFYING	4.40	.68	Dreadful	4.11	.76			
Punishment									
	PUNISHING	3.45	.69	Racking	3.33	1.03	PUNISHING	−.07	.75
	GRUELLING	3.60	.75	PUNISHING	3.50	.79	GRUELLING	.17	.79
	Racking	3.70	.86	GRUELLING	3.73	.80	CRUEL	.22	.70
	CRUEL	3.95	.76	CRUEL	3.95	.89	VICIOUS	.71	.61
	VICIOUS	4.10	.72	VICIOUS	4.26	.99	Racking	.89	.91
	Torturing	4.45	.60	KILLING	4.50	.61	KILLING	.96	.82
	KILLING	4.45	.82	Torturing	4.53	.70			
Affective–evaluative–sensory: miscellaneous									
	Grinding	2.70	.80	Grinding	3.10	1.12	Awful	−.07	.71
	WRETCHED	3.30	1.22	WRETCHED	3.16	.83	WRETCHED	.02	.80
	Awful	3.35	.88	Awful	3.40	1.05	Wicked	.17	.76
	Wicked	3.75	.79	BLINDING	3.45	1.00	Grinding	.38	.90
	BLINDING	4.05	.82	Wicked	4.00	.74	BLINDING	1.67	1.01
EVALUATIVE									
	Distracting	1.60	.60	ANNOYING	1.89	.76	Mild	−2.03	.44
	ANNOYING	1.70	.57	Bearable	2.35	1.14	Bearable	−1.65	.72
	TROUBLESOME	1.85	.34	TROUBLESOME	2.42	.69	ANNOYING	−1.52	.63
	Bearable	2.15	.67	MISERABLE	2.85	.96	Distracting	−1.39	.73
	MISERABLE	2.95	.66	Distracting	2.89	.99	TROUBLESOME	−1.34	.56
	Ugly	3.00	1.00	Agonizing	3.20	1.67	Discomforting	−1.33	.59
	INTENSE	3.85	.59	Ugly	3.60	.99	Distressing	−.73	.69
	Violent	4.32	.48	INTENSE	3.75	1.12	Ugly	−.23	.79
	Agonizing	4.35	.59	Intolerable	4.18	.88	MISERABLE	−.21	.62
	Savage	4.58	1.65	UNBEARABLE	4.42	1.07	Horrible	.43	.66
	UNBEARABLE	4.63	.50	Savage	4.44	.98	INTENSE	.60	.68
	Intolerable	4.70	.47	Violent	4.55	.60	Agonizing	.93	.72
								Savage	.94	.74
								Violent	1.03	.78
								Intolerable	1.20	1.00
								UNBEARABLE	1.39	1.08
								Excruciating	1.65	.84

*In each category, capitalized words have same rank order in all three groups of subjects. Absence of one or more words in several subclasses reflects minor variations in lists during course of study.

asked to rate the words on a scale from least to most pain. The data were analyzed by Thurstone's categorical judgment model. Several words within each subclass were found to have the same relation in all three sets.

There are many words in English to describe pain, which may be classified as representing particular dimensions or properties of pain. Substantial numbers of words have about the same relative positions on a common intensity scale for persons with widely divergent backgrounds. This points the way toward eventual determination of the dimensions of the pain experience in analogy to visual and auditory experiences. Besides the words themselves, general anchor points in patients' usage of words must be determined, as must the spatial distribution of pain on or in the body and the temporal variation.

► [Those proposing a pain study will surely want to read this carefully.— Eds.]

Capillary Po₂ as Measure of Sympathetic Blockade. Many surgeons prefer to have a diagnostic sympathetic blockade with a local anesthetic agent done before performing surgical sympathectomy. The problem with chemical blockade is in proving that the sympathetic fibers have really been blocked and that a lack of beneficial effect is not due to a missed block. Phillip O. Bridenbaugh, Daniel C. Moore and L. Donald Bridenbaugh[7] (Seattle, Wash.) used the Astrup microtechnic to study skin capillary Po₂ before and after sympathetic blockade with local anesthetic agents. Elective surgical patients had sciatic or femoral block of the lower limb or brachial plexus block of the upper extremity. All were adults, and most underwent orthopedic procedures. Arterial, venous and skin capillary samples were taken from both extremities, the unblocked limb serving as control for the blocked one. Sampling was repeated in the post-block anesthetic period.

Data were obtained from 36 patients having femorosciatic block, 15 having supraclavicular brachial plexus block and 10 having axillary block. The mean difference in capillary Po₂ in the two feet was −1.2 mm. Hg before and 14.6 mm. Hg after femorosciatic block, comparing the blocked to the unblocked limb. No significant change occurred in the control limb after the block. The mean difference between the upper extremities was 0.6 mm. Hg before and 9.5 mm. Hg after the block, comparing the blocked to the unblocked extremity. The mean difference after the block was 6.5 mm. Hg in the blocked extremity and −3.4 mm. Hg in the unblocked one. The Pao₂ increased slightly in the upper extremity after the block, but no significant change occurred in the lower extremity. Venous Po₂ was significantly elevated in the blocked extremity but did not change significantly in unblocked extremities.

An improvement in the Po₂ of over 8 mm. Hg after regional

(7) Anesth. & Analg. 50:26-30, Jan.-Feb., 1971.

blockade is probably indicative of blockade of sympathetic activity. A unilateral nerve block is preferred if sympathetic blockade is required in only one extremity. It permits ambulation on crutches without orthostatic hypotension when the lower limb is operated on and allows comparison of the two limbs to evaluate the presence or absence of sympathetic activity. This comparison considerably increases the accuracy of predicting over the arbitrary 8-mm. Hg increase.

▶ [Interesting observations, but many surgeons have found that surgical sympathectomy will yield better than predicted results because the duration of the block may be more important than the quality of the block.—Eds.]

Therapeutic Epidural Block with Combination of Weak Local Anesthetic and Steroids in Management of Complicated Low Back Pain. Epidural block has been used only sporadically with steroids in treating low back pain. Kenneth O. Cho[8] (Georgetown Univ.) studied 5 men and 3 women, aged 29-58, who had lumbar laminectomy for the removal of a herniated intervertebral disk, and subsequent spinal fusion or repeated fusion for the repair of pseudarthrosis.

No patient had recurrent disk herniation at the same or a different level. All had severe persistent postoperative pain. Most often, multiple trigger points were found in the lower back, with tenderness at the sciatic notch and the posterior superior iliac spine. Straight-leg raising was limited, with or without sciatic pain. The pain had been present for 1-10 years since operation and conservative treatment had not given relief. Seven patients with recently herniated disks were also studied.

The L2-3 interspace is entered with the patient sitting or lying on his side and the epidural space is penetrated. From 20 to 30 ml. of 0.5% Xylocaine with 1 ml. Aristocort and Decadron is injected at a rate of about 5 ml. per minute. The patient is examined after the procedure.

No patient had objective motor or sensory changes. Straight-leg raising was increased and trigger points were markedly reduced or absent. All patients but 1 showed increased straight-leg raising from 20-70 to 60-90 degrees after epidural block. One patient had three blocks at 2-week intervals, with adequate relief. Relative relief from pain lasted 3-10 months except in 2 patients treated recently. All patients were significantly improved, although most had a recurrence of some pain 2-3 weeks after the block.

<hr>

(8)   Am. Surgeon 36:303-308, May, 1970.

Two of 7 patients with recent disk herniations did not improve at all; 1 had adenocarcinoma in the epidural space and 1 had a ruptured incarcerated disk with complete block. Two patients with large herniated disks improved only minimally. Three improved markedly after epidural blockade. The subarachnoid space was inadvertently entered in 2 patients, both of whom had headache. One patient had shortness of breath and hypotension. Three had temporary dizziness without appreciable changes in blood pressure.

Epidural block with 0.5% Xylocaine and steroids is recommended in patients with persistent residual low back pain after lumbar disk removal, especially when other treatment has been ineffective. Epidural block can differentiate surgical and nonsurgical conditions. Patients who do not respond favorably rarely improve significantly after continued conservative treatment and should be considered early surgical candidates.

Postdiscectomy pain may be related to a delay in reversing existing inflammatory changes in the nerve roots preoperatively, as well as scar tissue involvement of sensitive peridural structures. The block anesthetizes only fine recurrent meningeal nerve fibers temporarily and may break up periradicular adhesions as well as suppressing inflammatory nerve root changes to a tolerable level.

▶ [Several years ago, one of us (JWD) reviewed hundreds of postdisk surgical patients. Pain in these patients is complex. One must persist for long periods if one is to help these patients and relief may only be psychotherapeutic. Caution is advised before becoming too enthusiastic over the recommended treatment.—Eds.]

Subarachnoidal Injection Therapy in Chronic Cases of the So-Called Whiplash Syndrome. With the increase in whiplash injuries, treatment of the chronic sequelae is becoming important in clinics. Yasuo Tsumura and Takaaki Hoshiga[9] (Toyonaka, Japan) have developed an effective method for treating chronic posttraumatic cervical syndromes. The technic, called Tsumura's total spinal blocking method, consists of the subarachnoid infusion of an anesthetic at a high level to produce total spinal blockade. The drugs used were 18 ml. of 1.5% mepivacaine with 1:200,000 epinephrine, 4 mg. dexamethasone and 50 mg. thiamine pyrophosphate in a mixed solution of specific gravity 1.018. Drug amounts were adjusted by age and size of the patient. The injection was made with the patient lateral and the affected side down. The site was C7-T1 in pa-

(9)   Acta anaesth. scandinav. 15: 61-64, 1971.

tients with symptoms mainly in the upper region and L1-L2 in those with symptoms in the lower region.

The treatment was given to 113 men and 34 women, aged 21-52, all injured more than 5 months previously. Obvious organic changes were present in 31 cases, the commonest being narrowed intervertebral disks and osteophytosis. The principal complaints were headache, nuchal pain, neck and shoulder pain and numbness of the extremities. All symptoms disappeared within 1 week after spinal blockade in 22 of these patients (71%), but partial recurrence was apparent in 21 patients 1 month later. Forty of 106 patients without organic changes but with psychogenic complaints noted disappearance of all symptoms for 1 month; another 42 had marked improvement. There was no response in 7.7% of this group. Headache disappeared completely in 35.8% of the cases and to a considerable degree in another 32.1%. Nuchal pain was completely relieved in 27.7% of the cases and markedly improved in 38.4%. Numbness of the extremities disappeared in 53 (85.5%) of 62 cases and improved satisfactorily in 9. Tinnitus disappeared completely in 6 of 27 patients. Dizziness and nausea resolved completely in 6 of 21 cases.

Patients with whiplash syndrome and no organic changes, except for those with the Guillain-Barré syndrome, responded satisfactorily to total spinal blockade. The block was not satisfactory in most cases with ineffective therapy. This treatment is remarkably effective for chronic whiplash injury. The general condition of patients is unaltered. In using total spinal anesthesia with 1.5% mepivacaine with epinephrine for hysterectomy and other operations, there was a slight difficulty in adjusting the duration of anesthesia, but there were no disadvantages in regard to muscle relaxation, blood pressure, etc.

▶ [At first glance this seems like witchcraft, but one must acknowledge our current use of intrathecal saline and the great variability of the whiplash syndrome.—Eds.]

Civilian Experience with Causalgia. "Minor" causalgia or "reflex sympathetic dystrophy" is a misunderstood, often misdiagnosed clinical entity. Fremont P. Wirth, Jr., and Robert B. Rutherford[1] (Johns Hopkins Hosp.) reviewed the records of 32 patients with minor causalgia seen during 10 years, during which period there were 4 cases of "major" causalgia.

The median age of the 22 women and 10 men was 46 years.

(1)　Arch. Surg. 100:633-638, June, 1970.

The most common inciting events were fracture, operation, sprain and crush injury. Symptoms occurred in the lower limb in 23 cases and the upper limb in 9. The median delay between onset and treatment was 2 years. Osteoporosis was present in 7 of the 12 involved limbs examined by x-ray. The most common clinical features were burning pain, edema, increased sensitivity to touch and pressure, impaired motor function and muscle atrophy. Nineteen patients had been treated previously.

Neurolysis had a good effect in the only patient so treated. Sympathetic block had a temporary beneficial effect in 19 patients and a lasting effect in 3. Sympathectomy gave good relief in 24 of 27 patients; 16 of the 24 patients benefited had been relieved by a previous sympathetic block.

Fifteen patients who had undergone sympathectomy responded to a follow-up questionnaire; the average follow-up was $5\frac{1}{2}$ years. Thirteen patients reported complete relief from pain or gratifying improvement; 5 of these had had some return or increase in residual symptoms. Two of the 15 patients reported continued symptoms, but these did not resemble the original causalgic pain as described in their charts. All 6 patients in whom compensation was known to have been involved were relieved by sympathectomy. Twelve patients were considered to have a psychiatric disturbance, but only 2 of them had persisting emotional problems after pain was relieved.

Minor causalgia is more common than major causalgia in civilian practice. Early recognition is important as it is readily treated. The degree of pain is out of proportion to severity of the inciting cause or injury. The most reliable diagnostic test is paravertebral sympathetic block. Surgical sympathectomy relieves the pain. Failure to achieve satisfactory long-term results is generally due to incorrect diagnosis, long delay in treatment, incomplete sympathectomy or collateral reinnervation.

▶ [We doubt if anyone who has had much experience with this syndrome would argue with the conclusions.—Eds.]

Cord Paralysis Following Injection into Traumatic Cervical Meningocele: Complication of Stellate Ganglion Block is reported by Hugo Adam Keim[2] (Columbia-Presbyterian Med. Center). This was an unusual and serious complication.

Man, 44, incurred multiple fractures in a motorcycle accident, including fracture-dislocation of a hip, forearm fractures, and fracture-dislocation of the right humerus with a brachial plexus deficit. The hip fracture was reduced. The right arm and hand were devoid of

(2) New York J. Med. 70:2115-2116, Aug. 15, 1970.

motor control, but sensation remained in the medial aspect of the upper arm. Causalgia developed in the entire right arm and hand and required opiates. A right stellate ganglion block was attempted at 3 weeks, using a paratracheal approach. After two attempts at aspiration, 12 ml. of 1% lidocaine was injected. The patient became unable to speak and quickly lost all respiratory control. A resuscitator was applied, and then an endotracheal tube was inserted. The heart stopped after about 35 minutes. After about 45 seconds of cardiac standstill, the patient sat up and pulled the endotracheal tube from his mouth. The causalgic pain was greatly relieved. A Pantopaque cervical myelogram showed an avulsed nerve root sleeve at the C6-C7 level, the exact area where lidocaine had been injected.

The paratracheal approach is considered the safest for stellate ganglion block because of a lower risk of pneumothorax and the ease of execution. Such blocks should always be done where anesthetic assistance is available. The injecting needle should be completely rotated when aspiration is attempted, and a test dose should be injected. Bilateral blocks should be avoided. If no results are obtained, there should be at least an hour delay before the injection is repeated. Stellate ganglion blocks should be done by a skilled operator who is also familiar with emergency resuscitative procedures.

▶ [Some articles get very unusual titles. In this one, does "cord paralysis" refer to the vocal cord? Spinal cord? Spermatic cord? Although spinal anesthesia is not common after cervical sympathetic block, it is a constant potential danger.—Eds.]

MISCELLANEOUS

Enzyme Histochemical Studies of Liver during Immunosuppressive Treatment in Dogs. Azathioprine, the most widely used immunosuppressive agent in transplant surgery, is known to be hepatotoxic, but the effects of antilymphocyte serum and globulin on the liver are unknown. K. F. Aronson, B. Husberg, I. Hägerstrand, J. G. Nordén and B. Pihl[3] (Univ. of Lund) used enzyme histochemical technics to study the hepatotoxicity of these materials in beagles. Azathioprine and antilymphocyte IgG were given alone or in combination to groups of dogs. The dose of antilymphocyte globulin was 250 units (20 mg. antibody protein per kg.) twice daily for 5 days preoperatively and for 27 days postoperatively. Only one dose was given for the next week, and 125 units were given once daily for the next week. Azathioprine was given in a dose of 25 mg. per day postopera-

----

(3) Acta chir. scandinav. 136:529-536, 1970.

tively; some dogs received 50 mg. daily instead. The dose was temporarily reduced if the white blood cell count fell below 5,000/cu. mm. Liver biopsies were obtained after treatment.

Four of 5 dogs given azathioprine and antilymphocyte globulin showed small clusters of neutrophils with disruption of hepatic plates and single necrotic hepatocytes, usually after 2 or 3 weeks of treatment. Four had signs of biliary stasis after 3-7 weeks, but only 1 had marked cholestasis. Two of 5 dogs given azathioprine alone had discrete inflammatory foci, and 1 had bile thrombi after 9 weeks of treatment. Moderate vacuolation of hepatocyte cytoplasm resulted from treatment with antilymphocyte globulin alone in 2 dogs, as did cholestasis. Control dogs showed no necrosis or cholestasis. Succinate dehydrogenase changed inconsistently. Monamine oxidase, ATP and nonspecific esterase showed no consistent treatment-related changes. Acid phosphatase was increased in pericanalicular areas with bile thrombi and Kupffer cells stained more intensely than normally inside small inflammatory foci in some dogs. A stronger canalicular alkaline phosphatase reaction was seen in dogs given either agent. The γ-glutamyl transpeptidase reaction was reduced periportally in treated dogs. Dogs given azathioprine showed pathologic serum levels of serum glutamic pyruvic transaminase and alkaline phosphatase and, sometimes, bilirubin. Serum γ-glutamyl transpeptidase decreased in all treated dogs, often to zero.

The combination of a small dose of azathioprine with antilymphocyte globulin appears to be preferable to a large dose of azathioprine alone, but both agents cause cholestasis and increased alkaline phosphatase activity in hepatic tissue.

► [When evaluating possible liver toxicity of anesthetic agents given to patients receiving these drugs, studies such as these must be borne in mind.—Eds.]

Ventilatory Lung Scan in Diagnosis of Pulmonary Embolism. Gerald L. DeNardo, David A. Goodwin, Ruggero Ravasini and Peter A. Dietrich[4] assessed regional pulmonary blood-flow and ventilation in 10 patients with pulmonary embolism, 5 patients with other pulmonary diseases and 5 normal subjects by a dual perfusion-ventilation lung scan.

METHOD.—Patients, sitting or recumbent, were studied by Anger scintillation camera with the use of a diverging multichanneled collimator. Posterior, lateral and sometimes anterior views of the chest were obtained. Regional distribution of pulmonary blood flow was

(4) New England J. Med. 282:1334-1336, June 11, 1970.

determined after intravenous administration of 300 μCi macroaggregated human serum albumin-^{131}I or 3 mCi iron hydroxide particles-[113m]In. Particles, chiefly 25-50 μ in diameter, are trapped for a time in alveolar capillaries and precapillary arterioles and so permit images of perfused parts of the pulmonary arteriolar bed to be obtained. For each perfusion image, 100,000-300,000 counts were collected in 3-8 minutes. Regional distribution of ventilation was estimated after the patient fully expired to residual volume and then maximally inspired to total lung capacity from a spirometer containing 50 mCi (5 mCi/L.) radioactive xenon (^{133}Xe) in air. Since most patients inspired 2-5 L. of the mixture, 10-25 mCi ^{133}Xe was transferred temporarily to the lungs. In 5-15 seconds of breath holding, images with 100,000 counts were obtained. These high-resolution images of ventilation distribution within each lung were compared with the subject's perfusion scans. Perfusion scanning takes about 45 minutes and ventilation scanning, 30 minutes or less.

In normal lung perfusion or ventilation, radioactivity is uniformly distributed throughout both lung fields. On anterior projections, the heart, mediastinum and sometimes hili are areas of diminished or absent radioactivity. On posterior projections, vertebrae show no radioactivity. The left lateral view may show decreased radioactivity at the anteroinferior aspect in the heart area. The conventional scan pattern of major pulmonary embolism shows decreased or absent perfusion in areas served by the involved artery (Fig. 49, A). All involved areas

Fig. 49.—Anterior views of lungs of woman, 42, who suddenly had hemoptysis and pleuritic pain on the right side of chest 1 day before this study. Perfusion scan (A) reveals markedly decreased blood flow to most of right lung. Ventilation scan (B) is normal. Perfusion scan 19 days later (C) shows almost normal blood flow to right lung. The patient had received anticoagulants in the interval. Serial x-rays and determinations of serum lactic dehydrogenase gave normal results. (Courtesy of DeNardo, G. L., et al.: New England J. Med. 282:1334-1336, June 11, 1970.)

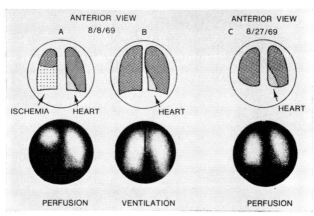

tend to be broader at the lung periphery and have an apex pointing toward the hilus. In the normal ventilatory scan, the lung outline is usually larger because the scintophoto is exposed after maximal inspiration. The 10 patients with embolism showed 10-50% perfusion abnormality, but only 1 of these 10 showed an abnormal ventilation distribution (5%). The other 9 ventilation scans were normal (Fig. 49, *B*). In 5 patients with other pulmonary diseases, mostly chronic obstructive disease, the abnormality in ventilatory pattern was equal to or greater than that of the perfusion pattern.

The dual perfusion-ventilation lung scan has proved to be a sensitive and specific approach to the diagnosis of pulmonary embolism. Since the radiation dose to the patient is low, the examination may be repeated to follow the course of the disease or the efficacy of treatment.

▶ [This technic appears to be the definitive way to diagnose pulmonary embolism. It does take time, but if the patient cannot endure this, he'd not be likely to survive any attempt at therapy.—Eds.]

Evoked Nerve Conduction after Nerve Block by Chemical Means. Phenol is still widely used to control spasticity, and reports on its mechanisms of action are inconclusive and contradictory. Ernst Fischer, Robert H. Cress, Gerald Haines, Nicholas Panin and Boris J. Paul[5] (Albany Med. College) examined the physiologic changes induced by the application of phenol and other chemical blocking agents in rabbits. An electrode was placed on the sciatic nerve of rabbits anesthetized with Nembutal, and the action potential at the posterior tibial nerve was recorded. Prolonged stimuli were used to activate slower fibers. Electroneurograms were recorded before and after partial nerve block with dilute aqueous phenol solutions.

The recording showed unequivocally that the entire spectrum of nerve fibers, with regard to diameter and conduction velocity, are affected essentially equally by this form of chemical blockade. Using dilute solutions of procaine, a distinct preference for the smaller diameter, slower conducting nerve fibers, including the gamma efferent fibers, was evident. Using weak ethanol solutions, no discrimination was noted according to fiber diameter or conduction velocity.

A blocking action on the gamma motor fibers can no longer be invoked as the mechanism by which partial phenol block reduces spasticity without significantly affecting voluntary motor control. Dilute aqueous phenol solutions do not specifically

(5) Am. J. Phys. Med. 49:333-347, December, 1970.

block only the smaller diameter gamma fibers of the rabbit sciatic nerve. Clinical depression of spasticity with relative preservation of volitional movement, noted after partial block of motor nerves by phenol, can be attributed to at least three mechanisms: (1) higher resistance to phenol by cutaneous sensory fibers than by proprioceptive afferent fibers; (2) a diminished afferent influence on alpha motor neuron activity in the spinal cord, restoring normal reciprocal innervation and reducing spasticity while retaining volitional movement; and (3) some reduction in the number of functioning alpha motor fibers that can affect spasticity relatively more than volitional movements.

▶ [Until this study was performed, most workers considered procaine, alcohol and phenol to have a selective blocking action in small-diameter, slow-conducting nerve fibers. Reduction of spasticity with preservation of volitional motion was explained on the basis of selective block of gamma motor fibers. This study shows that only procaine has this selective action and that phenol and alcohol lack it. The authors state that the explanation of the beneficial effects that follow phenol and dilute alcohol blocks are "still somewhat obscure."—Eds.]

Familial Dysautonomia is an inherited disease with protean manifestations largely attributable to abnormal nervous system function. The diagnosis may be made by noting a lack of fungiform papillae on the tongue, or by an impaired response to intradermal histamine injection, without a "flare" occurring. The crucial anesthetic problem, hypotension followed by bradycardia and cardiac standstill, has been attributed to deficient catecholamine release; normal subjects can compensate for the stress of anesthesia and operation by increased catecholamine secretion. Johannes Bartels and Valentino D. B. Mazzia[6] (New York Univ.) report data on a patient who underwent pulmonary lobectomy in whom application of this hypothesis underlay the anesthetic management.

Boy, 3, with classic symptoms of familial dysautonomia, was admitted with recurrent pneumonia and persistent collapse of the right middle lung lobe. A bronchogram was scheduled using general anesthesia. Chlorpromazine and meperidine were given intravenously, permitting induction of topical analgesia with 1% tetracaine; the trachea was intubated. Anesthesia was maintained with 2:1 nitrous oxide-oxygen. The patient recovered uneventfully. The affected lobe was removed 2 months later, using similar anesthetic preparation. Chlorpromazine and meperidine were used for premedication and to facilitate induction with N_2O-O_2. Intubation was done easily without muscle relaxant. Two doses of curare were given during the procedure. The arterial pressure dropped precipitously after the chest

(6)   J.A.M.A. 212:318-319, Apr. 13, 1970.

was opened, and the pulse dropped from 120 to 88. Epinephrine was given intravenously in doses of 10 and then 50 μg., restoring the pressure and pulse to normal. They again fell during hilar dissection, and an epinephrine infusion maintained a normal pressure and pulse for the next hour. The infusion was stopped completely, well before the end of the operation. Recovery was uneventful.

Patients with familial dysautonomia are relatively unresponsive to hypoxia and hypercarbia. During sedation and anesthesia, the failure of premonitory signs to occur could result in brain damage or cardiac arrest before the anesthetist became aware of asphyxia. Alveolar ventilation should be controlled with an adequate inspired oxygen concentration, and the arterial Po_2, Pco_2, pH and hematocrit should be monitored. The bradycardic and hypotensive crises during anesthesia result from an inability to release catecholamines. The defect can be corrected by giving epinephrine and/or levarterenol, but the dose must be carefully regulated from moment to moment, since the patients are unusually sensitive to catecholamines. Epinephrine infusion is begun at a rate of about 0.1 μg./kg./minute at the first sign of falling arterial pressure.

▶ [An unusual case handled well because the anesthesiologist treated the patient within the frame of limitations imposed by the disease. This separates the consultants from the cookbook copiers.—Eds.]

Magnesium Ion Blockade of Regional Vasoconstriction. Bernard S. Levowitz, Howard Goldson, Alan Rashkin, Harold Kay, Andre Valcin, Ambrish Mathur and Joseph N. LaGuerre[7] (Brooklyn) studied magnesium ion blockade of adrenergic and nonadrenergic constriction of the renal and mesenteric arterial systems, with a view toward restoring effective regional circulation through reducing vasomotor tone when vasoconstriction is refractory to the usual measures. Magnesium ion as the hydrated sulfate salt was instilled into the arterial trunk vessel as a bolus or by infusion, and flow was measured proximal to the infusion site. Studies were done on 20 dogs anesthetized with pentobarbital. Flow was reduced by over 50% in 14 dogs by potassium ion, Neosynephrine, norepinephrine, epinephrine, angiotensin or Pitressin injected into the renal or superior mesenteric artery; magnesium ion was injected simultaneously until the vasoconstriction was reversed. In 6 studies a vasopressor was given intravenously and magnesium was infused into one renal artery before or after pressor administration at rates of 0.8-4 mEq./ml.

(7)   Ann. Surg. 172:33-40, July, 1970.

Magnesium ion blocked kalemic constriction of both the renal and mesenteric vascular beds. Sympathetic amine constriction and that mediated by angiotensin and Pitressin was similarly blocked by magnesium ion. The amount required did not appreciably change systemic pressures. Magnesium infused into the renal artery promptly reversed the constriction induced by intravenous angiotensin. Findings were similar when renal flow was reduced by norepinephrine or Pitressin given intravenously.

Magnesium ion is a potent inhibitor of vascular constriction due to adrenergic and nonadrenergic mediators. A continuous regional infusion of magnesium was required for sustained local inhibition of systemic vasopressors. Advantages of magnesium as an agent to inhibit regional vasoconstriction include rapid onset of action, brief duration of action, effectiveness against a variety of vasoconstricting agents and ability to control the blockade.

▶ [Magnesium ion is a surprisingly potent vascular relaxant, but just how do the authors propose to use it regionally without getting undesirable effects?—Eds.]

Clinical and Laboratory Evaluation of an Expired Anesthetic Gas Monitor (Narko-Test) is reported by Harry J. Lowe and Karl Hagler[8] (Univ. of Chicago). A recently developed halothane analyzer, the Narko-Test, operates on the principle of relaxation of elasticity of silicon rubber bands in the presence of halothane vapor. It is recommended for monitoring dry inspired halothane only, but its use to continuously monitor end-expired gas provides a more meaningful index of anesthetic depth.

Selected concentrations of various anesthetics were delivered to the analyzer from kettle vaporizers. Delivered concentrations were analyzed with a hydrogen flame detector. An anesthetic circuit was modified with two three-way breathing valves and two T tubes to permit analysis of either inspired or expired gas concentrations during semiclosed- and closed-circuit anesthesia. Retention times of the anesthetics relative to the retention time of halothane on chromatographic columns of silicon or conductive rubber were compared with the response of the Narko-Test to each agent.

The instrument dial readings were directly proportional to the concentrations of each agent. The Narko-Test had a linear

(8) Anesthesiology 34: 378-382, April, 1971.

response to cyclopropane, fluroxene, enflurane, diethyl ether, halothane and methoxyflurane. Factors were derived to convert analyzer scale readings to agent concentrations. Corrections for saturated water vapor at room temperature and 100% nitrous oxide were both 0.3 scale unit.

When the Narko-Test was used to monitor mixed expired gas in semiclosed or closed systems, the analyzer response was a measure of the anesthetic potency of a single agent or of the combined potency of a mixture of agents. The response to each agent was proportional to its solubility in silicon rubber or brain lipids. The scale units may be considered multiples of minimum alveolar concentration. When a true analysis of a single agent is desired, disposable polyethylene breathing tubes should be used.

Oxygenation by Ventilation with Fluorocarbon Liquid (FX-80). Clark and Gollan (1966) found that mice and cats could breathe liquid fluorocarbon. In 1970, Modell *et al.* reported that adult dogs can survive after being ventilated with oxygenated fluorocarbon liquid. However, the animals had hypoxemia and ventilatory difficulty for about a week after liquid ventilation. Jerome H. Modell, C. Ian Hood, Earlene J. Kuck and Bruce C. Ruiz[9] studied the nature of the ventilatory insufficiency observed in the earlier study.

METHOD.—Thirty mongrel dogs were anesthetized with pentobarbital, and 15 were paralyzed with succinylcholine and their endotracheal tubes connected to a chamber containing 1,200 ml. fluorocarbon fluid. Oxygen was bubbled through the liquid at a rate of 3-5 L. per minute, and the dogs' lungs were then ventilated with a tidal volume of 300-400 ml. liquid. The other 15 dogs were ventilated with fluorocarbon liquid but did not receive succinylcholine. Fluorocarbon was drained from the lungs after an hour of continuous ventilation, and the animals breathed pure oxygen for 3 hours. A volume-limited respirator was used in the paralyzed group.

Six other dogs, not paralyzed, were killed 1 or 2 months after ventilation with fluorocarbon liquid.

All animals survived ventilation with oxygenated fluorocarbon liquid and reconversion to breathing gaseous oxygen. The Pao_2 on breathing air was less than control value for several days afterward but had returned to control levels within 10 days. Examination of the lungs 3 hours after termination of liquid ventilation showed an acute exudative inflammatory reaction, largely confined to the bronchioles. By 72 hours, the acute reaction had subsided and the dominant change was

(9) Anesthesiology 34:312-320, April, 1971.

vacuolated intra-alveolar macrophages, presumably containing fluorocarbon. Macrophages persisted at 10 days but in much smaller numbers, and only scattered small groups were present after a month. At 18 months, the lungs were normal.

Mammals can breathe fluorocarbon liquid for an hour, with reconversion to breathing oxygen in gaseous form. The low Pao_2 during air breathing seen for a few days after ventilation with fluorocarbon liquid is attributed to a reduced diffusion rate of oxygen across residual fluorocarbon liquid in the lung and/ or partial airway closure.

SUBJECT INDEX

Ventricle
  arrhythmia, and diazepam for
    cardioversion, 189
  function (in dog)
    after alcohol, 98
    diazepam and, 43
  tachycardia, reverting, chest
    thump for, 185
Vertebra: prevertebral surgery,
  complications of, 347
Vessels
  cerebral (*see* Cerebrum, vessels)
  changes in vaginal deliveries and
    cesarean section, 239
  effects
    of diethyl ether, 21
    of halothane, fluroxene, ether
      and cyclopropane, 20

  of oxytocics, postpartum, 244
  function, and glucagon, 297
  resistance, vasopressin and angio-
    tensin (in cat), 22
  responsiveness, and hypoxia, 76
  revascularization with coronary
    gas endarterectomy, 348
Vocal cord paralysis: after tracheal
  intubation, 169

W

Whiplash syndrome: subarachnoidal injections in, 371
Wound tensile strength: oxygen and
  carbon dioxide (in rat), 236

X

X-ray (*see* Radiation)

INDEX TO AUTHORS